Multimodal Therapy of Upper Gastrointestinal Malignancies

Multimodal Therapy of Upper Gastrointestinal Malignancies

Editor

Ulrich Ronellenfitsch

MDPI • Basel • Beijing • Wuhan • Barcelona • Belgrade • Manchester • Tokyo • Cluj • Tianjin

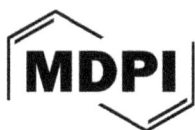

Editor
Ulrich Ronellenfitsch
University Hospital Halle (Saale)
Germany

Editorial Office
MDPI
St. Alban-Anlage 66
4052 Basel, Switzerland

This is a reprint of articles from the Special Issue published online in the open access journal *Cancers* (ISSN 2072-6694) (available at: https://www.mdpi.com/journal/cancers/special_issues/MTUGM_cancer).

For citation purposes, cite each article independently as indicated on the article page online and as indicated below:

LastName, A.A.; LastName, B.B.; LastName, C.C. Article Title. *Journal Name* **Year**, *Volume Number*, Page Range.

ISBN 978-3-0365-0920-4 (Hbk)
ISBN 978-3-0365-0921-1 (PDF)

© 2021 by the authors. Articles in this book are Open Access and distributed under the Creative Commons Attribution (CC BY) license, which allows users to download, copy and build upon published articles, as long as the author and publisher are properly credited, which ensures maximum dissemination and a wider impact of our publications.

The book as a whole is distributed by MDPI under the terms and conditions of the Creative Commons license CC BY-NC-ND.

Contents

About the Editor ix

Preface to "Multimodal Therapy of Upper Gastrointestinal Malignancies" xi

Ulrich Ronellenfitsch, Johannes Klose and Jörg Kleeff
Multimodal Therapy of Upper Gastrointestinal Malignancies
Reprinted from: *Cancers* **2021**, *13*, 793, doi:10.3390/cancers13040793 1

Donelle Cummings, Joyce Wong, Russell Palm, Sarah Hoffe, Khaldoun Almhanna and Shivakumar Vignesh
Epidemiology, Diagnosis, Staging and Multimodal Therapy of Esophageal and Gastric Tumors
Reprinted from: *Cancers* **2021**, *13*, 582, doi:10.3390/cancers13030582 7

Franz Ludwig Dumoulin, Ralf Hildenbrand, Tsuneo Oyama and Ingo Steinbrück
Current Trends in Endoscopic Diagnosis and Treatment of Early Esophageal Cancer
Reprinted from: *Cancers* **2021**, *13*, , doi:10.3390/cancers13040752 41

Karol Rawicz-Pruszyński, Bogumiła Ciseł, Radosław Mlak, Jerzy Mielko, Magdalena Skórzewska, Magdalena Kwietniewska, Agnieszka Pikuła, Katarzyna Gęca, Katarzyna Sędlak, Andrzej Kurylcio and Wojciech P. Polkowski
The Role of the Lymph Node Ratio in Advanced Gastric Cancer After Neoadjuvant Chemotherapy
Reprinted from: *Cancers* **2019**, *11*, 1914, doi:10.3390/cancers11121914 55

Rebekka Schirren, Alexander Novotny, Helmut Friess and Daniel Reim
Histopathologic Response Is a Positive Predictor of Overall Survival in Patients Undergoing Neoadjuvant/Perioperative Chemotherapy for Locally Advanced Gastric or Gastroesophageal Junction Cancers—Analysis from a Large Single Center Cohort in Germany
Reprinted from: *Cancers* **2020**, *12*, 2244, doi:10.3390/cancers12082244 67

Nicola Simoni, Michele Pavarana, Renato Micera, Jacopo Weindelmayer, Valentina Mengardo, Gabriella Rossi, Daniela Cenzi, Anna Tomezzoli, Paola Del Bianco, Simone Giacopuzzi, Giovanni De Manzoni and Renzo Mazzarotto
Long-Term Outcomes of Induction Chemotherapy Followed by Chemo-Radiotherapy as Intensive Neoadjuvant Protocol in Patients with Esophageal Cancer
Reprinted from: *Cancers* **2020**, *12*, 3614, doi:10.3390/cancers12123614 79

Rebekka Schirren, Alexander Novotny, Christian Oesterlin, Julia Slotta-Huspenina, Helmut Friess and Daniel Reim
Significance of Lauren Classification in Patients Undergoing Neoadjuvant/Perioperative Chemotherapy for Locally Advanced Gastric or Gastroesophageal Junction Cancers—Analysis from a Large Single Center Cohort in Germany
Reprinted from: *Cancers* **2021**, *13*, 290, doi:10.3390/cancers13020290 93

Kazuo Koyanagi, Kohei Kanamori, Yamato Ninomiya, Kentaro Yatabe, Tadashi Higuchi, Miho Yamamoto, Kohei Tajima and Soji Ozawa
Progress in Multimodal Treatment for Advanced Esophageal Squamous Cell Carcinoma: Results of Multi-Institutional Trials Conducted in Japan
Reprinted from: *Cancers* **2021**, *13*, 51, doi:10.3390/cancers13010051 111

**Christian Galata, Susanne Blank, Christel Weiss, Ulrich Ronellenfitsch,
Christoph Reissfelder and Julia Hardt**
Role of Postoperative Complications in Overall Survival after Radical Resection for Gastric
Cancer: A Retrospective Single-Center Analysis of 1107 Patients
Reprinted from: *Cancers* **2019**, *11*, 1890, doi:10.3390/cancers11121890 . . . . **129**

**Patrick Téoule, Emrullah Birgin, Christina Mertens, Matthias Schwarzbach, Stefan Post,
Nuh N. Rahbari, Christoph Reißfelder and Ulrich Ronellenfitsch**
Clinical Pathways for Oncological Gastrectomy: Are They a Suitable Instrument for
Process Standardization to Improve Process and Outcome Quality for Patients Undergoing
Gastrectomy? A Retrospective Cohort Study
Reprinted from: *Cancers* **2020**, *12*, 434, doi:10.3390/cancers12020434 . . . . **141**

**Johanna Grün, Lea Elfinger, Han Le, Christel Weiß, Mirko Otto, Christoph Reißfelder and
Susanne Blank**
The Influence of Pretherapeutic and Preoperative Sarcopenia on Short-Term Outcome
after Esophagectomy
Reprinted from: *Cancers* **2020**, *12*, 3409, doi:10.3390/cancers12113409 . . . . **155**

**Christian Galata, Ulrich Ronellenfitsch, Susanne Blank, Christoph Reißfelder
and Julia Hardt**
Postoperative Morbidity and Failure to Rescue in Surgery for Gastric Cancer: A Single Center
Retrospective Cohort Study of 1107 Patients from 1972 to 2014
Reprinted from: *Cancers* **2020**, *12*, 1953, doi:10.3390/cancers12071953 . . . . **167**

**Dolores T. Müller, Benjamin Babic, Veronika Herbst, Florian Gebauer, Hans Schlößer, Lars
Schiffmann, Seung-Hun Chon, Wolfgang Schröder, Christiane J. Bruns and Hans F Fuchs**
Does Circular Stapler Size in Surgical Management of Esophageal Cancer Affect Anastomotic
Leak Rate? 4-Year Experience of a European High-Volume Center
Reprinted from: *Cancers* **2020**, *12*, 3474, doi:10.3390/cancers12113474 . . . . **177**

**Jeong Il Yu, Hee Chul Park, Jeeyun Lee, Changhoon Choi, Won Ki Kang, Se Hoon Park,
Seung Tae Kim, Tae Sung Sohn, Jun Ho Lee, Ji Yeong An, Min Gew Choi, Jae Moon Bae,
Kyoung-Mee Kim, Heewon Han, Kyunga Kim, Sung Kim and Do Hoon Lim**
Outcomes of Radiotherapy for Mesenchymal and Non-Mesenchymal Subtypes of
Gastric Cancer
Reprinted from: *Cancers* **2020**, *12*, 943, doi:10.3390/cancers12040943 . . . . **189**

**Hun Jee Choe, Jin Won Kim, Song-Hee Han, Ju Hyun Lee, Sang-Hoon Ahn, Do Joong Park,
Ji-Won Kim, Yu Jung Kim, Hye Seung Lee, Jee Hyun Kim, Hyung-Ho Kim
and Keun-Wook Lee**
Conversion Surgery in Metastatic Gastric Cancer and Cancer Dormancy as a
Prognostic Biomarker
Reprinted from: *Cancers* **2020**, *12*, 86, doi:10.3390/cancers12010086 . . . . **201**

**Giulia Accordino, Sara Lettieri, Chandra Bortolotto, Silvia Benvenuti, Anna Gallotti,
Elisabetta Gattoni, Francesco Agustoni, Emma Pozzi, Pietro Rinaldi, Cristiano Primiceri,
Patrizia Morbini, Andrea Lancia and Giulia Maria Stella**
From Interconnection between Genes and Microenvironment to Novel Immunotherapeutic
Approaches in Upper Gastro-Intestinal Cancers—A Multidisciplinary Perspective
Reprinted from: *Cancers* **2020**, *12*, 2105, doi:10.3390/cancers12082105 . . . . **215**

**Nikolaos Vassos, Jens Jakob, Georg Kähler, Peter Reichardt, Alexander Marx, Antonia
Dimitrakopoulou-Strauss, Nils Rathmann, Eva Wardelmann and Peter Hohenberger**
Preservation of Organ Function in Locally Advanced Non-Metastatic Gastrointestinal Stromal
Tumors (GIST) of the Stomach by Neoadjuvant Imatinib Therapy
Reprinted from: *Cancers* **2021**, *13*, 586, doi:10.3390/cancers13040586 . . . . **245**

About the Editor

Ulrich Ronellenfitsch is Associate Professor of Surgery at the Medical Faculty of the Martin-Luther-University Halle-Wittenberg (Germany). He studied medicine at the University of Heidelberg (Germany), Complutense University Madrid (Spain), and University of Basel (Switzerland). After having earned his medical degree, he specialized in General Surgery and Vascular Surgery at the University Medical Center Mannheim (Germany) and Medical Faculty Mannheim of the University of Heidelberg (Germany). Currently, he is a fellow in Visceral Surgery and Advanced Clinician Scientist at the Department of Visceral, Vascular, and Endocrine Surgery of the University Hospital Halle (Germany) and the Medical Faculty of the Martin-Luther-University Halle-Wittenberg (Germany). His research interests include multimodal treatment of gastrointestinal cancers and quality of care in surgery and he is PI of several clinical trials and meta-analyses on these topics.

Preface to "Multimodal Therapy of Upper Gastrointestinal Malignancies"

Recent decades have seen remarkable advances in the treatment of upper gastrointestinal malignancies, i.e., adenocarcinoma and squamous cell carcinoma as well as gastrointestinal stromal and other rare tumors of the esophagus and stomach. While, historically, surgical resection has been the sole treatment for these tumors, multimodal therapies have meanwhile proven their efficacy. At present, pre- and postoperative chemotherapy and radiotherapy, targeted drug therapy, and stage-specific surgical approaches are all indispensable cornerstones of an individualized treatment for upper gastrointestinal malignancies. With such multimodal treatment, better outcomes comprising improved quality of life and prolonged survival have been achieved for patients. However, for many tumor entities and stages, the ideal combination and sequence of treatments is still being evaluated in clinical trials. Moreover, the value of novel approaches such as immunotherapy or robotic surgery remains a matter of research.

In this Special Issue of Cancers, up-to-date original research, short communications, and comprehensive review articles on all modalities playing a role in the treatment of upper gastrointestinal malignancies have been published. I wish you a thoughtful reading and appreciation of the contents.

Ulrich Ronellenfitsch
Editor

Editorial

Multimodal Therapy of Upper Gastrointestinal Malignancies

Ulrich Ronellenfitsch *, Johannes Klose and Jörg Kleeff

Department of Visceral, Vascular and Endocrine Surgery, Martin-Luther-University Halle-Wittenberg, University Medical Center Halle (Saale), Ernst-Grube-Str. 40, 06120 Halle (Saale), Germany; johannes.klose@uk-halle.de (J.K.); joerg.kleeff@uk-halle.de (J.K.)
* Correspondence: ulrich.ronellenfitsch@uk-halle.de; Tel.: +49-345-557-2327

Upper gastrointestinal carcinomas comprise squamous cell carcinoma (SCC) and adenocarcinoma (AC) of the esophagus, as well as gastric AC. There are regionally different epidemiological trends for the diseases. While in many Asian countries, esophageal SCC and distal gastric AC are still the most common upper gastrointestinal carcinomas, their incidence has declined and the incidence of esophageal AC and proximal gastric AC has risen in many Western countries [1,2]. All of these tumor entities have in common that only multimodal treatment, i.e., a combination of chemotherapy, radiotherapy, and surgery tailored to the individual characteristics of the patient and the tumor, can achieve optimal outcomes and improve the hitherto often poor prognosis. The original research and review articles in this Special Issue of *Cancers* provide a comprehensive overview of the diagnosis—preoperative, surgical, postoperative—as well as systemic treatment for upper gastrointestinal carcinoma.

Correct and timely diagnosis is the foundation for any therapy. This holds particularly true for an oncological disease in which the exact tumor stage and histopathological tumor characteristics determine the appropriate treatment. As described in the reviews by Dumoulin et al. and Cummings et al. [3,4], high definition and virtual or dye chromoendoscopy can greatly enhance the diagnostic yield for early tumors. This holds particularly true in repeat endoscopy for Barrett's esophagus and in screening for SCC, which is recommended in certain high-risk populations. Tumor stage should be ascertained by a combination of computed tomography (CT), endosonography, and, in selected patients, positron emission tomography-computed tomography (PET-CT).

While early esophageal and gastric cancers can be treated by advanced endoscopic techniques such as endoscopic submucosal dissection, there is now consistent evidence that for locally advanced cancers, neoadjuvant therapy is associated with survival benefits compared to surgery alone. For gastroesophageal AC, both neoadjuvant chemotherapy and chemoradiotherapy are viable options [5], with none of the two modalities having shown superiority over the other and randomized head-to-head comparisons still ongoing [6,7]. For esophageal SCC, neoadjuvant chemotherapy without radiotherapy has no role any longer, given the substantial survival benefit attained by neoadjuvant chemoradiotherapy [8]. The survival advantage could possibly be further augmented by administering intensified induction chemotherapy prior to chemoradiotherapy. This approach is used in ongoing trials comparing neoadjuvant chemoradiotherapy to chemotherapy for esophageal AC [6,7], but has also proven feasible and effective outside a population of selected trial participants, as shown in the retrospective study by Simoni et al. [9]. To achieve the best oncological outcomes, it is crucial to distinguish beforehand patients who will likely benefit from neoadjuvant therapy from those who will not. The histological subtype according to the Laurén classification might play an important role in this association. Schirren et al. showed that in patients with a diffuse type tumor, neoadjuvant chemotherapy is not associated with longer survival compared to surgery alone, as opposed to patients with intestinal- and mixed-type tumors, in whom neoadjuvant chemotherapy leads to a relevant survival benefit [10]. Patients might also be stratified according to HER2neu expression.

A phase II/III trial comparing dual HER2neu blockade in combination with docetaxel, oxaliplatin, and fluorouracil/leucovorin (FLOT) versus FLOT alone for HER2-positive tumors showed promising results regarding histopathological response, which will now need to be corroborated regarding survival outcomes [11]. For esophageal SCC, following promising results and drug registration for unresectable tumors, neoadjuvant immune checkpoint inhibitor therapy is currently being tested in a phase III trial by the Japanese Esophageal Oncology Group, as described in the review article by Koyanagi et al. [12].

Schirren et al. demonstrated for gastroesophageal AC that histopathological response of the primary tumor, expressed in the proportion of remaining viable tumor cells, is an independent predictor of survival [13]. Besides, the histopathological TNM stage upon resection following neoadjuvant therapy has been shown to be predictive for survival [14,15]. A specific predictor could be the lymph node ratio, i.e., the number of metastatic lymph nodes divided by the number of lymph nodes harvested in total. Rawicz-Pruszyński et al. showed in their analysis that the ratio was inversely associated with survival in patients who had undergone neoadjuvant chemotherapy, with statistical significance being reached in the subgroups of patients with intestinal type tumors and those with no response of the primary tumor to neoadjuvant therapy [16].

Although postoperative mortality has substantially decreased in recent decades, as shown in a study by Galata et al. comprising gastrectomies conducted over a 40-year period, upper gastrointestinal cancer surgery still carries a relevant morbidity risk [17]. Preoperative risk stratification and preparation of patients is therefore important. Interestingly, pretherapeutic and preoperative sarcopenia measured by CT as one measure of nutritional status was not associated with postoperative complications in patients undergoing thoracoabdominal esophagectomy in a relatively small study by Grün et al. [18]. Yet, a potential effect of poor nutritional status in the cohort might have been offset by nutritional assessment and therapy, which was offered to all patients. This underlines the importance of appropriate prehabilitation prior to surgery for upper gastrointestinal cancers [19]. To achieve the best possible postoperative outcomes, both intra- and perioperative treatment are important. Technical details such as anastomotic techniques supposedly play a role. A retrospective study by Müller et al. found no association between the diameter of the stapler used for creating the anastomosis and the incidence of anastomotic leak and other complications [20]. Of note, in the study population, stapler size was chosen individually according to the size of the esophageal remnant. Therefore, the result is most likely rather an expression of the need for individually tailored surgical techniques than of the fact that technical details are of lower importance. Teoule et al. showed in their study that using a dedicated clinical pathway for patients undergoing oncological gastrectomy improved process quality outcomes, such as nutritional management and spirometer therapy, which are both known to be important contributors to postoperative recovery [21]. However, probably due to the relatively small study population, no significant effects on postoperative morbidity and mortality could be observed. An important factor contributing to fatal postoperative outcomes is the so-called failure to rescue, i.e., the inability to avert death in a patient suffering a postoperative complication. While the incidence of complications has remained unchanged, such failure has become less frequent in recent decades, probably due to advances in emergency perioperative care. This explains the decline in postoperative mortality shown by Galata et al. [17]. Averting postoperative mortality does not only have short-term effects. In the same cohort, patients who had survived a complication did not have different overall survival from those who did not suffer complications [22].

Although it has proven beneficial regarding long-term outcomes compared to surgery alone [23,24], postoperative chemotherapy or chemoradiotherapy has by now lost importance. It is generally aimed to administer these treatments preoperatively, especially if chemoradiotherapy is applied [8]. The standard chemotherapy schemes for gastroesophageal AC stipulate postoperative continuation of chemotherapy [25], but this requires a good and timely recovery from surgery. Given that this is not always feasible, usually only slightly more than half of patients proceed to the adjuvant part of chemotherapy.

Adding postoperative radiotherapy to perioperative chemotherapy for gastric cancer has not been shown to increase survival and is thus not generally recommended [26,27]. Certain subgroups might still benefit from this approach. Yu et al. however failed to show in the population of the randomized ARTIST trial that a mesenchymal subtype (microsatellite-stable with epithelial-to-mesenchymal transition phenotype) was predisposed to higher susceptibility to postoperative chemoradiotherapy [28]. Adjuvant therapy does however have a stand in patients with an advanced histopathological tumor stage who were initially understaged and thus erroneously proceeded to upfront surgery. This once again emphasizes the importance of accurate pretherapeutic staging, as described above.

Treatment for metastatic or non-resectable upper gastrointestinal cancers poses a challenge, as described in the review by Accordino et al. [29]. First-line chemotherapy is usually platinum-based and consists of a doublet or triplet combination depending on the physical status of the patient. Some targeted therapies such as trastuzumab for HER2neu-overexpressing AC or ramucirumab for AC in second-line treatment are available. The immune checkpoint inhibitor nivolumab has recently been approved for second-line treatment of PD-L1 positive esophageal SCC, based on the results of a multi-national trial. For gastroesophageal AC, trials with immune checkpoint inhibitors have yielded heterogeneous results and no approval of a corresponding drug has been made so far. Other therapeutic approaches such as cancer vaccines or CAR-T cell therapy are still in early clinical testing. Surgery in metastatic disease might have a circumscribed role in gastroesophageal AC. A German phase II trial showed that oligometastatic patients, who proceeded to tumor resection after intensive chemotherapy, showed a favorable overall survival, almost reaching that of a non-metastatic control group [25]. The retrospective study by Choe et al. compared patients with oligometastatic disease undergoing resection of the primary and metastases to similar patients who did not proceed to surgery and found a survival benefit for the former [30]. Results from both studies are promising, but cannot be generalized because their non-randomized study designs were predisposed to selection bias. Therefore, the concept of surgical clearance of oligometastatic disease is currently being further tested and compared to non-surgical treatment in a randomized trial [31].

In summary, the articles in this Special Issue give proof of the many facets and challenges associated with upper gastrointestinal cancers. Both the patient and the tumor need to be assessed and treated individually and with a meaningful combination of the best available methods. Only by doing so, the prognosis of patients with these diseases can further be improved.

Funding: This research received no external funding.

Conflicts of Interest: The authors declare no conflict of interest.

References

1. Gupta, B.; Kumar, N. Worldwide incidence, mortality and time trends for cancer of the oesophagus. *Eur. J. Cancer Prev.* **2017**, *26*, 107–118. [CrossRef] [PubMed]
2. Lyons, K.; Le, L.C.; Pham, Y.T.-H.; Borron, C.; Park, J.Y.; Tran, C.T.; Tran, T.V.; Tran, H.T.-T.; Vu, K.T.; Do, C.D.; et al. Gastric cancer: Epidemiology, biology, and prevention: A mini review. *Eur. J. Cancer Prev.* **2019**, *28*, 397–412. [CrossRef]
3. Cummings, D.; Wong, J.; Palm, R.; Hoffe, S.; Almhanna, K.; Vignesh, S. Epidemiology, Diagnosis, Staging and Multimodal Therapy of Esophageal and Gastric Tumors. *Cancers* **2021**, *13*, 582. [CrossRef]
4. Dumoulin, F.L.; Hildenbrand, R.; Oyama, T.; Steinbrück, I. Current Trends in Endoscopic Diagnosis and Treatment of Early Esophageal Cancer. *Cancers* **2021**, *13*, 752. [CrossRef]
5. Ronellenfitsch, U.; Schwarzbach, M.; Hofheinz, R.; Kienle, P.; Kieser, M.; Slanger, T.E.; Burmeister, B.; Kelsen, D.; Niedzwiecki, N.; Schuhmacher, C.; et al. Preoperative chemo(radio)therapy versus primary surgery for gastroesophageal adenocarcinoma: Systematic review with meta-analysis combining individual patient and aggregate data. *Eur. J. Cancer* **2013**, *49*, 3149–3158. [CrossRef] [PubMed]

6. Leong, T.; Smithers, B.M.; Haustermans, K.; Michael, M.; Gebski, V.; Miller, D.; Zalcberg, J.; Boussioutas, A.; Findlay, M.; O'Connell, R.L.; et al. TOPGEAR: A Randomized, Phase III Trial of Perioperative ECF Chemotherapy with or Without Preoperative Chemoradiation for Resectable Gastric Cancer: Interim Results from an International, Intergroup Trial of the AGITG, TROG, EORTC and CCTG. *Ann. Surg. Oncol.* **2017**, *24*, 2252–2258. [CrossRef] [PubMed]
7. Lorenzen, S.; Biederstädt, A.; Ronellenfitsch, U.; Reißfelder, C.; Mönig, S.; Wenz, F.; Pauligk, C.; Walker, M.; Al-Batran, S.-E.; Haller, B.; et al. RACE-trial: Neoadjuvant radiochemotherapy versus chemotherapy for patients with locally advanced, potentially resectable adenocarcinoma of the gastroesophageal junction - a randomized phase III joint study of the AIO, ARO and DGAV. *BMC Cancer* **2020**, *20*, 1–9. [CrossRef]
8. Van Hagen, P.; Hulshof, M.; Van Lanschot, J.; Steyerberg, E.; Henegouwen, M.V.B.; Wijnhoven, B.; Richel, D.; Nieuwenhuijzen, G.A.; Hospers, G.A.P.; Bonenkamp, J.; et al. Preoperative Chemoradiotherapy for Esophageal or Junctional Cancer. *N. Engl. J. Med.* **2012**, *366*, 2074–2084. [CrossRef] [PubMed]
9. Simoni, N.; Pavarana, M.; Micera, R.; Weindelmayer, J.; Mengardo, V.; Rossi, G.; Cenzi, D.; Tomezzoli, A.; Del Bianco, P.; Giacopuzzi, S.; et al. Long-Term Outcomes of Induction Chemotherapy Followed by Chemo-Radiotherapy as Intensive Neoadjuvant Protocol in Patients with Esophageal Cancer. *Cancers* **2020**, *12*, 3614. [CrossRef]
10. Schirren, R.; Novotny, A.; Oesterlin, C.; Slotta-Huspenina, J.; Friess, H.; Reim, D. Significance of Lauren Classification in Patients Undergoing Neoadjuvant/Perioperative Chemotherapy for Locally Advanced Gastric or Gastroesophageal Junction Cancers—Analysis from a Large Single Center Cohort in Germany. *Cancers* **2021**, *13*, 290. [CrossRef]
11. Hofheinz, R.D.; Haag, G.M.; Ettrich, T.J.; Borchert, K.; Kretzschmar, A.; Teschendorf, C.; Siegler, G.M.; Ebert, M.P.; Goekkurt, E.; Welslau, M.; et al. Perioperative trastuzumab and pertuzumab in combination with FLOT versus FLOT alone for HER2-positive resectable esophagogastric adenocarcinoma: Final results of the PETRARCA multicenter randomized phase II trial of the AIO. *J. Clin. Oncol.* **2020**, *38*, 4502. [CrossRef]
12. Koyanagi, K.; Kanamori, K.; Ninomiya, Y.; Yatabe, K.; Higuchi, T.; Yamamoto, M.; Tajima, K.; Ozawa, S. Progress in Multimodal Treatment for Advanced Esophageal Squamous Cell Carcinoma: Results of Multi-Institutional Trials Conducted in Japan. *Cancers* **2020**, *13*, 51. [CrossRef]
13. Schirren, R.; Novotny, A.; Friess, H.; Reim, D. Histopathologic Response Is a Positive Predictor of Overall Survival in Patients Undergoing Neoadjuvant/Perioperative Chemotherapy for Locally Advanced Gastric or Gastroesophageal Junction Cancers—Analysis from a Large Single Center Cohort in Germany. *Cancers* **2020**, *12*, 2244. [CrossRef] [PubMed]
14. Davies, A.R.; Gossage, J.A.; Zylstra, J.; Mattsson, F.; Lagergren, J.; Maisey, N.; Smyth, E.C.; Cunningham, D.; Allum, W.H.; Mason, R.C. Tumor Stage After Neoadjuvant Chemotherapy Determines Survival After Surgery for Adenocarcinoma of the Esophagus and Esophagogastric Junction. *J. Clin. Oncol.* **2014**, *32*, 2983–2990. [CrossRef]
15. Ronellenfitsch, U.; Schwarzbach, M.; Hofheinz, R.; Kienle, P.; Nowak, K.; Kieser, M.; Slanger, T.; Burmeister, B.; Kelsen, D.; Niedzwiecki, D.; et al. Predictors of overall and recurrence-free survival after neoadjuvant chemotherapy for gastroesophageal adenocarcinoma: Pooled analysis of individual patient data (IPD) from randomized controlled trials (RCTs). *Eur. J. Surg. Oncol. (EJSO)* **2017**, *43*, 1550–1558. [CrossRef]
16. Rawicz-Pruszyński, K.; Cisel, B.; Mlak, R.; Mielko, J.; Skórzewska, M.; Kwietniewska, M.; Pikuła, A.; Gęca, K.; Sędłak, K.; Kurylcio, A.; et al. The Role of the Lymph Node Ratio in Advanced Gastric Cancer After Neoadjuvant Chemotherapy. *Cancers* **2019**, *11*, 1914. [CrossRef]
17. Galata, C.; Ronellenfitsch, U.; Blank, S.; Reißfelder, C.; Hardt, J. Postoperative Morbidity and Failure to Rescue in Surgery for Gastric Cancer: A Single Center Retrospective Cohort Study of 1107 Patients from 1972 to 2014. *Cancers* **2020**, *12*, 1953. [CrossRef] [PubMed]
18. Grün, J.; Elfinger, L.; Le, H.; Weiß, C.; Otto, M.; Reißfelder, C.; Blank, S. The Influence of Pretherapeutic and Preoperative Sarcopenia on Short-Term Outcome after Esophagectomy. *Cancers* **2020**, *12*, 3409. [CrossRef] [PubMed]
19. Hughes, M.J.; Hackney, R.J.; Lamb, P.J.; Wigmore, S.J.; Deans, D.A.C.; Skipworth, R.J.E. Prehabilitation Before Major Abdominal Surgery: A Systematic Review and Meta-analysis. *World J. Surg.* **2019**, *43*, 1661–1668. [CrossRef]
20. Müller, D.T.; Babic, B.; Herbst, V.; Gebauer, F.; Schlößer, H.; Schiffmann, L.; Chon, S.-H.; Schröder, W.; Bruns, C.J.; Fuchs, H.F. Does Circular Stapler Size in Surgical Management of Esophageal Cancer Affect Anastomotic Leak Rate? 4-Year Experience of a European High-Volume Center. *Cancers* **2020**, *12*, 3474. [CrossRef] [PubMed]
21. Téoule, P.; Birgin, E.; Mertens, C.; Schwarzbach, M.; Post, S.; Rahbari, N.N.; Reißfelder, C.; Ronellenfitsch, U. Clinical Pathways for Oncological Gastrectomy: Are They a Suitable Instrument for Process Standardization to Improve Process and Outcome Quality for Patients Undergoing Gastrectomy? A Retrospective Cohort Study. *Cancers* **2020**, *12*, 434. [CrossRef]
22. Galata, C.; Blank, S.; Weiss, C.; Ronellenfitsch, U.; Reissfelder, C.; Hardt, J. Role of Postoperative Complications in Overall Survival after Radical Resection for Gastric Cancer: A Retrospective Single-Center Analysis of 1107 Patients. *Cancers* **2019**, *11*, 1890. [CrossRef]
23. gastric global advanced; Paoletti, X.; Koji GASTRIC (Global Advanced/Adjuvant Stomach Tumor Research International Collaboration) Group; Burzykowski, T.; Michiels, S.; Ohashi, Y.; Pignon, J.-P.; Rougier, P.; Sakamoto, J.; Sargent, D.; et al. Benefit of Adjuvant Chemotherapy for Resectable Gastric Cancer. *JAMA* **2010**, *303*, 1729–1737. [CrossRef]
24. Smalley, S.R.; Benedetti, J.K.; Haller, D.G.; Hundahl, S.A.; Estes, N.C.; Ajani, J.A.; Gunderson, L.L.; Goldman, B.; Martenson, J.A.; Jessup, J.M.; et al. Updated Analysis of SWOG-Directed Intergroup Study 0116: A Phase III Trial of Adjuvant Radiochemotherapy Versus Observation After Curative Gastric Cancer Resection. *J. Clin. Oncol.* **2012**, *30*, 2327–2333. [CrossRef]

25. Al-Batran, S.-E.; Homann, N.; Pauligk, C.; O Goetze, T.; Meiler, J.; Kasper, S.; Kopp, H.-G.; Mayer, F.; Haag, G.M.; Luley, K.; et al. Perioperative chemotherapy with fluorouracil plus leucovorin, oxaliplatin, and docetaxel versus fluorouracil or capecitabine plus cisplatin and epirubicin for locally advanced, resectable gastric or gastro-oesophageal junction adenocarcinoma (FLOT4): A randomised, phase 2/3 trial. *Lancet* **2019**, *393*, 1948–1957. [CrossRef] [PubMed]
26. Cats, A.; Jansen, E.P.M.; Van Grieken, N.C.T.; Sikorska, K.; Lind, P.; Nordsmark, M.; Kranenbarg, E.M.-K.; Boot, H.; Trip, A.K.; Swellengrebel, H.A.M.; et al. Chemotherapy versus chemoradiotherapy after surgery and preoperative chemotherapy for resectable gastric cancer (CRITICS): An international, open-label, randomised phase 3 trial. *Lancet Oncol.* **2018**, *19*, 616–628. [CrossRef]
27. Park, S.H.; Sohn, T.S.; Lee, J.; Lim, D.H.; Hong, M.E.; Kim, K.-M.; Sohn, I.; Jung, S.H.; Choi, M.G.; Lee, J.H.; et al. Phase III Trial to Compare Adjuvant Chemotherapy with Capecitabine and Cisplatin Versus Concurrent Chemoradiotherapy in Gastric Cancer: Final Report of the Adjuvant Chemoradiotherapy in Stomach Tumors Trial, Including Survival and Subset Analyses. *J. Clin. Oncol.* **2015**, *33*, 3130–3136. [CrossRef]
28. Yu, J.I.; Park, H.C.; Lee, J.; Choi, C.; Kang, W.K.; Park, S.H.; Kim, S.T.; Sohn, T.S.; Lee, J.H.; An, J.Y.; et al. Outcomes of Radiotherapy for Mesenchymal and Non-Mesenchymal Subtypes of Gastric Cancer. *Cancers* **2020**, *12*, 943. [CrossRef]
29. Accordino, G.; Lettieri, S.; Bortolotto, C.; Benvenuti, S.; Gallotti, A.; Gattoni, E.; Agustoni, F.; Pozzi, E.; Rinaldi, P.; Primiceri, C.; et al. From Interconnection between Genes and Microenvironment to Novel Immunotherapeutic Approaches in Upper Gastro-Intestinal Cancers—A Multidisciplinary Perspective. *Cancers* **2020**, *12*, 2105. [CrossRef]
30. Choe, H.J.; Kim, J.W.; Han, S.-H.; Lee, J.H.; Ahn, S.-H.; Park, D.J.; Kim, Y.J.; Lee, H.S.; Kim, J.H.; Kim, H.-H.; et al. Conversion Surgery in Metastatic Gastric Cancer and Cancer Dormancy as a Prognostic Biomarker. *Cancers* **2019**, *12*, 86. [CrossRef] [PubMed]
31. Al-Batran, S.-E.; Goetze, T.O.; Mueller, D.W.; Vogel, A.; Winkler, M.; Lorenzen, S.; Novotny, A.; Pauligk, C.; Homann, N.; Jungbluth, T.; et al. The RENAISSANCE (AIO-FLOT5) trial: Effect of chemotherapy alone vs. chemotherapy followed by surgical resection on survival and quality of life in patients with limited-metastatic adenocarcinoma of the stomach or esophagogastric junction—a phase III trial of the German AIO/CAO-V/CAOGI. *BMC Cancer* **2017**, *17*, 1–7. [CrossRef]

Review

Epidemiology, Diagnosis, Staging and Multimodal Therapy of Esophageal and Gastric Tumors

Donelle Cummings [1], Joyce Wong [2], Russell Palm [3], Sarah Hoffe [3], Khaldoun Almhanna [4] and Shivakumar Vignesh [5,*]

[1] Division of Gastroenterology and Hepatology, Department of Medicine, New York Medical College, New York City Health and Hospitals Corporation-Metropolitan Hospital Center, 1901 First Avenue, New York, NY 10029, USA; cummingd2@nychhc.org
[2] Division of Surgery, Mid Atlantic Kaiser Permanente, 700 2nd St. NE, 6th Floor, Washington, DC 20002, USA; Joyce.x.wong@kp.org
[3] Department of Radiation Oncology, Moffitt Cancer Center, 12902 USF Magnolia Drive, Tampa, FL 33612, USA; russell.palm@moffitt.org (R.P.); sarah.hoffe@moffitt.org (S.H.)
[4] Division of Hematology/Oncology, Lifespan Cancer Institute, Rhode Island Hospital, The Warren Alpert Medical School of Brown University, 593 Eddy St, George 312, Providence, RI 02903, USA; Kalmhanna@lifespan.org
[5] Division of Gastroenterology and Hepatology, Department of Medicine, SUNY Downstate Health Sciences University, MSC 1196, 450 Clarkson Avenue, Brooklyn, NY 11203, USA
* Correspondence: shivakumar.vignesh@downstate.edu

Simple Summary: Upper gastrointestinal tumors involve the tubular organs from the upper esophagus, the stomach, and the first part of the small intestine. Esophageal and gastric cancers are responsible for high rates of disease, morbidity, and mortality throughout the world. Diagnosis of these tumors involves a combination of clinical symptoms, endoscopy, endoscopic ultrasound, and radiological studies. Treatment depends on input from many medical doctors including gastroenterologists, surgeons, pathologists, medical oncologists, radiologists, and radiation oncologists. Treatment may include endoscopy, surgery, chemotherapy, radiation therapy, or a combination of these approaches. Future directions of diagnosis may include improvements in endoscopy, endoscopic ultrasound, blood testing, and tissue testing.

Abstract: Gastric and esophageal tumors are diverse neoplasms that involve mucosal and submucosal tissue layers and include squamous cell carcinomas, adenocarcinomas, spindle cell neoplasms, neuroendocrine tumors, marginal B cell lymphomas, along with less common tumors. The worldwide burden of esophageal and gastric malignancies is significant, with esophageal and gastric cancer representing the ninth and fifth most common cancers, respectively. The approach to diagnosis and staging of these lesions is multimodal and includes a combination of gastrointestinal endoscopy, endoscopic ultrasound, and cross-sectional imaging. Likewise, therapy is multidisciplinary and combines therapeutic endoscopy, surgery, radiotherapy, and systemic chemotherapeutic tools. Future directions for diagnosis of esophageal and gastric malignancies are evolving rapidly and will involve advances in endoscopic and endosonographic techniques including tethered capsules, optical coherence tomography, along with targeted cytologic and serological analyses.

Keywords: esophageal cancer; gastric cancer; gastrointestinal stromal tumor; neuroendocrine tumor; MALT lymphoma; mucosal resection; submucosal dissection

1. Introduction

1.1. Anatomic Principles

Upper gastrointestinal neoplasia is a complex disease process of the digestive organs of the foregut involving structures from the upper esophageal sphincter to the duodenum at the ligament of Treitz. These lesions originate from the mucosal or submucosal tissue layers of the esophagus, stomach, and duodenum and involve numerous cell types, including squamous cell carcinomas, adenocarcinomas, spindle-cell neoplasms, lymphomas, neuroendocrine tumors, and several less common tumors.

1.2. Epidemiology

Available WHO statistics indicate that upper gastrointestinal malignancies are responsible for a significant disease burden globally. Esophageal cancer (including adenocarcinoma and squamous cell carcinoma) is the ninth most common malignancy worldwide and has the sixth-highest cancer mortality [1]. Squamous cell cancer of the esophagus accounts for approximately 90% of incident esophageal cancers all over the world. It is much less common than adenocarcinoma in the United States. Gastric cancer (adenocarcinoma) represents an even greater disease burden, and is the fifth most common cancer, representing the fourth-highest cause of cancer mortality worldwide [2]. Gastric adenocarcinoma exhibits a unique geographic predilection, with a high incidence documented in Asian countries, particularly in Japan and South Korea (41 cases per 100,000 persons) and lowest in North America (below 5 cases per 100,000 persons) [3]. Gastric adenocarcinoma is subdivided into the intestinal and diffuse subgroups based on the Lauren classification, which includes intestinal, diffuse, mixed, and indeterminate histological variants. Alternatively, the WHO classification is based upon histology and subdivides gastric adenocarcinoma into tubular, papillary, mucinous, poorly cohesive, and rare variants [2,4].

Gastric lymphomas account for 1–6% of gastric neoplasms diagnosed annually. Infection with *H. pylori* is known to be an important factor in carcinogenesis. Chronic *H. pylori* infection is thought to promote clonal expansion of gastric lymphocytes, leading to gastric lymphoma. Approximately 40–50% of cases are gastric marginal zone lymphoma of mucosa-associated lymphoid tissue (MALT) and 20–40% are extra-nodal lymphomas [5].

Gastrointestinal stromal tumors (GISTs) are rare mesenchymal tumors. They may occur anywhere along the digestive tract, but they are most commonly located in the stomach and small intestine. Within the US, the incidence is estimated at 4000 to 6000 cases per year [6].

Gastrointestinal neuroendocrine tumors (NET) are uncommon and may occur anywhere along the gastrointestinal tract or within the pancreaticobiliary system. There are four subtypes of gastric neuroendocrine tumors (I, II, III, and IV). Type I tumors are associated with atrophic chronic gastritis. They may be well-differentiated and multifocal. Smaller type I lesions may be amenable to endoscopic resection and surveillance. Type II NETs are associated with Zollinger Ellison Syndrome (as part of Multiple Endocrine Neoplasia I) and have an increased malignant potential. Type III and Type IV neuroendocrine tumors have a higher malignant potential and may be metastatic on presentation. In the US, from 2000 to 2012, SEER 18 Registry data indicated a neuroendocrine tumor incidence of 3.56 per 100,000 in gastroenteropancreatic sites. It is estimated that only 7–8% of NETS are found in the stomach [6].

1.3. Natural History

Adenocarcinomas, squamous cell carcinomas, neuroendocrine tumors, and spindle-cell neoplasms of the upper GI tract each demonstrate a characteristic natural history. The therapeutic approach is determined by numerous factors. These factors include tissue of origin, histology, anatomic location, size, and anatomic stage. It is important to consider precursor conditions (e.g., Barrett's esophagus, intestinal metaplasia) in the approach to surveillance, diagnosis, and ultimately therapy of upper GI malignancies.

Barrett's esophagus is a premalignant condition characterized by specialized intestinal metaplasia (SIM) within the distal esophagus. It is considered a precursor lesion in the development of esophageal adenocarcinoma and is related to numerous factors, including chronic reflux of gastric acid and bile salts into the lower esophagus [7,8]. Similarly, intestinal metaplasia within the stomach can lead to the development of intestinal-type gastric adenocarcinoma over time. Risk factors include chronic bile reflux, high dietary salt intake, smoking, alcohol consumption, and consumption of nitrates or smoked foods [9]. *H. pylori* gastritis is also an important risk factor in the development of gastric intestinal metaplasia, with some studies showing that individuals with associated *H. pylori* infection have a six-fold increase in developing gastric cancer [10,11].

1.4. Approaches to Diagnosis, Staging, and Therapy

Endoscopy with high-definition white light imaging is recommended and is the standard for detecting and documenting the presence of mucosal or submucosal lesions, as shown in Figure 1. Non-invasive approaches to screening for premalignant lesions of the esophagus include devices such as the "EsophaCap" [12] and cytosponge -TFF3 that detect genetic and epigenetic alterations on samples gathered non-invasively and can be used by primary care physicians to screen for Barrett's esophagus [13]. Non-invasive diagnostic modalities, using molecular biomarkers from a variety of body fluids to diagnose early gastric cancer, have been developed. These include "liquid-based biopsy," which uses circulating nucleic acids. This is an exciting area of research that may change the diagnostic landscape [14].

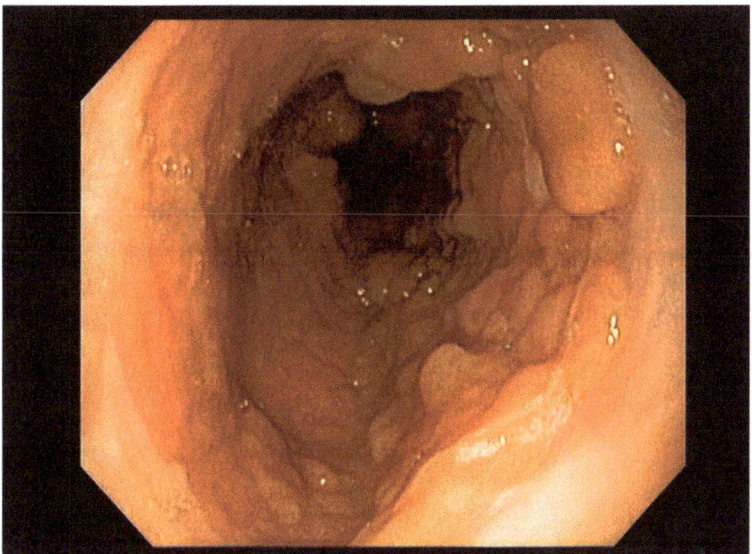

Figure 1. Barrett's esophagus with Nodules White Light Endoscopy.

Early endoscopic detection of premalignant lesions such as Barrett's esophagus, gastric intestinal metaplasia, and mucosal cancer using optical chromoendoscopy techniques such as narrow-band imaging (NBI) combined with high-definition white light imaging (HD-WLE) is becoming routine across the world. Targeted biopsies from endoscopically suspicious areas or using the updated Sydney protocol are important for successful diagnosis [15,16]. In the presence of dysplasia with visible lesions or carcinoma, endoscopic ultrasound (EUS), a minimally invasive procedure, has a well-established role in the early diagnosis and locoregional staging of non-metastatic foregut malignancies [17–19], see Figure 2.

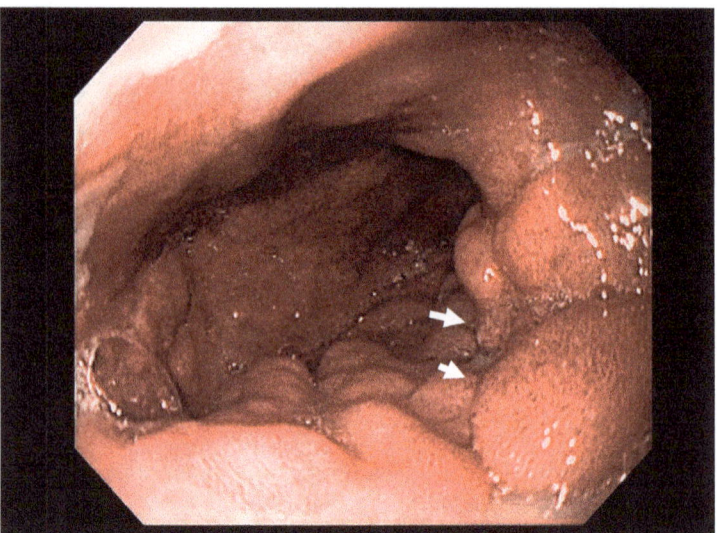

Figure 2. Barrett's esophagus with nodules under narrow band imaging (NBI) (arrows).

1.5. Endoscopic Approaches to Therapy

Factors including lesion size, histological features, anatomical stage, and esophageal location are important variables for determining favorability of endoscopic therapy, demonstrating curative resection in some studies [20]. Adenocarcinoma of the esophagus, limited to the mucosa (T1a)—see Figure 3—is amenable to endoscopic resection, with excellent long-term outcomes. Other tumors such as neuroendocrine tumors of the foregut may also be amenable to endoscopic therapy, including endoscopic mucosal resection (EMR) or endoscopic submucosal dissection (ESD). Specifically, these therapeutic approaches are used for resection of mucosal-based lesions, depending on the size, location, submucosal involvement, and complexity.

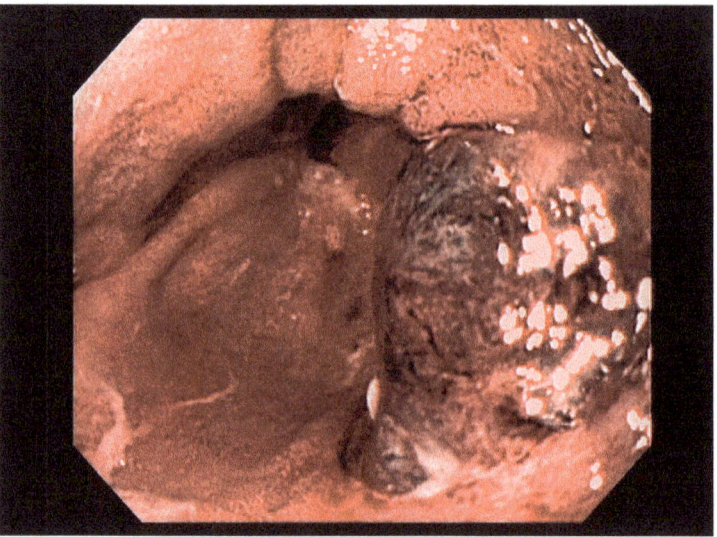

Figure 3. T1a esophageal cancer in Barrett's Esophagus.

1.6. Role of Multidisciplinary Care

Treatment of upper gastrointestinal malignancies must be individualized and based on an interdisciplinary discussion in a tumor board setting, facilitated by National Comprehensive Cancer Network (NCCN) guidelines and institutional clinical pathways. In a Dutch study, the diagnostic or treatment plan was altered after a multidisciplinary tumor board discussion in over one third of cases [21]. A recent systematic review has endorsed the importance and impact of a multidisciplinary tumor board discussion in the diagnosis and management of patients with GI malignancies [22].

In addition to patient and clinical factors (e.g., functional status, comorbidities, and patient preferences), the therapeutic strategy is highly dependent on histological parameters (e.g., type of neoplasm, grade/differentiation, mitotic rate/Ki 67%, and other unique histological markers of response to certain therapies such as HER2/neu expression), anatomy/location, and, most importantly, the stage of the tumor [23,24]. The management approach may therefore involve a combination of chemotherapy, radiotherapy, endoscopic therapy, and surgery.

2. Esophageal Malignancies

2.1. Epidemiology/Pathophysiology

(i) Esophageal squamous cell carcinoma (SCC) arises proximal to the squamocolumnar junction and its pathogenesis is multifactorial in nature. It results from inflammation or other carcinogenic or mutagenic factors leading to dysplasia in situ and eventual malignant transformation. Alcohol, tobacco, caustic strictures, tylosis, thoracic radiation, and achalasia are important risk factors [25]. Dietary exposures including betel nuts and hot beverages should also be considered [26]. Areas with the highest global incidence of esophageal SCC are East Asia and Central Asia, followed by areas in Africa along the Great Rift Valley and in Uruguay in South America [27]. In the United States, Black men and women were seen to have an incidence of esophageal SCC twice that of white men and women. Between the years 1977 and 2005, SCC accounted for 87% of esophageal cancers in Black patients and 43% of white patients [28].

(ii) Esophageal adenocarcinoma (EAC) is more common in the distal and mid-esophagus and is thought to develop from specialized intestinal epithelium as a result of chronic exposure to bile, pancreatic juice, pepsin, and gastric acid. This may lead squamous cells to transform into specialized intestinal epithelium and possible dysplasia and malignancy. EAC is the predominant histological subtype of esophageal cancer in Europe and North America, with a global incidence of 0.7 cases per 100,000. Esophageal AC has surpassed SCC in a number of Western countries, including the United Kingdom, Ireland, Denmark, New Zealand, Canada, and the United States. In the United States, there are notable ethnic variations in AC incidence, with rates being higher in non-Hispanic white individuals, followed by Hispanic white, Native American, and Black American individuals, and lowest in Asian Pacific Islanders [29].

(iii) Barrett's esophagus is a premalignant condition of the tubular esophagus, associated with gastroesophageal reflux disease, characterized endoscopically by abnormal salmon-colored mucosa located at least 1 cm proximal to the gastroesophageal junction (GEJ) and confirmed histologically as specialized intestinal metaplasia [30]. Such findings are suspicious for metaplastic change of the typical squamous epithelial lining of the esophagus to specialized intestinal epithelium with goblet cells called specialized intestinal metaplasia (SIM). Risk factors for the development of Barrett's esophagus include male gender, Caucasian ethnicity, smoking, central obesity, increasing age, and chronic heartburn symptoms [31]. Barrett's esophagus associated dysplasia is regarded as a precursor lesion to esophageal adenocarcinoma [8]. In patients with SIM, the risk of cancer is significantly elevated under the following circumstances: patients with specialized intestinal epithelium at index biopsy versus those without (0.38% per year vs. 0.07% per year; hazard ratio (HR) = 3.54, 95% CI = 2.09 to 6.00, $p < 0.001$), in men compared with women (0.28% per year vs. 0.13% per year; HR = 2.11, 95% CI = 1.41 to 3.16, $p < 0.001$), and in patients with low-grade dysplasia compared with no dysplasia (1.40% per year vs 0.17% per year; HR = 5.67, 95% CI = 3.77 to 8.53, $p < 0.001$) [32]. The risk of progression to adenocarcinoma may be as high as 6% per year when high-grade dysplasia is seen [33,34]. Endoscopic surveillance of Barrett's esophagus is a powerful tool for detecting low- or high-grade dysplasia for ablative therapies or T1a adenocarcinoma which may be amenable to endoscopic resection [8,35]. High-definition white light endoscopy (HD-WLE) examination using the Seattle protocol for biopsies is the standard of care and has the same detection rate for Barrett's intestinal metaplasia as optical chromoendoscopy techniques such as narrow-band imaging (NBI). NBI-targeted biopsies detected more areas with dysplasia, required fewer biopsies, and were therefore cost-effective [18,36]. A newer advanced endoscopic imaging modality, confocal laser endomicroscopy (CLE), has demonstrated higher sensitivity but a lower specificity when compared to NBI for detection of Barrett's esophagus and related dysplasia in a meta-analysis of five studies [37].

2.2. Distant and Locoregional Staging

Staging esophageal malignancies is a crucial practice that provides prognostic information and stratifies patients to appropriate treatment modalities including endoscopic resection, surgery, radiation therapy, chemotherapy, or a combination thereof [38]. Once a lesion is identified, cross-sectional imaging with contrast-enhanced CT imaging or PET imaging is important to evaluate for metastatic disease.

Endoscopic ultrasound is a useful modality to assess the depth of invasion (T stage) of mucosa, the layer of origin of submucosal tumors and regional nodal involvement (N stage) of foregut tumors, and in some cases metastatic adenopathy. EUS is a minimally invasive procedure that allows for high-resolution imaging of the esophageal wall layers and has a diagnostic accuracy of over 80% [39]. In a meta-analysis, EUS had a high pooled sensitivity to diagnose T2 stage esophageal cancer (81.4%), T3 stage cancer (91.4%), and T4 stage cancer (92.4). EUS has a lower sensitivity in diagnosing T1 stage esophageal cancer, with a pooled sensitivity of 81.6% [38]. A recent meta-analysis looking at the ability of EUS in differentiating mucosal from submucosal cancers concluded that EUS has good accuracy (area under the curve ≥ 0.93) in staging superficial esophageal cancers [40], see Figure 4.

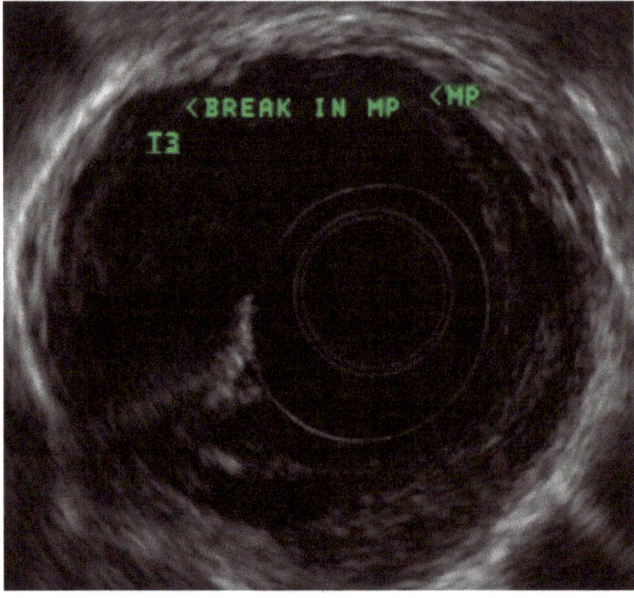

Figure 4. Esophageal cancer endoscopic ultrasound (EUS) image T3.

Another meta-analysis of 44 studies on EUS for staging squamous esophageal cancer showed that the overall accuracy of EUS for T staging was 79%, and for N staging, 71% [41]. In terms of N staging, EUS has acceptable accuracy, with a pooled sensitivity for diagnosing esophageal cancer of 85% and EUS fine needle aspiration (FNA) increasing the sensitivity for diagnosing esophageal cancer to 97% (95% CI: 0.92–0.99) [38].

For patients with invasive disease, imaging for staging should include PET/CT as 15% of patients present with occult metastatic disease after conventional staging with EUS or CT imaging and improved specificity of regional lymph nodes [42]. The role of PET imaging in adaptive treatment planning and assessment of tumor response is still investigational and only preliminary results have been published [43].

3. Treatment

3.1. Endoscopic Therapeutic Options for Barrett's Esophagus Associated Dysplasia

Therapeutic options are based upon the stage of the disease at diagnosis.

Barrett's esophagus with low- or high-grade dysplasia (HGD) without visible lesions can be treated with radio-frequency ablation (RFA) or cryoablation therapies [34,44]. A randomized, controlled trial demonstrated that (RFA) for Barrett's esophagus with HGD was superior to surveillance with respect to the outcome of progression to esophageal adenocarcinoma but did not find any difference in progression to cancer among patients with low-grade dysplasia (LGD) [34]. A European, multicenter, randomized, controlled trial in a large group of patients with Barrett's esophagus and LGD proved that RFA prevents progression to cancer in patients with LGD [45]. After RFA for BE dysplasia, there is >30% chance of recurrence within 5 years, but most recurrences are responsive to further endoscopic therapy [46].

Visible, discrete mucosal lesions within the Barrett's segment, including high-grade dysplasia, T1a adenocarcinoma, and T1b adenocarcinoma with favorable histological features [47], can be approached with endoscopic resection techniques. EMR is a widely utilized endoscopic resection technique, performed using either the "Cap-assisted EMR (Cap-EMR)" technique or multiband mucosectomy (MBM) techniques with the primary goal of assessing the depth of invasion (pathological T-stage) of a visible lesion that is suspicious for intramucosal adenocarcinoma or high-grade dysplasia; see Figure 5. EMR and ESD are performed with intent of "staging" but can indeed be curative if the resection margins are "negative" or free of cancer, but the primary goal in Barrett's esophagus is to obtain an accurate pathological T-stage of the lesion. This concept of "Staging-EMR" is demonstrated by studies that have shown a change in pathological diagnosis and/or T-staging noted in 20–30% of patients, both upstaging and downstaging, based on the pathology from the EMR specimen [48], see Figure 6.

3.2. Endoscopic Resection Techniques for Early-Stage Esophageal Cancer (T1a and T1b)

Endoscopic resection techniques applied to T1a and T1b mucosal cancer with favorable histological features include EMR or ESD. As mentioned earlier, EMR is primarily a "staging procedure" that provides the most accurate T-stage for mucosal lesions that are likely T1 based on EUS and/or optical chromoendoscopy [49,50]. EMR is a technique that involves submucosal injection of saline or a colloidal solution mixed with a dye such as methylene blue to create a "submucosal cushion", followed by resection using a snare, and may be considered for lesions less than 20 mm. Techniques such as Cap-EMR, MBM, and ESD may be employed depending on anatomical location [51,52].

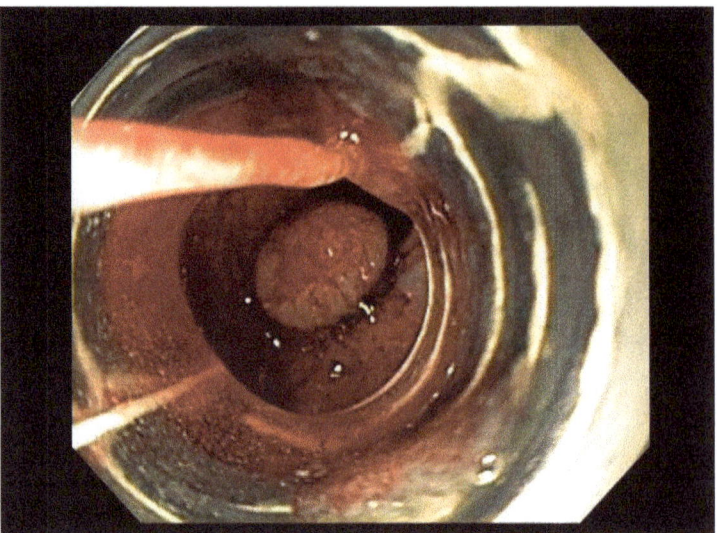

Figure 5. Band-assisted mucosectomy.

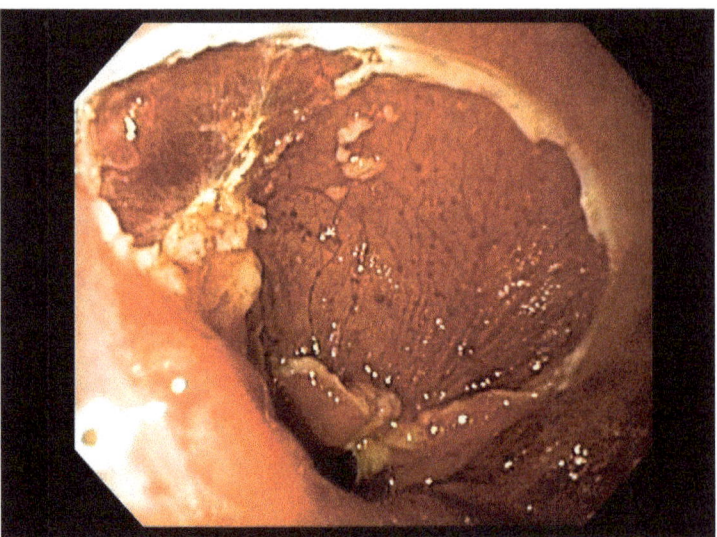

Figure 6. Endoscopic Mucosal Rejection (EMR) T1 esophageal cancer; resection site.

Cap-assisted EMR involves submucosal injection to lift the target lesion from the mucosa, isolating the lesion within a transparent "cap" mounted on the tip of the endoscope, gentle suction, followed by resection of the lesion using the pre-deployed snare within the cap using electrocautery [53]. MBM involves suction of target tissue into an endoscopic band-ligation device and deployment of a band over the target lesion followed by resection of the tissue with electrocautery snaring [54]. EMR can be either stepwise/complete (sEMR) or focal (fEMR), with focal EMR often combined with RFA. Piecemeal EMR has a high local recurrence and therefore is combined with RFA to ablate the residual BE epithelium [55]. In theory, ESD is an en-bloc resection technique with the goal being an R0 resection and is therefore a more appealing endoscopic therapeutic option.

ESD is a more complex technique that may be considered for lesions less than 20 mm. Larger lesions may be amenable to this technique depending on availability of advanced expertise and resources [56]. Specifically, this technique involves the creation of a submucosal tract to dissect lesions restricted to the mucosa (T1a or selected T1b), for complete resection. Factors including lesion size less than approximately 20 mm, anatomical stage (T1a), and middle thoracic and lower thoracic esophageal locations are favorable variables for successful ESD, demonstrating curative resection in some studies [20,56]. Additionally, T1a m2, T1a m3, and select T1b lesions with favorable histological features [57] are amenable to ESD, with comparable outcomes to esophagectomy [58,59]. For these types of lesions, current evidence shows that EMR and ESD are comparable in terms of complication rates, referral to surgery, positive margins, lymph node positivity, local recurrence, and metachronous cancer. When compared to piecemeal EMR resection, ESD may offer some advantages, but data are limited [60,61]. Meta-analyses comparing both of these therapies revealed comparable outcomes in terms of Barrett's eradication, low rates of recurrence, and have shown non-inferiority of EMR to ESD for therapy of Barrett's related cancer or GEJ neoplasia, with similar complication rates [15,62].

3.3. Multimodality Therapy for Locally Advanced Esophageal Cancer

For locally advanced tumors (T2 or with nodal involvement), a combination of neoadjuvant chemoradiation therapy and surgical therapy can be used, with systemic chemotherapy being reserved for metastatic disease (Stage IV) with possible consolidation chemoradiation to sites of disease involvement if the patient responds well [63].

Based on current guidelines, esophagectomy for operable non-metastatic patients with T1b or greater primary lesions and/or any nodal disease should be performed with one of several techniques including: transhiatal, transthoracic, three field, and, increasingly, minimally invasive approaches [64]. Meta-analyses of minimally invasive esophagectomy, which includes laparoscopic/thoracoscopic and robotic approaches, have shown no difference in survival and improved or no difference in complications. Robotic-assisted esophagectomy is becoming increasingly popular, with demonstrated reduction in cardiac and pulmonary complications when compared with open esophagectomy. Technologic advances in the minimally invasive and robotic platforms are also rapidly developing and may allow for further innovation with these techniques [65,66]. While surgery alone can be considered for early-stage, low-risk adenocarcinoma (<3 cm and well differentiated) and early-stage squamous cell carcinoma, trimodality therapy with neoadjuvant chemoradiation followed by surgery is now a preferred treatment pathway for more advanced disease and requires multidisciplinary management [67]. Less commonly, postoperative chemoradiation for pathologic T3 and/or node positive disease may be indicated if a GEJ cancer was treated with preoperative chemotherapy, while palliative radiotherapy may be indicated for treatment of significant dysphagia or bleeding. In definitive treatment of inoperable patients or those who decline esophagectomy, concurrent chemoradiation should be prioritized, followed by imaging and endoscopic surveillance to determine clinical complete response [68]. While clinical outcomes and morbidity for these patients are still suboptimal, there are a growing number of long-term survivors after definitive chemoradiation and investigations are being made into radiotherapy dose escalation, proton therapy, and inclusion of targeted therapy [69–72].

Three-dimensional conformal planning for radiation therapy can be utilized; however, more institutions have implemented intensity-modulated radiation therapy (IMRT) to reduce cardiac and lung dosing, which allows for a simultaneous integrated boost (SIB) or sequential boost techniques [73–75]. This approach is important as cardiac dose is increasingly seen as an independent risk factor for reduced survival [76] and has been correlated with excess G3+ cardiac toxicity [77,78].

Fiducial markers can be placed endoscopically to delineate the extent of disease with high technical success with a small risk of migration [79–81]. Stable fiducial markers improve the reliability of target volume delineation and assessment of respiratory tumor motion with four-dimensional CT (4D-CT) simulation as a direct visual correlate of tumor extent. Combined with fused PET/CT, fiducials reduce the margins for treatment planning due to improved confidence of accurately defined gross tumor volumes (GTVs) [82] and facilitate daily image-guided radiation therapy (IGRT) during treatment [83], see Figures 7 and 8. Moreover, 4D-CT imaging at simulation has a greater benefit in GEJ and gastric tumors due to the propensity of respiratory motion [84] and aids in internal target volume construction and planning target volume expansions during treatment planning. Radiation treatments generally are conventionally fractionated (1.8–2.0 Gy daily); however, previously mentioned SIB techniques treating at 2.2–2.25 Gy daily can push dose to gross disease past 60 Gy. If given sequential neoadjuvant chemotherapy, the extent of original disease is often included in the clinical target volume receiving 4500–5040 cGy and boost is only directed to residual gross disease. Clinical target volumes extend 3–4 cm craniocaudal and 1 cm radially and are edited off anatomical structures that are clinically uninvolved such as vertebral bodies, trachea, aorta, lung, and pericardium. For middle and upper thoracic tumors, the at-risk periesophageal and adjacent mediastinal lymph nodes and, for distal esophageal and GEJ tumors, the celiac lymph nodes are covered. Multi-institutional consensus contouring guidelines for IMRT in esophageal and gastroesophageal tumors have been published [85].

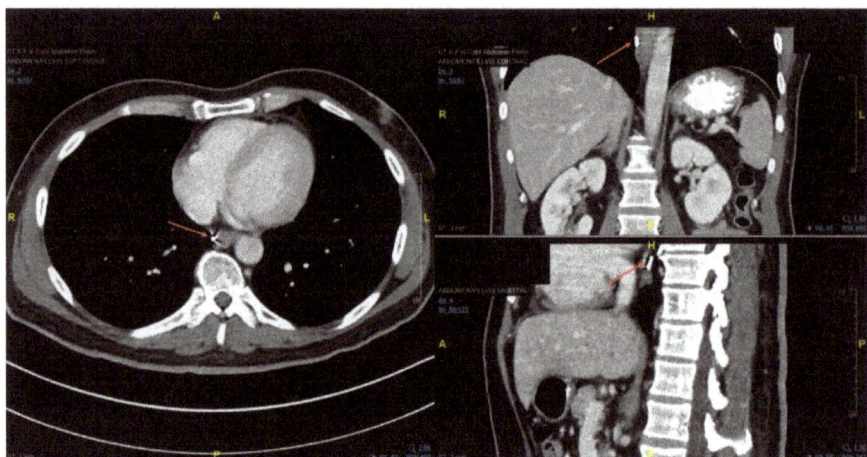

Figure 7. Axial, coronal, and sagittal CT images demonstrating EUS-placed fiducial (red arrow) proximal to esophageal tumor.

3.4. Neoadjuvant Radiation Therapy Alone and Adjuvant Therapy

Neoadjuvant treatment carries the theoretical gains of tumor downstaging, margin attenuation, and improved control of regional disease. However, limited benefit has been observed across several randomized trials investigating the role of radiotherapy alone in preoperative or adjuvant treatment of esophageal cancer. Early studies on patients who received 4000 cGy followed by surgery 1–4 weeks after found no difference in resectability or survival compared to surgery alone [86,87]. A trial from the European Organization for Research and Treatment of Cancer (EORTC) also demonstrated no difference in survival, but noted a lower rate of local failure with the addition of radiotherapy to 46% from 67% [88]. More recent studies that reported improved survival included patients that received chemotherapy but had an imbalance of lower stage tumors conflicting the interpretation of the results [89]. These findings have been confirmed in meta-analyses that demonstrate no statistical difference in survival, or at best, the suggestion of a very modest clinical benefit of <4% with neoadjuvant radiotherapy alone [90,91].

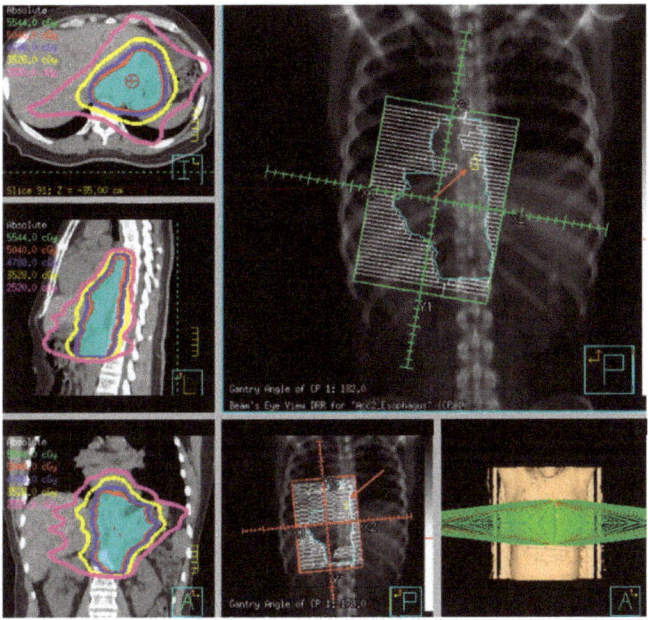

Figure 8. Example radiotherapy plan for image-guided treatment with fiducial contoured (red arrow) and within the planning target volume (PTV).

Recommendations for postoperative or adjuvant treatment are generally driven by adverse pathological features such as positive lymph nodes, positive margins, or locally advanced disease found at time of surgery. While the goal of local therapy is to reduce the risk of local recurrence, often, toxicity is greater due to larger treatment volumes, efficacy is reduced due to a hypoxic tumor bed, and dose is limited by the surgical anastomosis. In two historic series, adjuvant radiotherapy alone showed no survival benefit compared to observation [92,93]. However, similar to preoperative treatment, there are trends towards improved local control after delivery of 4500–5500 cGy [93] after subtotal resection [92]. Retrospective data and population-level analyses show a benefit of adjuvant chemoradiation in pathologically node positive [94] but not node negative disease [95]. The benefit of the addition of chemotherapy to adjuvant radiation is currently being investigated in a phase II/III protocol seeking to add paclitaxel and cisplatin/nedaplatin to 50.4–54.0 Gy of radiotherapy for pathological stage IIB-III disease [96].

3.5. Preoperative Chemoradiation

For locally advanced resectable disease, the CROSS trial (Chemoradiotherapy for Oesophageal Cancer Followed by Surgery Study) established a new paradigm towards total neoadjuvant treatment with chemoradiation followed by surgical resection in esophageal cancer [97]. Other comparisons to neoadjuvant chemotherapy alone in the German POET trial [98] and the NeoRes trial [99] demonstrated improvements, with pathological downstaging with the addition of 30 and 40 Gy of chemoradiation, but did not translate to statistically significant survival differences, likely limited by increased toxicity in the experimental arms with concurrent cisplatin/flurouracil. Within CROSS, radiation therapy was delivered to 4140 in 1.8 daily fractions with concurrent paclitaxel/carboplatin and was compared to surgery alone. Neoadjuvant chemoradiation was associated with a 25-month improvement in median overall survival (49 vs. 24 months) and was notable for a 47% 5-year survival rate and 29% overall pCR rate that was significantly different between histologies (28% adenocarcinoma vs. 49% squamous) [100]. Additionally, preoperative chemoradiation reduced hematogenous metastases (35% vs. 29%) and peritoneal carcinomatosis (14% vs. 4%). There was no difference in operative mortality between the arms or long-term quality of life, with all endpoints declining after surgery and subsequently improved and stabilized between 6 and 12 months afterwards [101].

The CROSS trial excluded patients with tumor diameter greater than 8 cm and patients who had lost more than 10% of their original body weight. In these patients, upfront chemotherapy alone can be considered as they are at high risk of clinical decline during chemoradiation. Therapeutic response to chemotherapy may enable a reduction in irradiation volumes to mitigate pulmonary toxicity with concurrent taxols or motivate one to switch to an alternative regimen before or during chemoradiation. This strategy may also be considered in patients with advanced primary tumor (T4) or regional nodal burden (bulky nodes or cN2+ disease) as they are at higher risk of distant progression and theoretically may derive greater benefit from intensification of systemic therapy. The outcomes from the CROSS trial remain some of the best to date with this strategy, and similar patterns were noted in the Chinese multicenter NEOCRTEC5010 trial that demonstrated improved median survival (66 vs. 100 months), disease-free survival, and R0 resection rate with neoadjuvant vinorelbine/cisplatin with 40 Gy compared to surgery alone [102]. Future strategies seek to compare FOLFOX to paclitaxel-carboplatin with concurrent neoadjuvant radiation for both squamous and adenocarcinoma in the PROTECT-1402 trial (Preoperative Chemoradiation for Resectable Esophageal and Junctional Cancer) [103]. Given the advances in surgical and radiotherapy techniques and corresponding declines in perioperative morbidity and mortality, trimodality therapy is now a preferred approach.

3.6. Definitive Radiation and Chemoradiation

Historically, definitively treated patients generally carry significant comorbidities precluding surgery or are opposed to the morbidity of resection. Alternatively, the surgical options for patients diagnosed with cervical esophageal cancer are often limited and these patients are treated within the paradigm of head and neck cancer with definitive chemoradiation. The use of radiation alone in the modern era is generally considered to be palliative, with 5-year survival of <10% [104,105], while the importance of concurrent chemotherapy has been demonstrated historically by RTOG 8501 where, at 5 years, no survival was noted with dose escalated 64 Gy radiotherapy alone versus 27% survival with 50 Gy and concurrent four cycles of fluorouracil and cisplatin [106]. Initial forays of radiotherapy dose escalation in the definitive treatment of esophageal cancer showed disappointing clinical results. INT 0123 investigated chemoradiation with cisplatin/fluorouracil and compared 5040 cGy to dose escalation to 6480 cGy [107]. A total of 236 patients were enrolled with T1-4, N0-1 disease with 85% squamous cell carcinoma. Overall, the target volumes for this trial were relatively large, with 5-cm superior/inferior and 2-cm radial esophageal expansion as well as a 2-cm isometric expansion from tumor for the boost to gross disease. The dose escalation arm experienced a 10% treatment-related G5 toxicity rate; however, 64% of the mortality occurred prior to surpassing the dose of the control arm, potentially implicating the toxic combination of cisplatin and fluorouracil. Median survival approximated 15 months; however, 2-year locoregional failure was greater than 50%. RTOG 9207 was a phase I/II study that utilized the same control arm as INT 0123 but dose-escalated through the use of predominantly high dose rate (HDR) brachytherapy with iridium-192 to 15 Gy in three weekly fractions [108]. Unfortunately, toxicity from this strategy was high, with 12% fistula rates, 24% G4 toxicity, and 10% treatment-related deaths. Subsequently, the brachytherapy dose was dropped to 10 Gy in two weekly fractions and no fistulas were noted in the 10 patients treated with the intermediate dose. However, overall clinical outcomes remained poor, with 1-year survival of 50% and 37% local control.

With a goal of improving on the near 50% local failure rate seen in previous studies as well as overcoming high rates of persistent disease [107–109], dose escalation in the modern era appears to be more tolerable but still carries an elevated risk of toxicity as well as minimal evidence of clinical benefit. In preliminary results, both a sequential boost to

60 Gy with cisplatin/docetaxel [110] and simultaneous integrated boost to 61.2 Gy with carboplatin/paclitaxel [111] failed to show improvement in overall or progression free survival, despite the latter regimen carrying a 13% rate of G4 toxicity and 10% treatment-related toxicity in the high dose arm. MD Anderson has published results with their SIB technique of a high dose gross tumor volume (GTV) plus 3 mm and a planning target volume (PTV) margin of 5 mm with concurrent chemotherapy, demonstrating encouraging 66% local control at 2 years, acute G3 toxicity in 23%, and only stricture-related late G3 toxicity in 7% [112].

Newer strategies include proton therapy, which carries dosimetric benefits and higher relative biological effectiveness than photons due to the physical nature of the particle. Early retrospective data have not demonstrated an oncological benefit in comparison to photon therapy [113]; however, there is some evidence of a decrease in treatment-related toxicity which, in larger prospective studies, may carry clinical significance [114]. More work remains to further elucidate the benefits from these techniques.

3.7. Therapy for Metastatic Esophageal Cancer

Palliative radiotherapy is commonly delivered for esophageal obstruction in metastatic patients as a significant improvement in patient quality of life. Other indications are severe pain, chronic blood loss, or nausea due to tumor mass effect. While external beam radiotherapy and self-expanding metal stents (SEMS) to palliate dysphagia remain more common palliative techniques, growing literature supports the safe use of intraluminal brachytherapy for durable palliation with caution for fistulation or stenosis [115].

A meta-analysis of 53 studies (mostly RCTs) on palliation of dysphagia in inoperable esophageal cancer concluded that SEMS insertion is safe, effective, and quicker in palliating dysphagia compared to other modalities. The authors added that, "Brachytherapy might be a suitable alternative to SEMS in providing a survival advantage and possibly a better quality of life" [116].

The goal of chemotherapy in patients with stage IV metastatic esophageal cancer is to improve survival and quality of life; several chemotherapeutic agents have been tested and used in the past several decades and proven to be effective in achieving this goal. Unfortunately, survival has remained poor and rarely surpasses one year.

Combination of 5 fluorouracil (5 fu) and platinum agents is an acceptable first-line treatment option and is considered the standard of care in this setting; other regimens including paclitaxel with platinum regimen, irinotecan plus 5-fu are recommended as well. Three drug combinations such as modified DCF (Docetaxel, Cisplatin, 5 fu) are usually given to patients with high volume disease, young age, and good performance status who might benefit from a higher response rate. Single-agent treatment is recommended for patients with low volume disease and or poor performance status.

Several targeted therapies have been tested as front-line and in combination without significant improvement in overall survival until the ToGA trial was conducted. The ToGA trial was a randomized phase III trial where patients with Her-2 expressing tumors were randomized to chemotherapy with or without trastuzumab (Her-2 monoclonal antibody); patients who received the combination had better overall survival, leading to the approval of this combination in this patient population [117].

Recently, at the European Society of Medical oncology meeting in 2020 (ESMO 2020), three important trials were presented incorporating immune checkpoint inhibitors in the front-line treatment of esophageal and gastric cancer. The CheckMate 649 trial evaluated nivolumab plus chemotherapy versus chemotherapy alone as first-line treatment in patients with non-HER-2-positive advanced gastric and GE junction adenocarcinoma. The addition of Nivolumab improved overall survival and progression-free survival in patients with PD-L1 combined positive score (CPS) ≥ 5 tumors. Improvements were also observed in patients with PD-L1 CPS ≥ 1 tumors and in the overall patient population. In another study, the ATTRACTION 4 trial, which was performed only in Asian patients and the primary endpoints were designed for all-comers, rather than a specific CPS value, first-line treatment with nivolumab plus chemotherapy improved the co-primary progression-free survival endpoint, but not overall survival [118].

The third trial, presented at the same meeting, the KEYNOTE 590 trial, examined first-line chemotherapy with or without pembrolizumab in patients with squamous cell carcinoma of the esophagus, adenocarcinoma of the esophagus, or Siewert-type GE junction adenocarcinoma. It demonstrated that pembrolizumab plus chemotherapy improved overall survival in patients with squamous cell carcinoma of the esophagus with PD-L1 CPS $\geq$10 tumors, all squamous cell carcinomas, all patients with CPS $\geq$10, and the study population as a whole. Progression-free survival was also improved. It is expected that these trials will change the landscape of the treatment of esophageal cancer worldwide [118].

Several chemotherapy and targeted agents have been studied in the second-line treatment of esophageal and gastric cancer and beyond. Chemotherapy improves survival compared to placebo, single-agent paclitaxel with or without ramucirumab, a monoclonal antibody targeting the VEGF pathway, which is a commonly used second-line regimen with overall survival approaching 9 months. Single-agent ramucirumab, irinotecan, and immune checkpoint inhibitors are all approved for the second-line treatment as well, with modest benefits. Patients with microsatellite instable disease should be treated with immune check point inhibitors at any point during the course of their disease [118].

Several ongoing trials are testing other targeted therapies and are beyond the scope of this review.

Patients with inoperable esophageal cancer and with high-grade dysphagia were randomized to receive a self-expandable metal stent (SEMS) alone (Group I), versus a combination of SEMS followed by external beam radiation (over 2 weeks) (Group II). Dysphagia scores improved significantly in both groups following stent insertion. However, dysphagia relief was more sustained in Group II than in Group I (7 vs. 3 months, $p = 0.002$), and overall median survival was significantly higher in Group II than in Group I [119]. A recent meta-analysis of several RCTs evaluating the efficacy of SEMS alone vs. SEMS combined with radiotherapy concluded that the combination of SEMS and radiation significantly improves the overall survival as well as leading to improvements in quality of life scores [120].

In summary, the current trend in the literature shows that the best oncological outcomes are associated with trimodality therapy with neoadjuvant chemoradiation. This has been supported by recent meta-analyses that conclude that compared with neoadjuvant chemotherapy, neoadjuvant chemoradiotherapy should be recommended, with a significant long-term survival benefit in patients with cancer of the esophagus or the GEJ [121,122]. While treatments and outcomes are improving, a large proportion of patients fail locally, and addition of biologically targeted agents or local therapy intensification may prove to be beneficial.

For patients who are considered to be surgical candidates, neoadjuvant chemotherapy with weekly carboplatin and paclitaxel in combination with radiation followed by surgical resection is the standard of care. This treatment is based on the CROSS trial, where neoadjuvant therapy resulted in improved overall survival compared to esophagectomy alone [97]. Definitive chemotherapy and radiation is a reasonable option for patients who are not surgical candidates or with cervical/mid-esophageal SCC. On rare occasions, patients who are thought to have T1N0 disease are upstaged during esophagectomy; the role of adjuvant therapy in this setting is not clear and carries significant toxicity. The addition of Her-2 targeted therapy with trastuzumab (Her-2 antibody) to the neoadjuvant therapy did not result in improved outcome [123]. Several ongoing trials are currently evaluating the addition of immune checkpoint inhibitors in both the neoadjuvant and the adjuvant settings. These results are highly anticipated.

As previously described, neoadjuvant radiation therapy in addition to chemotherapy plays an important role in the multimodality treatment of locally advanced esophageal cancer. Fiducial markers have been integrated into the management of multiple malignancies to guide more precise delivery of radiation therapy (RT).

4. Gastric Malignancies

There are several gastric tumors, but we will focus our discussion on gastric adenocarcinoma, gastric GIST, NET, and MALT lymphoma.

4.1. Gastric Adenocarcinoma

Gastric adenocarcinoma, commonly referred to as gastric cancer (GC), represents the second-most common cancer worldwide and the fifth leading cause of cancer deaths. Men are observed to have approximately double the incidence of gastric cancer as women [124]. Globally, almost two thirds of cases are observed in East Asia, with China representing 43% of cases annually [2]. Gastric adenocarcinoma is histologically divided into intestinal and diffuse types. The intestinal type is distinguished by gland-like structures, whereas the diffuse type is characterized by poorly differentiated cells. Gastric adenocarcinomas arise as a result of a complex multifactorial process. Environmental factors include dietary exposures to sodium, nitrates, nitrites, nitrosamines, and lack of refrigeration. *H. pylori* infection and its associated proinflammatory milieu also represent important risk factors. There are multiple virulent strains of *H. pylori*; however, they are divided into two major subpopulations based on their ability to produce a 120–145 kDa immunodominant protein called cytotoxin-associated gene A (*CagA*) antigen. Strains that express the (*cagA*) pathogenicity island (PAI), a 40-kilobase DNA segment, are associated with increased inflammatory response and important clinical outcomes including peptic ulcers and gastric cancer [125]. Approximately 60% of *H. pylori* strains isolated in Western countries express *cagA* PAI whereas nearly all *H. pylori* from East Asian isolates express *cagA* PAI [126]. Additional predisposing conditions for gastric cancer include intestinal metaplasia and pernicious anemia. Rarely, genetic mutations such as CDH-1 contribute to familial predisposition to gastric adenocarcinoma [2].

4.2. Early Gastric Cancer (EGC)

Early Gastric Cancer: Endoscopic Diagnosis and Therapy

High-definition white light endoscopy (HD-WLE) combined with optical chromoendoscopy techniques such as narrow-band imaging (NBI) and targeted biopsies is the standard for early diagnosis of gastric cancer; see Figure 9. NBI increases the diagnostic yield for advanced gastric premalignant lesions compared to white light endoscopy [127]. The updated Sydney protocol is a standardized biopsy technique recommended for mapping the stomach to screen for atrophy and gastric intestinal metaplasia [128].

According to the Japanese Gastric Cancer Association, nonulcerated EGCs confined to the mucosa (T1a), with differentiated histology, and ≤20 mm, have low risk for lymph node metastasis and therefore are appropriate for endoscopic resection using the ESD technique. The criteria for ESD were expanded to include (1) nonulcerated differentiated EGCs of any size, (2) ulcerated differentiated EGCs <30 mm, or (3) differentiated EGCs <30 mm with superficial submucosal invasion (SM1; <500 μm below the muscularis mucosae) [129]; see Figure 10.

Asian endoscopists have applied the expanded criteria for EGC and have demonstrated that ESD has high curative rates comparable with those of traditional gastrectomy [113]. ESD is the standard of care for the management of EGC, meeting the expanded criteria as outlined by the Japanese guidelines [130]. The expanded Japanese criteria for resection were applied in the European setting with an en bloc resection rate of 98.4% for the standard guideline criteria and 89.0% for expanded criteria, and the R0 resection rate was 90.2% and 73.6%, respectively. Based on the excellent long-term outcome using the expanded criteria in EGCs in Western countries, ESD was recommended as the treatment of choice for intramucosal nonulcerated EGCs regardless of their diameter [131].

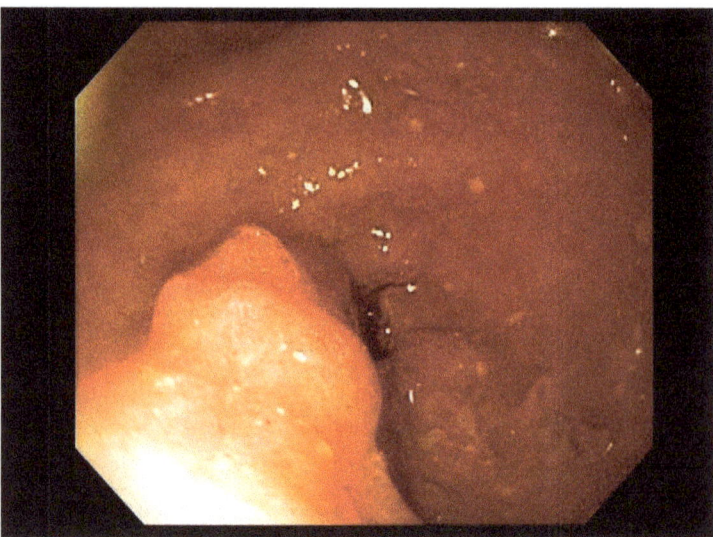

Figure 9. High-definition white light endoscopy (HD-WLE) combined with optical chromoendoscopy techniques such as narrow-band imaging (NBI) and targeted biopsies.

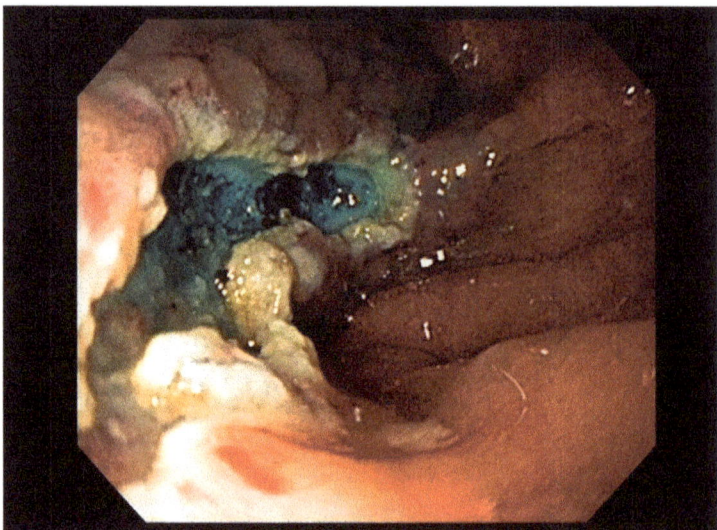

Figure 10. EMR of Early Gastric Cancer (EGC); submucosa stained with methylene blue.

However, the applicability of the current Japanese guidelines for endoscopic resection of EGC outside of Asia has been questioned based on differences in tumor characteristics and survival rates between Asian and Western populations [132,133]. The majority of undifferentiated intramucosal early gastric cancer (EGC) cases do not have lymph node metastasis but endoscopic resection has not been accepted as an alternative treatment to surgery for this subgroup of EGC.

Abe et al. have identified two independent risk factors for lymph node metastases: a tumor ≥20 mm and presence of lymphatic involvement on endoscopic resection specimens. They recommended that undifferentiated EGC <10 mm without lymphatic involvement may be treated by endoscopic resection primarily [134]. If lymphatic involvement is seen on the endoscopic resection specimen, additional surgery is warranted.

Others have suggested a size threshold of 20 mm or less in tumors without lymphatic-vascular capillary involvement or ulceration as suitable candidates for endoscopic resection based on low rate of lymphatic metastases, incidence of lymph node metastasis, and the feasibility of endoscopic resection for undifferentiated-type early gastric cancer [135].

4.3. Endoscopic Ultrasound in Staging of Gastric Cancer

EUS accuracy has historically been suboptimal in the preoperative staging of gastric cancer and it is recommended that EUS should be combined with other modalities for the preoperative staging of gastric cancer [136]. A meta-analysis evaluated the diagnostic accuracy of EUS for the preoperative locoregional staging of GC and the Cochrane Collaboration Group evaluated 66 articles on GC staged with EUS. EUS sensitivity and specificity to discriminate T1-T2 from T3-T4 lesions to be 86% and 90%, respectively [137]; see Figure 11. In a prospective study of patients with GC before and after neoadjuvant chemotherapy, the overall accuracy of EUS was around 80% and EUS performed better than PET-CT for N staging and restaging [138]. Similar to esophageal cancer, patients with potentially resectable GC with T2 disease and higher or any evidence of nodal involvement have significant benefits of adjuvant or neoadjuvant therapy compared to surgery alone. In patients with GC, a complete staging with laparoscopy and peritoneal washing is recommended if feasible, followed by perioperative treatment. Several regimens have been evaluated in large randomized trials for locally advanced potentially resectable gastric cancer including adjuvant chemoradiotherapy: Intergroup 0116(2) and Cancer and Leukemia Group B(3) (CALGB 80101), perioperative chemotherapy [139] and more recently the FLOT regimen [133], and adjuvant chemotherapy alone in Asia. All showed benefits of perioperative treatment. In the United States, the majority of patients receive perioperative chemotherapy with or without radiation. Similar to esophageal cancer, several targeted agents such as VEGFR antibodies and Her-2 antibodies have been integrated in the perioperative setting, with limited benefits. Several ongoing studies are evaluating the addition of immunotherapy to chemotherapy in this setting as well.

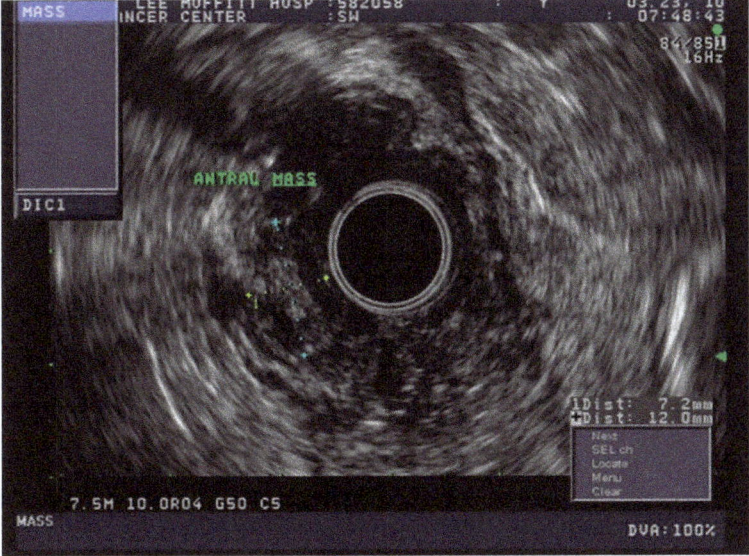

Figure 11. Early gastric cancer; EUS image polypoid lesion T1N0.

4.4. Gastrointestinal Stromal Tumor (GIST)

Gastrointestinal stromal tumors arise anywhere along the digestive tract and are thought to arise from the interstitial cells of Cajal or a common progenitor cell, based on common immunophenotypes. These are found in patients with advanced age and are most commonly found in the stomach, duodenum, jejunum, and ileum. Histologically, these may be spindle-cell, epithelioid, or mixed type. These tumors may express mutations in tyrosine kinase (TK), KIT receptor, or platelet-derived growth factor (PDGF). Histologically, these are distinguished with spindle-cell morphology. These may be localized or metastatic (peritoneum, liver). Disease progression is related to several key factors including location, size, and mitotic index [140]; see Figures 12 and 13.

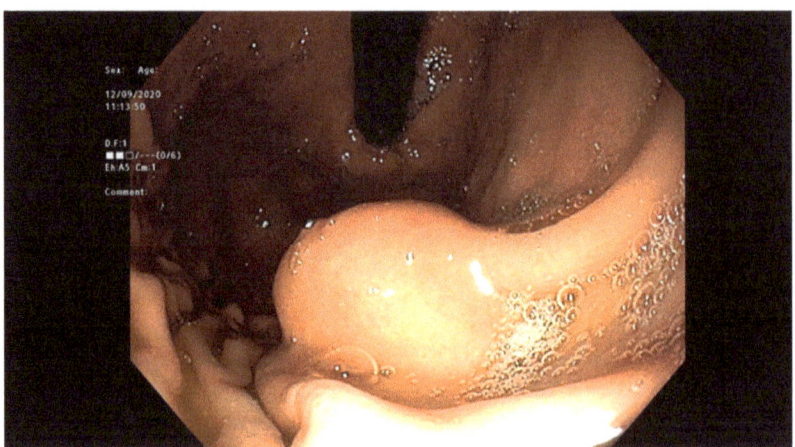

Figure 12. Gastrointestinal stromal tumor, as seen with high-definition white light endoscopy.

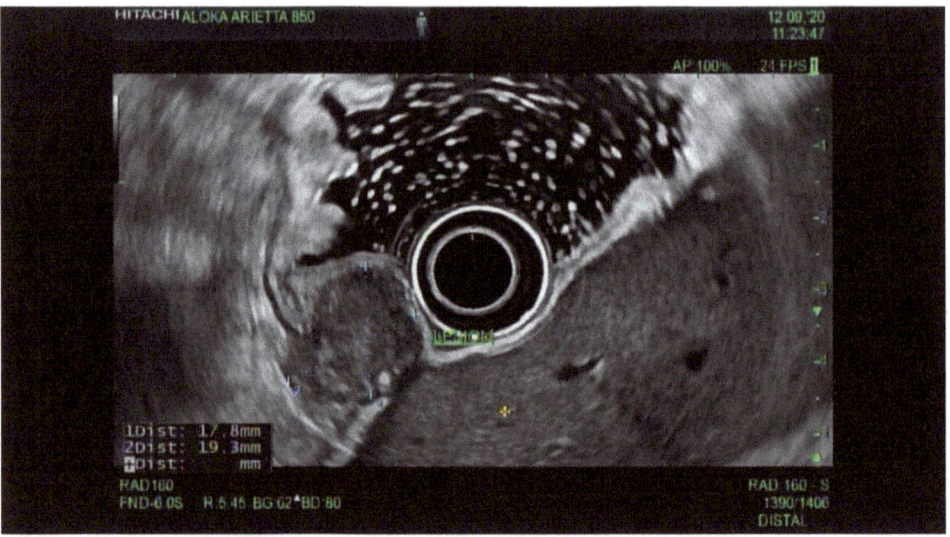

Figure 13. EUS images of a gastrointestinal stromal tumor originating from muscularis propria.

Surgical resection is the preferred treatment for localized GIST tumors. The goal of surgery is to achieve a negative margin resection without causing tumor rupture. For gastric GISTs, a wedge resection can be performed, avoiding formal gastrectomy. Lymphadenectomy is not indicated. Laparoscopic or minimally invasive resections have been associated with less blood loss, lower rates of complications, and shorter hospital stays without compromise of oncologic principles [141]. With some GIST tumors, either small or predominantly intraluminal ones, they may be difficult to fully visualize and anticipate margins by visualization laparoscopically. Endoscopic assistance in this circumstance can provide the added benefit of intraluminal assessment and delineation of margins; this combined endoscopic and laparoscopic approach (i.e., laparoscopic and endoscopic cooperative surgery) can help avoid more major gastric resections [142]. The goal of surgery is to achieve complete resection, and if feasible, then an upfront resection is recommended. If a highly morbid operation is required, or one requiring multivisceral resection, neoadjuvant imatinib can be considered [143]. This may allow for downsizing of the tumor, to avoid a more morbid operation [144]. A biopsy should be performed, and tumor genotype could help guide neoadjuvant treatment. Imatinib is the treatment of choice in this setting; however, tumors that have a platelet-derived growth factor receptor-alpha (*PDGFRA*) D842V mutation, or a succinate dehydrogenase (SDH)-deficient or neurofibromatosis (NF)-related GIST, are considered resistant to imatinib and will not benefit from neoadjuvant treatment; in these cases, upfront surgery is recommended. Tumors that harbor an exon 9 *KIT* mutation should be treated with an initial dose of 800 mg per day. Patients should be treated to the maximum response followed by surgical resection.

Based upon the results of the Scandinavian Sarcoma Group (SSG) XVIII adjuvant trial, daily imatinib treatment for 36 months is currently the standard of care for patients with high-risk disease [145]. Patients with metastatic disease are best treated with systemic therapy with imatinib and the other approved TKIs, with surgical debulking reserved for those who respond well and can achieve complete resection.

4.5. Neuroendocrine Tumors

Neuroendocrine tumors can arise throughout the digestive tract and other areas of the body. Gastric neuroendocrine tumors account for 7–8% of all neuroendocrine tumors [146]. These tumors are derived from the enterochromaffin-like cells in the stomach and are divided into three distinct types (I–III).

Type I neuroendocrine tumors are the most common and represent 70–80% of gastric neuroendocrine tumors. They can be seen in association with chronic atrophic gastritis. Due to resultant chronic achlorhydria, G-cell hyperplasia happens and results in increased gastrin secretion and hypergastrinemia. These tumors typically occur in the mucosa or submucosa and are more indolent. Smaller tumors (less than 1 cm) may be amenable to endoscopic resection (EMR and ESD) and surveillance via upper endoscopy, endoscopic ultrasound.

Type II neuroendocrine tumors are associated with Zollinger Ellison syndrome (Multiple Endocrine Neoplasia I). These are the least-frequently occurring, representing between 5% and 8% of cases. Metastatic potential is estimated at approximately 30% [147].

Type III and Type IV neuroendocrine tumors are more aggressive and may be metastatic at presentation. Therapeutic approaches may be more systemic.

The three types of gastric neuroendocrine tumors have previously been described, as well as their relationship to gastrin levels. Type II gastric neuroendocrine tumors are rare and found in the setting of increased acid production from hypergastrinemia secondary to gastrinoma. Type 2 gastric NET should be resected. Type III gastric NET are found in the setting of normal gastrin levels and exhibit a more aggressive behavior; they are treated surgically in a manner similar to adenocarcinoma: formal gastric resection and regional lymphadenectomy. Small, low-grade, Type III gastric NET without evidence of lymphovascular invasion can be treated with wedge or endoscopic resection [148].

Type I and II G-NETs appear either as small (<10 mm) polypoid lesions, or more frequently, as smooth hemispherical submucosal lesions, that may appear yellow or red in color. EUS is useful for assessing the depth of the gastric NETs and their location within the layers of the gastric wall. They usually arise from the second (deeper mucosal) or third (submucosal) echo layers and are identified as hypoechoic intramural structures [149].

EUS-FNB is a useful modality in the diagnosis of gastric NET and, in the appropriate settings, can provide adequate tissue for histological diagnosis [150]. Endoscopic resection using the band ligation or cap technique is an established technique for resection of gastric NETs <1 cm [151]. Currently, there is no role of adjuvant therapy following surgical resection in these patients per NCCN guidelines [152].

4.6. Gastric Lymphoma

There are two major types of primary gastric lymphoma: mucosa-associated lymphoid tissue (MALT) gastric lymphoma or diffuse large B-cell lymphoma (DLBCL) of the stomach. MALT lymphoma is a type of extra-nodal low-grade marginal-B cell lymphoma which may occur in the stomach, small bowel, and other organs. These lesions may present as erosions or nodular masses and are distinct from gastric adenocarcinoma [153]. *H. pylori* is noted as a causative factor for MALT lymphoma and eradication of *H. pylori* can result in remission in 50–90% of cases. Therefore, eradication of *H. pylori* is regarded as a first-line treatment for gastric MALT lymphoma, with remission favorably associated with early lesions, lesions limited to the mucosa, and absence of the *API2MALT1* mutation [154]. The role of endoscopy is one of diagnosis, response to therapy, and surveillance, with EUS demonstrating value in predicting submucosal and regional lymph node involvement [155].

4.7. Staging

Laparoscopic assessment of the peritoneal cavity for patients with advanced gastric cancer (T2+) is an established method of detecting radiographic-occult peritoneal disease, both in Eastern and Western countries. Over 30% of patients may be found to have peritoneal disease or positive peritoneal cytology [156,157]. Positive peritoneal disease or cytology renders a stage IV prognosis and diagnosis and can help temper treatment expectations. For those with Tis or T1a cancers that fit the Japanese guidelines, consideration of endoscopic resection techniques such as ESD is a reasonable approach. For distal tumors, subtotal distal gastrectomy is recommended. For proximal tumors, total gastrectomy with roux-y esophagojejunostomy is preferred. Concomitant splenectomy is no longer performed as morbidity is increased without any survival benefit [158]. For patients with localized or regional disease, total formal gastrectomy with modified D2 lymphadenectomy is recommended in the US, with the goal of examining at least 15 lymph nodes, following a multidisciplinary review for consideration of perioperative chemotherapy. In Eastern countries, modified D2 lymphadenectomy is considered standard of care. The 15-year follow-up of the Dutch D1D2 trial did not show any overall survival benefit; however, there was lower local and regional recurrence and gastric cancer-related deaths. This was not shown in other trials, thereby rendering modified D2 lymphadenectomy as a recommendation in NCCN guidelines [159,160]. Laparoscopic approaches to gastrectomy have also been investigated, mostly in Eastern countries, and have been shown to have similar oncologic outcomes to open gastrectomy [161,162].

4.8. Treatment

Primary gastric cancer encompasses tumors with an epicenter classification of Siewert III superiorly (>2 cm distal to GEJ) and extends inferiorly to tumors arising from the gastric antrum and pylorus. As in most upper intestinal GI malignancies, surgery by gastrectomy with lymph node dissection is considered the primary curative therapy. Similar to esophageal cancer, no adjuvant therapy is generally recommended for early-stage pT1N0 disease and these tumors may be adequately treated by endoscopic resection and close follow-up. However, if pT2+ or pN+, adjuvant chemotherapy is given with consideration for radiotherapy based on risk factors of positive margins or inadequate nodal dissection (D1, or <15 total LN). More recent evidence supports a survival benefit of neoadjuvant chemotherapy for resectable disease. In patients with locally advanced disease, neoadjuvant chemotherapy with or without chemoradiation can be considered [98]. For inoperable patients, definitive chemoradiation may be given; however, outcomes are generally poor.

Radiotherapy simulation and treatment planning for GC generally follows a similar paradigm to GEJ tumors with 4D-CT simulation and IGRT to EUS-placed fiducial markers or surgical clips. Contouring guidelines have been published to aid delineation in the setting of esophagogastrectomy, total gastrectomy, and subtotal gastrectomy [163]. Generally, dose in the adjuvant setting is conventionally fractionated to 45 Gy with a 5.4–9.0 Gy boost for microscopically positive disease or higher for gross residual disease. Nodal regions at risk are dependent on the primary site of disease as well as extent of invasion and commonly include the perigastric, celiac and celiac axis, SMA, as well as supra- and infra-pyloric nodal basins. The distal paraesophageal, porto-hepatic, and pancreaticoduodenal lymph nodes may be covered depending on primary tumor location. Elective node coverage can be omitted in patients with pT2-3N0 disease with D2 nodal dissection with ≥15 LN removed [164].

Acute toxicity during treatment may be significant with fatigue, nausea, vomiting, dyspepsia, or gastritis and may be particularly pronounced in the adjuvant setting after more extensive gastrectomies. Late toxicity including GI stricture, chronic kidney insufficiency, and secondary malignancies has been associated with gastric radiotherapy. These toxicities were particularly pronounced with two-dimensional fields as utilized in INT0116 that resulted in 33% G3+ GI toxicity and upwards of 50% hematologic G3+ toxicity [165]. Modern IMRT techniques have a dosimetric benefit in silico for tumor coverage as well as organ sparing [166,167], and early reports are favorable regarding toxicity in preoperative [168] and postoperative settings [169,170].

4.8.1. Adjuvant Chemoradiation

The use of adjuvant radiotherapy in the treatment of GC has historically been limited in dose due to organ and anastomosis tolerance as well as high toxicity rates. Furthermore, as our understanding of the impact of the extent and quality of surgical resection has broadened, patient selection and risk stratification has improved. The landmark INT0116 trial demonstrated a survival benefit of adjuvant chemoradiation versus observation after gastrectomy with D0/D1 lymph node dissection [165]. This population consisted of predominantly advanced disease with nearly 70% pT3-4 and 85% pN+, and with extended follow-up of 10.3 years, chemoradiation offered a survival benefit (HR 1.32, $p < 0.001$) and nearly halved locoregional relapses [171], while more extensive D2 lymph node dissection initially resulted in higher rates of surgical morbidity and postoperative mortality than D1 [172], long-term follow-up demonstrated improvements in locoregional recurrence and gastric cancer specific mortality [160]. Within this domain, the data to date mostly show no benefit in the addition of radiation to adjuvant chemotherapy due to the outcomes of the CRITICS [173] and ARTIST trials [174,175].

The ARTIST I trial enrolled 458 patients with pathologic stage IB-IV (M0) disease who underwent an R0 gastrectomy and D2 lymph node dissection to adjuvant capecitabine and cisplatin (XP) for six cycles alone vs. chemoradiation to 45 Gy with concurrent capecitabine sandwiched by two cycles of XP [174]. With extended follow-up, there was no significant difference in OS and DFS; however, on subgroup analysis, radiotherapy was associated with improvement in DFS in patients with pN+, high lymph node ratio and intestinal-type histology [175]. These findings were explored in ARTIST II in pathologically node positive patients; however, no benefit was noted with chemoradiation against combination chemotherapy alone (HR 0.91, $p = 0.667$) [176]. The trial was terminated early but final publication is anticipated.

Finally, CRITICS included 788 non-metastatic stage IB-IVA gastric cancer patients who were randomized upfront to adjuvant chemoradiation or chemotherapy alone [173]. All patients were given neoadjuvant chemotherapy consisting of epirubicin, capecitabine, cisplatin/oxaliplatin (ECF/ECX) for three cycles followed by gross total resection, with 79% D1+ resections and a median of 20 lymph nodes removed. After surgery, patients received either three cycles of chemotherapy or chemoradiation to 45 Gy with weekly cisplatin and capecitabine. Unfortunately, the dropout rate during adjuvant therapy was high in both arms, approximating 50%, limiting conclusions of the study, but median survival for adjuvant chemoradiotherapy was numerically less at 37 months vs. 43 months with adjuvant chemotherapy but not statistically different. Perioperative morbidity was high, with a pooled 66% G3+ toxicity rate with preoperative chemotherapy and similar G3+ GI toxicity rates near 40% between both adjuvant treatments, highlighting the toxicity of these regimens.

The authors of CRITICS concluded that in the era of delivery of intensive neoadjuvant therapy, the impact of adjuvant chemotherapy or chemoradiation may be minimalized, especially as rates of compliance with adjuvant therapy in modern series approximate 50% [133,139,173]. Furthermore, more recent data favor FLOT chemotherapy (docetaxel, oxaliplatin, leucovorin, fluorouracil), with demonstrated improved survival over the ECF/ECX regimen [133]. These findings, coupled with the results of the landmark MAGIC trial favoring delivery of neoadjuvant therapy [139], suggest that postoperative radiotherapy only has benefit in highly selected patients with significant adverse pathological features.

4.8.2. Neoadjuvant Chemoradiation

A few series have investigated the benefit of neoadjuvant therapy in gastric cancer. Early investigations included patients with gastric cardia tumors comparing surgery alone to multimodal therapy consisting of fluorouracil and cisplatin with concurrent 40 Gy in 15 fractions [177]. With a limited median follow-up of 10 months, they reported an improved median survival with multimodality therapy to 16 months compared to 11 months; however, these overall outcomes poorly compared to contemporary results implicating inferior surgical technique. However, of note, the pCR rate in resected patients treated with multimodality therapy was 25% and lymph node positivity was reduced by nearly 50%. The phase II RTOG 9904 further investigated this strategy in 49 patients with gastric cancer, treating patients with induction fluorouracil/cisplatin followed by chemoradiation to 45 Gy with weekly fluorouracil and paclitaxel and by surgical resection (50% D2) [178]. Despite major protocol deviations in 56% of radiotherapy treatment and 37% of surgery, a pCR rate of 26% was achieved that was associated with per protocol treatment ($p = 0.02$). More modern data are extrapolated from the POET trial where, despite elevated post-op mortality with combined modality treatment to 30 Gy, there was a trend for improved survival at 5 years [98].

Overall, these findings have driven interest in larger randomized trials investigating this strategy specifically for gastric cancer. Of particular interest is CRITICS II comparing three arms of neoadjuvant therapy including: standard chemotherapy with DOC × 4 cycles (docetaxel, oxaliplatin, capecitabine), neoadjuvant DOC × 2 cycles followed by chemoradiation to 45 Gy with concurrent weekly carboplatin and paclitaxel, and chemoradiation alone with the winner to be further assessed in a phase III format [179]. Finally, early safety outcomes of the TOPGEAR trial have been reported comparing perioperative ECF chemotherapy for six cycles to preoperative ECF for two cycles followed by neoadjuvant 45 Gy with concurrent fluorouracil or capecitabine and adjuvant ECF for three cycles [180]. Compliance with neoadjuvant therapy in both arms has been >90% with preoperative treatment and >85% of patients are able to proceed to surgery. However, 65% of the chemotherapy alone arm and 53% in the chemoradiation group have completed postoperative chemotherapy. Importantly, there have been no significant differences in toxicity or surgical morbidity between the two treatment arms. In contrast to esophageal cancer, a lack of high-level evidence exists for neoadjuvant chemoradiation in gastric cancer while the final results of these studies are awaited.

4.8.3. Unresectable Gastric Cancer

Inoperable patients or unresectable gastric cancer, including linitis plastica, are classically thought to be incurable; however, durable local control and an associated improvement in quality of life or palliation may be achieved with chemoradiation; see Figures 14 and 15. Historic radiotherapy techniques had significant early mortality associated with chemoradiation to 50 Gy but improved 4-year survival of 17% vs. 6% with chemotherapy alone [181]. Similar outcomes have been noted in a retrospective analysis of the MD Anderson experience, demonstrating 5-year survival rates of 18% in 71 unresected patients with improved outcomes associated with chemoradiation (HR 0.25, 95%CI 0.06–1.01) with a median dose of 45 Gy (range: 36–50.4 Gy) [182]. At the population level, an analysis of the NCDB demonstrated a 7% improvement in 2-year survival with chemoradiation as opposed to chemotherapy alone [183]. Alternatively, there have been case reports of the use of proton therapy in Japan for inoperable patients treated to 61–83 Gy with at least one clinical complete response 2 years after treatment [184,185]. Undoubtedly, this is an area ripe for further inquiry as interest and utilization of particle therapy increases. The role of chemotherapy in the treatment of metastatic gastric cancer is very similar to esophageal cancer (see Section 3.3). Several of the metastatic esophageal adenocarcinoma trials included gastric cancer trials and vice versa.

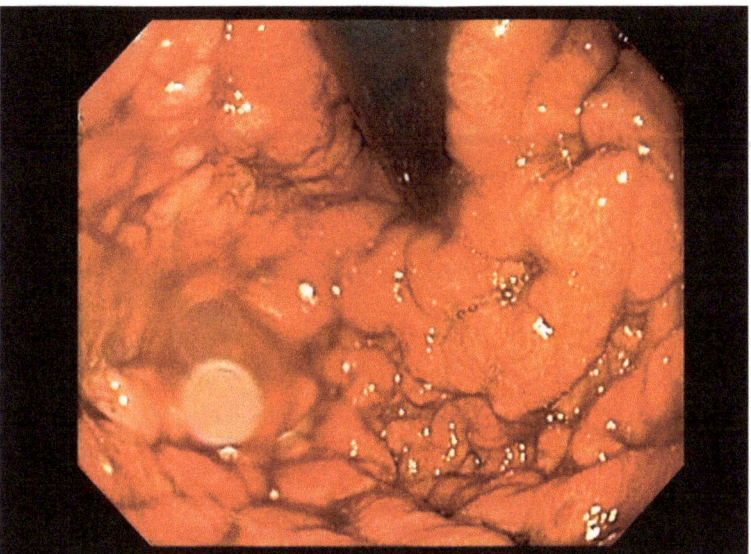

Figure 14. Gastric linitis plastica, submucosal infiltrating cancer; white light endoscopy.

4.8.4. Gastric Neuroendocrine Tumors

The role of radiation therapy for neuroendocrine tumors is generally limited to palliation of symptomatic or oligometastatic disease. To this end, hypofractionated regimens offer patient convenience and the ability to achieve high biological equivalent doses to improve local control [186,187]. There is some limited evidence that SBRT may be an effective option for treatment of functional neuroendocrine tumors, with clinical and biochemical responses reported in four patients [188].

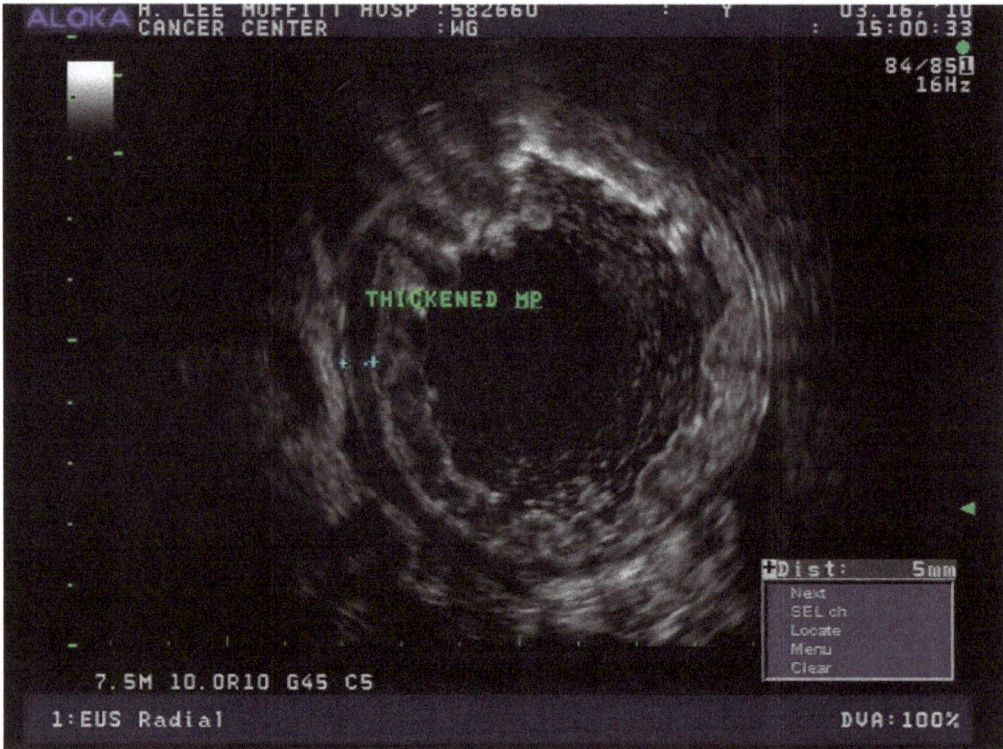

Figure 15. EUS Linitis plastica with significant wall thickening.

5. Future Directions in Diagnosis of Esophageal and Gastric Tumors

Novel methylated DNA markers assayed from plasma can detect esophageal cancer with moderate accuracy [189]. Serum markers to detect early esophageal and gastric cancer may be the first step to identifying patients at higher risk to undergo more invasive endoscopic screening. A non-endoscopic test, Cytosponge-trefoil factor 3 (TFF3), has demonstrated improved detection of Barrett esophagus compared with standard screening in a primary care setting [13]. Tethered capsule optical coherence tomography (OCT) is a non-endoscopic technique that has been developed and can volumetrically image esophageal mucosa and detect BE in unsedated patients in the outpatient setting [190].

In addition to advances in optical chromoendoscopy and endoscopic ultrasound, new modalities of image enhanced endoscopy are being studied. Techniques such as volumetric laser endomicroscopy (VLE) and confocal laser endomicroscopy have been shown to improve the detection of dysplasia associated with Barrett's esophagus [191]. The addition of wide-area transepithelial sampling to an already thorough examination with HDWLE-NBI-VLE-SP may increase the yield of dysplasia detection. The future will likely involve using a combination of diagnostic methodologies to improve the accuracy of detection of preneoplastic lesions.

Endoscopic resection techniques such as ESD, submucosal tunnel endoscopic resection (STER), and full thickness resection devices (FTRD) will become more refined and the design of devices will likely improve as well, making this the primary treatment of choice for early-stage/mucosal cancer of the esophagus and the stomach.

There has been interest in developing and studying drug-eluting stents and stents combined with brachytherapy delivery for treatment and palliation of unresectable, obstructing gastrointestinal cancers. It is likely that we will see the development of such stents that facilitate delivery of brachytherapy or local chemotherapy for esophageal cancer in the future.

6. Chemotherapy and Radiation

In the last decade, a major breakthrough in cancer treatment was the discovery of immune checkpoint proteins, which effectively inhibit the immune system through various mechanisms. Immune checkpoint inhibitors are currently approved in several tumors in the metastatic and adjuvant setting. In the upper GI malignancies, approval is currently restricted to the metastatic setting and beyond the first line. Recent studies have shown promising activities in the front-line setting and in the adjuvant setting at least in a subset of patients and approval is expected in the upcoming months. Currently, several ongoing trials are evaluating the integration of immune checkpoint inhibitors in the neoadjuvant setting in combination with chemotherapy and radiation as well as following surgical resection. Combining immune checkpoint inhibitors with other targeted therapies (Her-2 and VEGF) has shown some promising activity as well and is currently being tested. Advances in image-guided radiation and proton beam therapy to improve precision are promising as well to decrease toxicity and improve patient tolerance.

Several new tyrosine kinase inhibitors have shown promising activity in GIST and they will be tested in the adjuvant and the neoadjuvant setting as well. Several novel agents have been approved for neuroendocrine tumors in the last 5 years and several treatment combination trials are ongoing.

7. Conclusions

Upper GI neoplasia is a complex process involving the organs of the upper digestive tract with a multifactorial etiology and represents a significant burden of disease worldwide. Diagnosis and staging require a multimodal approach, involving endoscopy, endoscopic ultrasonography, endoscopic mucosal resection and submucosal dissection techniques, and imaging CT/PET imaging modalities. Once diagnosis and staging are achieved, treatment involves careful multidisciplinary planning involving gastrointestinal endoscopists, medical oncologists, surgical oncologists, and radiation oncologists to determine the most appropriate therapeutic approach. For early lesions, therapeutic endoscopic approaches include endoscopic mucosal resection and endoscopic submucosal dissection. For locally advanced lesions, adjuvant or neoadjuvant chemotherapy therapy may be required based on staging, prior to surgical resection. Image-guided radiotherapy represents an important adjuvant or neoadjuvant therapy, again depending on stage and anatomy.

Future directions in screening may involve office-based tissue sampling strategies along with serological "liquid biopsy" assays. Advances in the diagnosis and staging of gastrointestinal malignancy will rely upon advances in endoscopic imaging, including optical coherence tomography and endoscopic ultrasound. Improvements in endosurgical techniques represent an area of promise for the therapy of early lesions, while advances in surgical oncology, novel chemotherapeutics, and tailored radiotherapy will hopefully allow for decreased disease morbidity and mortality over time.

Funding: This research received no external funding.

Conflicts of Interest: The authors declare no conflict of interest.

References

1. Bray, F.; Ferlay, J.; Soerjomataram, I.; Siegel, R.L.; Torre, L.A.; Jemal, A. Global cancer statistics 2018: GLOBOCAN estimates of incidence and mortality worldwide for 36 cancers in 185 countries. *CA Cancer J. Clin.* **2018**, *68*, 394–424. [CrossRef]
2. Van Cutsem, E.; Sagaert, X.; Topal, B.; Haustermans, K.; Prenen, H. Gastric cancer. *Lancet* **2016**, *388*, 2654–2664. [CrossRef]
3. Arnold, M.; Park, J.Y.; Camargo, M.C.; Lunet, N.; Forman, D.; Soerjomataram, I. Is gastric cancer becoming a rare disease? A global assessment of predicted incidence trends to 2035. *Gut* **2020**, *69*, 823–829. [CrossRef] [PubMed]
4. Laurén, P. The two histological main types of gastric carcinoma: diffuse and so-called intestinal-type carcinoma. *Acta Pathol. Microbiol. Scand.* **1965**, *64*, 31–49. [CrossRef]

5. Adam, B.; Pech, O.; Steckstor, M.; Tannapfel, A.; Riphaus, A. Gastric Mucosa-Associated Lymphoid Tissue Lymphoma. *Video J. Encycl. GI Endosc.* **2013**, *1*, 174–175. [CrossRef]
6. Sanon, M.; Taylor, D.C.; Coombs, J.D.; Sirulnik, L.; Rubin, J.L.; Bollu, V. Epidemiology, survival, and costs of localized gastrointestinal stromal tumors. *Int. J. Gen. Med.* **2011**, *4*, 121–130. [CrossRef] [PubMed]
7. Que, J.; Garman, K.S.; Souza, R.F.; Spechler, S.J. Pathogenesis and Cells of Origin of Barrett's Esophagus. *Gastroenterology* **2019**, *157*, 349–364.e1. [CrossRef]
8. Shaheen, N.J.; E Richter, J. Barrett's oesophagus. *Lancet* **2009**, *373*, 850–861. [CrossRef]
9. Correa, P.; Piazuelo, M.B.; Wilson, K.T. Pathology of Gastric Intestinal Metaplasia: Clinical Implications. *Am. J. Gastroenterol.* **2010**, *105*, 493–498. [CrossRef]
10. Leung, W.K. Risk Factors Associated with the Development of Intestinal Metaplasia in First-Degree Relatives of Gastric Cancer Patients. *Cancer Epidemiol. Biomark. Prev.* **2005**, *14*, 2982–2986. [CrossRef]
11. Uemura, N.; Okamoto, S.; Yamamoto, S.; Matsumura, N.; Yamaguchi, S.; Yamakido, M.; Taniyama, K.; Sasaki, N.; Schlemper, R.J. Helicobacter pyloriInfection and the Development of Gastric Cancer. *N. Engl. J. Med.* **2001**, *345*, 784–789. [CrossRef] [PubMed]
12. Wang, Z.; Kambhampati, S.; Cheng, Y.; Ma, K.; Simsek, C.; Tieu, A.H.; Abraham, J.M.; Liu, X.; Prasath, V.; Duncan, M.; et al. Methylation Biomarker Panel Performance in EsophaCap Cytology Samples for Diagnosing Barrett's Esophagus: A Prospective Validation Study. *Clin. Cancer Res.* **2019**, *25*, 2127–2135. [CrossRef] [PubMed]
13. Fitzgerald, R.C.; Di Pietro, M.; O'Donovan, M.; Maroni, R.; Muldrew, B.; Debiram-Beecham, I.; Gehrung, M.; Offman, J.; Tripathi, M.; Smith, S.G.; et al. Cytosponge-trefoil factor 3 versus usual care to identify Barrett's oesophagus in a primary care setting: A multicentre, pragmatic, randomised controlled trial. *Lancet* **2020**, *396*, 333–344. [CrossRef]
14. Yamamoto, H.; Watanabe, Y.; Sato, Y.; Maehata, T.; Itoh, F. Non-Invasive Early Molecular Detection of Gastric Cancers. *Cancers* **2020**, *12*, 2880. [CrossRef] [PubMed]
15. Desai, M.; Saligram, S.; Gupta, N.; Vennalaganti, P.; Bansal, A.; Choudhary, A.; Vennelaganti, S.; He, J.; Titi, M.; Maselli, R.; et al. Efficacy and safety outcomes of multimodal endoscopic eradication therapy in Barrett's esophagus-related neoplasia: A systematic review and pooled analysis. *Gastrointest. Endosc.* **2017**, *85*, 482–495.e4. [CrossRef] [PubMed]
16. Waddingham, W.; Nieuwenburg, S.A.V.; Carlson, S.; Rodriguez-Justo, M.; Spaander, M.; Kuipers, E.J.; Jansen, M.; Graham, D.G.; Banks, M. Recent advances in the detection and management of early gastric cancer and its precursors. *Front. Gastroenterol.* **2020**. [CrossRef]
17. Pimentel-Nunes, P.; Dinis-Ribeiro, M.; Soares, J.B.; Marcos-Pinto, R.; Santos, C.; Rolanda, C.; Bastos, R.P.; Areia, M.; Afonso, L.; Bergman, J.; et al. A multicenter validation of an endoscopic classification with narrow band imaging for gastric precancerous and cancerous lesions. *Endoscopy* **2012**, *44*, 236–246. [CrossRef]
18. Sharma, P.; Hawes, R.H.; Bansal, A.; Gupta, N.; Curvers, W.; Rastogi, A.; Singh, M.; Hall, M.; Mathur, S.C.; Wani, S.; et al. Standard endoscopy with random biopsies versus narrow band imaging targeted biopsies in Barrett's oesophagus: a prospective, international, randomised controlled trial. *Gut* **2012**, *62*, 15–21. [CrossRef]
19. Ajani, J.A.; D'Amico, T.A.; Bentrem, D.J.; Chao, J.; Corvera, C.; Das, P.; Denlinger, C.S.; Enzinger, P.C.; Fanta, P.; Farjah, F.; et al. Esophageal and Esophagogastric Junction Cancers, Version 2.2019, NCCN Clinical Practice Guidelines in Oncology. *J. Natl. Compr. Cancer Netw.* **2019**, *17*, 855–883. [CrossRef]
20. Song, B.G.; Min, Y.W.; Cha, R.R.; Lee, H.; Min, B.-H.; Lee, J.H.; Rhee, P.-L.; Kim, J.J. Endoscopic submucosal dissection under general anesthesia for superficial esophageal squamous cell carcinoma is associated with better clinical outcomes. *BMC Gastroenterol.* **2018**, *18*, 80. [CrossRef]
21. Van Hagen, P.; Spaander, M.C.W.; Van Der Gaast, A.; Van Rij, C.M.; Tilanus, H.W.; Van Lanschot, J.J.B.; Wijnhoven, B.P.L. Impact of a multidisciplinary tumour board meeting for upper-GI malignancies on clinical decision making: A prospective cohort study. *Int. J. Clin. Oncol.* **2011**, *18*, 214–219. [CrossRef] [PubMed]
22. Basta, Y.L.; Bolle, S.; Fockens, P.; Tytgat, K.M.A.J. The Value of Multidisciplinary Team Meetings for Patients with Gastrointestinal Malignancies: A Systematic Review. *Ann. Surg. Oncol.* **2017**, *24*, 2669–2678. [CrossRef] [PubMed]
23. Subasinghe, D.; Acott, N.; Kumarasinghe, M.P. A survival guide to HER2 testing in gastric/gastroesophageal junction carcinoma. *Gastrointest. Endosc.* **2019**, *90*, 44–54. [CrossRef] [PubMed]
24. Turner, E.S.; Turner, J.R. Expanding the Lauren Classification: A New Gastric Cancer Subtype? *Gastroenterology* **2013**, *145*, 505–508. [CrossRef] [PubMed]
25. Watanabe, M. Risk factors and molecular mechanisms of esophageal cancer: differences between the histologic subtype. *J. Cancer Metastasis Treat.* **2015**. [CrossRef]
26. Abnet, C.C.; Arnold, M.; Wei, W. Epidemiology of Esophageal Squamous Cell Carcinoma. *Gastroenterology* **2018**, *154*, 360–373. [CrossRef] [PubMed]
27. Arnold, M.; Soerjomataram, I.; Ferlay, J.; Forman, D. Global incidence of oesophageal cancer by histological subtype in 2012. *Gut* **2015**, *64*, 381–387. [CrossRef]
28. Cook, M.B.; Chow, W.-H.; Devesa, S.S. Oesophageal cancer incidence in the United States by race, sex, and histologic type, 1977–2005. *Br. J. Cancer* **2009**, *101*, 855–859. [CrossRef]
29. Coleman, H.G.; Xie, S.-H.; Lagergren, J. The Epidemiology of Esophageal Adenocarcinoma. *Gastroenterology* **2018**, *154*, 390–405. [CrossRef]
30. Eluri, S.; Shaheen, N.J. Barrett's esophagus: Diagnosis and management. *Gastrointest. Endosc.* **2017**, *85*, 889–903. [CrossRef]

31. Ireland, C.J.; Thompson, S.K.; Laws, T.A.; Esterman, A. Risk factors for Barrett's esophagus: A scoping review. *Cancer Causes Control.* **2016**, *27*, 301–323. [CrossRef] [PubMed]
32. Sharma, P.; Shaheen, N.J.; Katzka, D.; Bergman, J.J. AGA Clinical Practice Update on Endoscopic Treatment of Barrett's Esophagus With Dysplasia and/or Early Cancer: Expert Review. *Gastroenterology* **2020**, *158*, 760–769. [CrossRef] [PubMed]
33. Bhat, S.; Coleman, H.G.; Yousef, F.; Johnston, B.T.; McManus, D.T.; Gavin, A.T.; Murray, L.J. Risk of Malignant Progression in Barrett's Esophagus Patients: Results from a Large Population-Based Study. *J. Natl. Cancer Inst.* **2011**, *103*, 1049–1057. [CrossRef] [PubMed]
34. Shaheen, N.J.; Sharma, P.; Overholt, B.F.; Wolfsen, H.C.; Sampliner, R.E.; Wang, K.K.; Galanko, J.A.; Bronner, M.P.; Goldblum, J.R.; Bennett, A.E.; et al. Radiofrequency Ablation in Barrett's Esophagus with Dysplasia. *N. Engl. J. Med.* **2009**, *360*, 2277–2288. [CrossRef] [PubMed]
35. Shaheen, N.J.; Falk, G.W.; Iyer, P.G.; Gerson, L.B. ACG Clinical Guideline: Diagnosis and Management of Barrett's Esophagus. *Am. J. Gastroenterol.* **2016**, *111*, 30–50. [CrossRef] [PubMed]
36. Furneri, G.; Klausnitzer, R.; Haycock, L.; Ihara, Z. Economic value of narrow-band imaging versus white light endoscopy for the diagnosis and surveillance of Barrett's esophagus: Cost-consequence model. *PLOS ONE* **2019**, *14*, e0212916. [CrossRef]
37. Xiong, Y.-Q.; Ma, S.-J.; Hu, H.-Y.; Ge, J.; Zhou, L.-Z.; Huo, S.-T.; Qiu, M.; Chen, Q. Comparison of narrow-band imaging and confocal laser endomicroscopy for the detection of neoplasia in Barrett's esophagus: A meta-analysis. *Clin. Res. Hepatol. Gastroenterol.* **2018**, *42*, 31–39. [CrossRef]
38. Puli, S.R.; Reddy, J.B.; Bechtold, M.L.; Antillon, D.; A Ibdah, J.; Antillon, M.R. Staging accuracy of esophageal cancer by endoscopic ultrasound: A meta-analysis and systematic review. *World J. Gastroenterol.* **2008**, *14*, 1479–1490. [CrossRef]
39. Qumseya, B.J.; Wolfsen, H.C. The Role of Endoscopic Ultrasound in the Management of Patients with Barrett's Esophagus and Superficial Neoplasia. *Gastrointest. Endosc. Clin. North Am.* **2017**, *27*, 471–480. [CrossRef]
40. Thosani, N.; Singh, H.; Kapadia, A.; Ochi, N.; Lee, J.H.; Ajani, J.; Swisher, S.G.; Hofstetter, W.L.; Guha, S.; Bhutani, M.S. Diagnostic accuracy of EUS in differentiating mucosal versus submucosal invasion of superficial esophageal cancers: a systematic review and meta-analysis. *Gastrointest. Endosc.* **2012**, *75*, 242–253. [CrossRef]
41. Luo, L.-N.; He, L.-J.; Gao, X.-Y.; Huang, X.-X.; Shan, H.-B.; Luo, G.-Y.; Li, Y.; Lin, S.-Y.; Wang, G.-B.; Zhang, R.; et al. Endoscopic Ultrasound for Preoperative Esophageal Squamous Cell Carcinoma: A Meta-Analysis. *PLOS ONE* **2016**, *11*, e0158373. [CrossRef] [PubMed]
42. Flamen, P.; Lerut, A.; Van Cutsem, E.; De Wever, W.; Peeters, M.; Stroobants, S.; Dupont, P.; Bormans, G.; Hiele, M.; De Leyn, P.; et al. Utility of Positron Emission Tomography for the Staging of Patients With Potentially Operable Esophageal Carcinoma. *J. Clin. Oncol.* **2000**, *18*, 3202–3210. [CrossRef] [PubMed]
43. Goodman, K.A.; Niedzwiecki, D.; Hall, N.; Bekaii-Saab, T.S.; Ye, X.; Meyers, M.O.; Mitchell-Richards, K.; Boffa, D.J.; Frankel, W.L.; Venook, A.P.; et al. Initial results of CALGB 80803 (Alliance): A randomized phase II trial of PET scan-directed combined modality therapy for esophageal cancer. *J. Clin. Oncol.* **2017**, *35*, 1. [CrossRef]
44. Johnston, M.H.; Eastone, J.A.; Horwhat, J.; Cartledge, J.; Mathews, J.S.; Foggy, J.R. Cryoablation of Barrett's esophagus: A pilot study. *Gastrointest. Endosc.* **2005**, *62*, 842–848. [CrossRef] [PubMed]
45. Phoa, K.N.; Van Vilsteren, F.G.I.; Weusten, B.L.; Bisschops, R.; Schoon, E.J.; Ragunath, K.; Fullarton, G.; Di Pietro, M.; Ravi, N.; Visser, M.; et al. Radiofrequency Ablation vs Endoscopic Surveillance for Patients With Barrett Esophagus and Low-Grade Dysplasia. *JAMA* **2014**, *311*, 1209–1217. [CrossRef] [PubMed]
46. Cotton, C.C.; Wolf, W.A.; Overholt, B.F.; Li, N.; Lightdale, C.J.; Wolfsen, H.C.; Pasricha, S.; Wang, K.K.; Shaheen, N.J.; Sampliner, R.E.; et al. Late Recurrence of Barrett's Esophagus After Complete Eradication of Intestinal Metaplasia is Rare: Final Report From Ablation in Intestinal Metaplasia Containing Dysplasia Trial. *Gastroenterology* **2017**, *153*, 681–688.e2. [CrossRef]
47. Manner, H.; Pech, O.; Heldmann, Y.; May, A.; Pohl, J.; Behrens, A.; Gossner, L.; Stolte, M.; Vieth, M.; Ell, C. Efficacy, Safety, and Long-term Results of Endoscopic Treatment for Early Stage Adenocarcinoma of the Esophagus With Low-risk sm1 Invasion. *Clin. Gastroenterol. Hepatol.* **2013**, *11*, 630–635. [CrossRef]
48. Conio, M.; Repici, A.; Cestari, R.; Blanchi, S.; Lapertosa, G.; Missale, G.; Della Casa, D.; Villanacci, V.; Calandri, P.G.; Filiberti, R. Endoscopic mucosal resection for high-grade dysplasia and intramucosal carcinoma in Barrett's esophagus: An Italian experience. *World J. Gastroenterol.* **2005**, *11*, 6650–6655. [CrossRef]
49. Bourke, M.J. Mucosal resection in the upper gastrointestinal tract. *Tech. Gastrointest. Endosc.* **2010**, *12*, 18–25. [CrossRef]
50. Moss, A.; Bourke, M.J.; Hourigan, L.F.; Gupta, S.; Swan, M.P.; Hopper, A.D.; Kwan, V.; Bailey, A.; Williams, S.J. Endoscopic Mucosal Resection (EMR) for Barrett's High Grade Dysplasia (HGD) and Early Esophageal Adenocarcinoma (EAC): An Essential Staging Procedure with Long-Term Therapeutic Benefit. *Gastrointest. Endosc.* **2009**, *69*, AB348. [CrossRef]
51. Jin, X.-F.; Chai, T.-H.; Gai, W.; Chen, Z.-S.; Guo, J.-Q. Multiband Mucosectomy Versus Endoscopic Submucosal Dissection for Treatment of Squamous Intraepithelial Neoplasia of the Esophagus. *Clin. Gastroenterol. Hepatol.* **2016**, *14*, 948–955. [CrossRef] [PubMed]
52. Rajaram, R.; Hofstetter, W.L. Mucosal Ablation Techniques for Barrett's Esophagus and Early Esophageal Cancer. *Thorac. Surg. Clin.* **2018**, *28*, 473–480. [CrossRef] [PubMed]
53. Inoue, H.; Endo, M.; Takeshita, K.; Yoshino, K.; Muraoka, Y.; Yoneshima, H. A new simplified technique of endoscopic esophageal mucosal resection using a cap-fitted panendoscope (EMRC). *Surg. Endosc.* **1992**, *6*, 264–265. [CrossRef] [PubMed]
54. Espinel, J.; Pinedo, E.; Ojeda, V.; Del Rio, M.G. Multiband mucosectomy for advanced dysplastic lesions in the upper digestive tract. *World J. Gastrointest. Endosc.* **2015**, *7*, 370–380. [CrossRef] [PubMed]

55. Wani, S.; Qumseya, B.; Sultan, S.; Agrawal, D.; Chandrasekhara, V.; Harnke, B.; Kothari, S.; McCarter, M.; Shaukat, A.; Wang, A.; et al. Endoscopic eradication therapy for patients with Barrett's esophagus–associated dysplasia and intramucosal cancer. *Gastrointest. Endosc.* **2018**, *87*, 907–931.e9. [CrossRef]
56. Ahmed, Y.; Othman, M. EMR/ESD: Techniques, Complications, and Evidence. *Curr. Gastroenterol. Rep.* **2020**, *22*, 1–12. [CrossRef]
57. Davison, J.M.; Landau, M.S.; Luketich, J.D.; McGrath, K.M.; Foxwell, T.J.; Landsittel, D.P.; Gibson, M.K.; Nason, K.S. A Model Based on Pathologic Features of Superficial Esophageal Adenocarcinoma Complements Clinical Node Staging in Determining Risk of Metastasis to Lymph Nodes. *Clin. Gastroenterol. Hepatol.* **2016**, *14*, 369–377.e3. [CrossRef]
58. Othman, M.O.; Lee, J.H.; Wang, K. AGA Clinical Practice Update on the Utility of Endoscopic Submucosal Dissection in T1b Esophageal Cancer: Expert Review. *Clin. Gastroenterol. Hepatol.* **2019**, *17*, 2161–2166. [CrossRef]
59. Zhang, Y.; Ding, H.; Chen, T.; Zhang, X.; Chen, W.-F.; Li, Q.; Yao, L.; Korrapati, P.; Jin, X.-J.; Zhang, Y.-X.; et al. Outcomes of Endoscopic Submucosal Dissection vs Esophagectomy for T1 Esophageal Squamous Cell Carcinoma in a Real-World Cohort. *Clin. Gastroenterol. Hepatol.* **2019**, *17*, 73–81.e3. [CrossRef]
60. Aadam, A.A.; Abe, S. Endoscopic submucosal dissection for superficial esophageal cancer. *Dis. Esophagus* **2018**, *31*. [CrossRef]
61. Sgourakis, G.; Gockel, I.; Lang, H. Endoscopic and surgical resection of T1a/T1b esophageal neoplasms: A systematic review. *World J. Gastroenterol.* **2013**, *19*, 1424–1437. [CrossRef] [PubMed]
62. Komeda, Y.; Bruno, M.; Koch, A. EMR is not inferior to ESD for early Barrett's and EGJ neoplasia: An extensive review on outcome, recurrence and complication rates. *Endosc. Int. Open* **2014**, *2*, E58–E64. [CrossRef] [PubMed]
63. Kaya, D.M.; Harada, K.; Das, P.; Weston, B.; Sagebiel, T.; Thomas, I.; Wang, X.; Murphy, M.A.B.; Minsky, B.D.; Estrella, J.S.; et al. 101 Long-Term Survivors Who Had Metastatic Gastroesophageal Cancer and Received Local Consolidative Therapy. *Oncology* **2017**, *93*, 243–248. [CrossRef] [PubMed]
64. Berry, M.F. Esophageal cancer: Staging system and guidelines for staging and treatment. *J. Thorac. Dis.* **2014**, *6*, S289–S297. [PubMed]
65. van Boxel, G.I.; Kingma, B.F.; Voskens, F.J.; Ruurda, J.P.; van Hillegersberg, R. Robotic-assisted minimally invasive esophagectomy: Past, present and future. *J. Thorac. Dis.* **2020**, *12*, 54–62. [CrossRef]
66. Van Der Sluis, P.C.; Schizas, D.; Liakakos, T.; Van Hillegersberg, R. Minimally Invasive Esophagectomy. *Dig. Surg.* **2020**, *37*, 93–100. [CrossRef] [PubMed]
67. Tepper, J.; Krasna, M.J.; Niedzwiecki, D.; Hollis, D.; Reed, C.E.; Goldberg, R.; Kiel, K.; Willett, C.; Sugarbaker, D.; Mayer, R. Phase III Trial of Trimodality Therapy With Cisplatin, Fluorouracil, Radiotherapy, and Surgery Compared With Surgery Alone for Esophageal Cancer: CALGB 9781. *J. Clin. Oncol.* **2008**, *26*, 1086–1092. [CrossRef]
68. Ohtsu, A. Chemoradiotherapy for esophageal cancer: current status and perspectives. *Int. J. Clin. Oncol.* **2004**, *9*, 444–450. [CrossRef]
69. Jethwa, K.R.; Haddock, M.G.; Tryggestad, E.J.; Hallemeier, C.L. The emerging role of proton therapy for esophagus cancer. *J. Gastrointest. Oncol.* **2020**, *11*, 144–156. [CrossRef]
70. Lindenmann, J.; Matzi, V.; Neuboeck, N.; Anegg, U.; Baumgartner, E.; Maier, A.; Smolle, J.; Smolle-Juettner, F.M. Individualized, multimodal palliative treatment of inoperable esophageal cancer: Clinical impact of photodynamic therapy resulting in prolonged survival. *Lasers Surg. Med.* **2012**, *44*, 189–198. [CrossRef]
71. Lloyd, S.; Chang, B. Current strategies in chemoradiation for esophageal cancer. *J. Gastrointest. Oncol.* **2014**, *5*, 156–165. [PubMed]
72. Xi, M.; Lin, S.H. Recent advances in intensity modulated radiotherapy and proton therapy for esophageal cancer. *Expert Rev. Anticancer. Ther.* **2017**, *17*, 635–646. [CrossRef] [PubMed]
73. Kole, T.P.; Aghayere, O.; Kwah, J.; Yorke, E.D.; Goodman, K.A. Comparison of Heart and Coronary Artery Doses Associated With Intensity-Modulated Radiotherapy Versus Three-Dimensional Conformal Radiotherapy for Distal Esophageal Cancer. *Int. J. Radiat. Oncol.* **2012**, *83*, 1580–1586. [CrossRef] [PubMed]
74. Nutting, C.M.; Bedford, J.L.; Cosgrove, V.P.; Tait, D.M.; Dearnaley, D.; Webb, S. A comparison of conformal and intensity-modulated techniques for oesophageal radiotherapy. *Radiother. Oncol.* **2001**, *61*, 157–163. [CrossRef]
75. Tonison, J.J.; Fischer, S.G.; Viehrig, M.; Welz, S.; Boeke, S.; Zwirner, K.; Klumpp, B.; Braun, L.H.; Zips, D.; Gani, C. Radiation Pneumonitis after Intensity-Modulated Radiotherapy for Esophageal Cancer: Institutional Data and a Systematic Review. *Sci. Rep.* **2019**, *9*, 2255. [CrossRef]
76. Pao, T.-H.; Chang, W.-L.; Chiang, N.-J.; Chang, J.S.-M.; Lin, C.-Y.; Lai, W.-W.; Tseng, Y.-L.; Yen, Y.-T.; Chung, T.-J.; Lin, F.-C. Cardiac radiation dose predicts survival in esophageal squamous cell carcinoma treated by definitive concurrent chemotherapy and intensity modulated radiotherapy. *Radiat. Oncol.* **2020**, *15*, 1–10. [CrossRef] [PubMed]
77. Ogino, I.; Watanabe, S.; Iwahashi, N.; Kosuge, M.; Sakamaki, K.; Kunisaki, C.; Kimura, K. Symptomatic radiation-induced cardiac disease in long-term survivors of esophageal cancer. *Strahlenther. Onkol.* **2016**, *192*, 359–367. [CrossRef]
78. Wang, X.; Palaskas, N.L.; Yusuf, S.W.; Abe, J.-I.; Lopez-Mattei, J.; Banchs, J.; Gladish, G.W.; Lee, P.; Liao, Z.; Deswal, A.; et al. Incidence and Onset of Severe Cardiac Events After Radiotherapy for Esophageal Cancer. *J. Thorac. Oncol.* **2020**, *15*, 1682–1690. [CrossRef]
79. Dhadham, G.C.; Hoffe, S.; Harris, C.L.; Klapman, J. Endoscopic ultrasound-guided fiducial marker placement for image-guided radiation therapy without fluoroscopy: Safety and technical feasibility. *Endosc. Int. Open* **2016**, *4*, E378–E382. [CrossRef]
80. DiMaio, C.J.; Nagula, S.; Goodman, K.A.; Ho, A.Y.; Markowitz, A.J.; Schattner, M.A.; Gerdes, H. EUS-guided fiducial placement for image-guided radiation therapy in GI malignancies by using a 22-gauge needle (with). *Gastrointest. Endosc.* **2010**, *71*, 1204–1210. [CrossRef]

81. Fernandez, D.C.; Hoffe, S.; Barthel, J.S.; Vignesh, S.; Klapman, J.B.; Harris, C.; Almhanna, K.; Biagioli, M.C.; Meredith, K.; Feygelman, V.; et al. Stability of endoscopic ultrasound-guided fiducial marker placement for esophageal cancer target delineation and image-guided radiation therapy. *Pr. Radiat. Oncol.* **2013**, *3*, 32–39. [CrossRef] [PubMed]
82. Oliver, J.A.; Venkat, P.; Frakes, J.M.; Klapman, J.; Harris, C.; Montilla-Soler, J.; Dhadham, G.C.; Altazi, B.A.; Zhang, G.G.; Moros, E.G.; et al. Fiducial markers coupled with 3D PET/CT offer more accurate radiation treatment delivery for locally advanced esophageal cancer. *Endosc. Int. Open* **2017**, *5*, E496–E504. [CrossRef] [PubMed]
83. Machiels, M.; Van Hooft, J.; Jin, P.; Henegouwen, M.I.V.B.; Van Laarhoven, H.M.; Alderliesten, T.; Hulshof, M.C. Endoscopy/EUS-guided fiducial marker placement in patients with esophageal cancer: A comparative analysis of 3 types of markers. *Gastrointest. Endosc.* **2015**, *82*, 641–649. [CrossRef] [PubMed]
84. Wang, J.; Lin, S.H.; Dong, L.; Balter, P.; Mohan, R.; Komaki, R.; Cox, J.D.; Starkschall, G. Quantifying the Interfractional Displacement of the Gastroesophageal Junction During Radiation Therapy for Esophageal Cancer. *Int. J. Radiat. Oncol.* **2012**, *83*, e273–e280. [CrossRef] [PubMed]
85. Wu, A.J.; Bosch, W.R.; Chang, D.T.; Hong, T.S.; Jabbour, S.K.; Kleinberg, L.R.; Mamon, H.J.; Thomas, C.R.; Goodman, K.A. Expert Consensus Contouring Guidelines for Intensity Modulated Radiation Therapy in Esophageal and Gastroesophageal Junction Cancer. *Int. J. Radiat. Oncol.* **2015**, *92*, 911–920. [CrossRef] [PubMed]
86. Launois, B.; Delarue, D.; Campion, J.P.; Kerbaol, M. Preoperative radiotherapy for carcinoma of the esophagus. *Surgery, Gynecol. Obstet.* **1981**, *153*, 690–692.
87. Wang, M.; Gu, X.Z.; Yin, W.B.; Huang, G.J.; Wang, L.J.; Zhang, D.W. Randomized clinical trial on the combination of preoper-ative irradiation and surgery in the treatment of esophageal carcinoma: Report on 206 patients. *Int. J. Radiat. Oncol. Biol. Phys.* **1989**, *16*, 325–327.
88. Gignoux, M.; Roussel, A.; Paillot, B.; Gillet, M.; Schlag, P.; Favre, J.-P.; Dalesio, O.; Buyse, M.; Duez, N. The value of preoperative radiotherapy in esophageal cancer: Results of a study of the E.O.R.T.C. *World J. Surg.* **1987**, *11*, 426–432. [CrossRef]
89. Nygaard, K.; Hagen, S.; Hansen, H.S.; Hatlevoll, R.; Hultborn, R.; Jakobsen, A.; Mäntyla, M.; Modig, H.; Munck-Wikland, E.; Rosengren, B.; et al. Pre-operative radiotherapy prolongs survival in operable esophageal carcinoma: A randomized, multicenter study of pre-operative radiotherapy and chemotherapy. The second scandinavian trial in esophageal cancer. *World J. Surg.* **1992**, *16*, 1104–1109. [CrossRef]
90. Arnott, S.J.; Duncan, W.; Gignoux, M.; Girling, D.J.; Hansen, H.S.; Launois, B.; Nygaard, K.; Parmar, M.K.; Roussel, A.; Spiliopoulos, G.; et al. Preoperative radiotherapy in esophageal carcinoma: A meta-analysis using individual patient data (oesophageal cancer collaborative group). *Int. J. Radiat. Oncol.* **1998**, *41*, 579–583. [CrossRef]
91. Batra, T.K.; Pai, E.; Singh, R.; Francis, N.J.; Pandey, M. Neoadjuvant strategies in resectable carcinoma esophagus: A meta-analysis of randomized trials. *World J. Surg. Oncol.* **2020**, *18*, 1–10. [CrossRef]
92. Fok, M.; Sham, J.S.; Choy, D.; Cheng, S.W.; Wong, J. Postoperative radiotherapy for carcinoma of the esophagus: a prospective, randomized controlled study. *Surgery* **1993**, *113*, 138–147. [PubMed]
93. Ténière, P.; Hay, J.M.; Fingerhut, A.; Fagniez, P.L. Postoperative radiation therapy does not increase survival after curative resection for squamous cell carcinoma of the middle and lower esophagus as shown by a multicenter controlled trial. French University Association for Surgical Research. *Surgery, Gynecol. Obstet.* **1991**, *173*, 123–130.
94. Hsu, P.-K.; Huang, C.-S.; Wang, B.-Y.; Wu, Y.-C.; Hsu, W.-H. Survival Benefits of Postoperative Chemoradiation for Lymph Node–Positive Esophageal Squamous Cell Carcinoma. *Ann. Thorac. Surg.* **2014**, *97*, 1734–1741. [CrossRef] [PubMed]
95. Rucker, A.J.; Raman, V.; Jawitz, O.K.; Voigt, S.L.; Harpole, D.H.; D'Amico, T.A.; Tong, B.C. The Impact of Adjuvant Therapy on Survival After Esophagectomy for Node-negative Esophageal Adenocarcinoma. *Ann. Surg.* **2020**. [CrossRef] [PubMed]
96. Ni, W.; Yu, S.; Zhang, W.; Xiao, Z.; Zhou, Z.; Chen, D.; Feng, Q.; Liang, J.; Lv, J.; Gao, S.; et al. A phase-II/III randomized controlled trial of adjuvant radiotherapy or concurrent chemoradiotherapy after surgery versus surgery alone in patients with stage-IIB/III esophageal squamous cell carcinoma. *BMC Cancer* **2020**, *20*, 1–8. [CrossRef] [PubMed]
97. Shapiro, J.; Van Lanschot, J.J.B.; Hulshof, M.C.C.M.; Van Hagen, P.; Henegouwen, M.I.V.B.; Wijnhoven, B.P.L.; Van Laarhoven, H.W.M.; Nieuwenhuijzen, G.A.P.; Hospers, G.A.P.; Bonenkamp, J.J.; et al. Neoadjuvant chemoradiotherapy plus surgery versus surgery alone for oesophageal or junctional cancer (CROSS): Long-term results of a randomised controlled trial. *Lancet Oncol.* **2015**, *16*, 1090–1098. [CrossRef]
98. Stahl, M.; Walz, M.K.; Riera-Knorrenschild, J.; Stuschke, M.; Sandermann, A.; Bitzer, M.; Wilke, H.; Budach, W. Preoperative chemotherapy versus chemoradiotherapy in locally advanced adenocarcinomas of the oesophagogastric junction (POET): Long-term results of a controlled randomised trial. *Eur. J. Cancer* **2017**, *81*, 183–190. [CrossRef]
99. Klevebro, F.; Von Döbeln, G.A.; Wang, N.; Johnsen, G.; Jacobsen, A.-B.; Friesland, S.; Hatlevoll, I.; Glenjen, N.I.; Lind, P.; Tsai, J.A.; et al. A randomized clinical trial of neoadjuvant chemotherapy versus neoadjuvant chemoradiotherapy for cancer of the oesophagus or gastro-oesophageal junction. *Ann. Oncol.* **2016**, *27*, 660–667. [CrossRef]
100. Oppedijk, V.; Van Der Gaast, A.; Van Lanschot, J.J.B.; Van Hagen, P.; Van Os, R.; Van Rij, C.M.; Van Der Sangen, M.J.; Beukema, J.C.; Rütten, H.; Spruit, P.H.; et al. Patterns of Recurrence After Surgery Alone Versus Preoperative Chemoradiotherapy and Surgery in the CROSS Trials. *J. Clin. Oncol.* **2014**, *32*, 385–391. [CrossRef]

101. Noordman, B.J.; Verdam, M.G.E.; Lagarde, S.M.; Hulshof, M.C.C.M.; Van Hagen, P.; Henegouwen, M.I.V.B.; Wijnhoven, B.P.L.; Van Laarhoven, H.W.M.; Nieuwenhuijzen, G.A.P.; Hospers, G.A.; et al. Effect of Neoadjuvant Chemoradiotherapy on Health-Related Quality of Life in Esophageal or Junctional Cancer: Results From the Randomized CROSS Trial. *J. Clin. Oncol.* **2018**, *36*, 268–275. [CrossRef] [PubMed]
102. Yang, H.; Liu, H.; Chen, Y.; Zhu, C.; Fang, W.; Yu, Z.; Mao, W.; Xiang, J.; Han, Y.; Chen, Z.; et al. Neoadjuvant Chemoradiotherapy Followed by Surgery Versus Surgery Alone for Locally Advanced Squamous Cell Carcinoma of the Esophagus (NEOCRTEC5010): A Phase III Multicenter, Randomized, Open-Label Clinical Trial. *J. Clin. Oncol.* **2018**, *36*, 2796–2803. [CrossRef] [PubMed]
103. Messager, M.; Mirabel, X.; Tresch, E.; Paumier, A.; Vendrely, V.; Dahan, L.; Glehen, O.; Vasseur, F.; Lacornerie, T.; Piessen, G.; et al. Preoperative chemoradiation with paclitaxel-carboplatin or with fluorouracil-oxaliplatin-folinic acid (FOLFOX) for resectable esophageal and junctional cancer: the PROTECT-1402, randomized phase 2 trial. *BMC Cancer* **2016**, *16*, 318. [CrossRef] [PubMed]
104. Okawa, T.; Kita, M.; Tanaka, M.; Ikeda, M. Results of radiotherapy for inoperable locally advanced esophageal cancer. *Int. J. Radiat. Oncol.* **1989**, *17*, 49–54. [CrossRef]
105. De-Ren, S.; Sun, D.R. Ten-year follow-up of esophageal cancer treated by radical radiation therapy: Analysis of 869 patients. *Int. J. Radiat. Oncol.* **1989**, *16*, 329–334. [CrossRef]
106. Herskovic, A.; Martz, K.; Al-Sarraf, M.; Leichman, L.; Brindle, J.; Vaitkevicius, V.; Cooper, J.; Byhardt, R.; Davis, L.; Emami, B. Combined Chemotherapy and Radiotherapy Compared with Radiotherapy Alone in Patients with Cancer of the Esophagus. *N. Engl. J. Med.* **1992**, *326*, 1593–1598. [CrossRef]
107. Minsky, B.D.; Pajak, T.F.; Ginsberg, R.J.; Pisansky, T.M.; Martenson, J.; Komaki, R.; Okawara, G.; Rosenthal, S.A.; Kelsen, D.P. INT 0123 (Radiation Therapy Oncology Group 94-05) Phase III Trial of Combined-Modality Therapy for Esophageal Cancer: High-Dose Versus Standard-Dose Radiation Therapy. *J. Clin. Oncol.* **2002**, *20*, 1167–1174. [CrossRef]
108. E Gaspar, L.; Winter, K.; I Kocha, W.; Coia, L.R.; Herskovic, A.; Graham, M. A phase I/II study of external beam radiation, brachytherapy, and concurrent chemotherapy for patients with localized carcinoma of the esophagus (Radiation Therapy Oncology Group Study 9207): Final report. *Cancer* **2000**, *88*, 988–995. [CrossRef]
109. Cooper, J.S.; Guo, M.D.; Herskovic, A.; Macdonald, J.S.; Martenson, J.J.A.; Al-Sarraf, M.; Byhardt, R.; Russell, A.H.; Beitler, J.J.; Spencer, S.; et al. Chemoradiotherapy of Locally Advanced Esophageal Cancer. *JAMA* **1999**, *281*, 1623–1627. [CrossRef]
110. Xu, Y.; Zhu, W.; Zheng, X.; Wang, W.; Li, J.; Huang, R.; He, H.; Chen, J.; Liu, L.; Sun, Z.; et al. A multi-center, randomized, prospective study evaluating the optimal radiation dose of definitive concurrent chemoradiation for inoperable esophageal squamous cell carcinoma. *J. Clin. Oncol.* **2018**, *36*, 4013. [CrossRef]
111. Hulshof, M.C.; Geijsen, D.; Rozema, T.; Oppedijk, V.; Buijsen, J.; Neelis, K.J.; Nuyttens, J.; Van Der Sangen, M.; Jeene, P.; Reinders, J.; et al. A randomized controlled phase III multicenter study on dose escalation in definitive chemoradiation for patients with locally advanced esophageal cancer: ARTDECO study. *J. Clin. Oncol.* **2020**, *38*, 281. [CrossRef]
112. Chen, D.; Menon, H.; Verma, V.; Seyedin, S.N.; Ajani, J.A.; Hofstetter, W.L.; Nguyen, Q.-N.; Chang, J.Y.; Gomez, D.R.; Amini, A.; et al. Results of a Phase 1/2 Trial of Chemoradiotherapy With Simultaneous Integrated Boost of Radiotherapy Dose in Unresectable Locally Advanced Esophageal Cancer. *JAMA Oncol.* **2019**, *5*, 1597–1604. [CrossRef] [PubMed]
113. Bhangoo, R.S.; DeWees, T.A.; Yu, N.Y.; Ding, J.X.; Liu, C.; Golafshar, M.A.; Rule, W.G.; Vora, S.A.; Ross, H.J.; Ahn, D.H.; et al. Acute Toxicities and Short-Term Patient Outcomes After Intensity-Modulated Proton Beam Radiation Therapy or Intensity-Modulated Photon Radiation Therapy for Esophageal Carcinoma: A Mayo Clinic Experience. *Adv. Radiat. Oncol.* **2020**, *5*, 871–879. [CrossRef] [PubMed]
114. DeCesaris, C.; Berger, M.; Choi, J.I.; Carr, S.R.; Burrows, W.M.; Regine, W.F.; Ii, C.B.S.; Molitoris, J.K. Pathologic complete response (pCR) rates and outcomes after neoadjuvant chemoradiotherapy with proton or photon radiation for adenocarcinomas of the esophagus and gastroesophageal junction. *J. Gastrointest. Oncol.* **2020**, *11*, 663–673. [CrossRef] [PubMed]
115. Lancellotta, V.; Cellini, F.; Fionda, B.; De Sanctis, V.; Vidali, C.; Fusco, V.; Barbera, F.; Gambacorta, M.A.; Corvò, R.; Magrini, S.M.; et al. The role of palliative interventional radiotherapy (brachytherapy) in esophageal cancer: An AIRO (Italian Association of Radiotherapy and Clinical Oncology) systematic review focused on dysphagia-free survival. *Brachytherapy* **2020**, *19*, 104–110. [CrossRef]
116. Dai, Y.; Li, C.; Xie, Y.; Liu, X.; Zhang, J.; Zhou, J.; Pan, X.; Yang, S. Interventions for dysphagia in oesophageal cancer. *Cochrane Database Syst. Rev.* **2014**. [CrossRef] [PubMed]
117. Bang, Y.-J.; Van Cutsem, E.; Feyereislova, A.; Chung, H.C.; Shen, L.; Sawaki, A.; Lordick, F.; Ohtsu, A.; Omuro, Y.; Satoh, T.; et al. Trastuzumab in combination with chemotherapy versus chemotherapy alone for treatment of HER2-positive advanced gastric or gastro-oesophageal junction cancer (ToGA): A phase 3, open-label, randomised controlled trial. *Lancet* **2010**, *376*, 687–697. [CrossRef]
118. Gourd, K.; Lai, C.; Reeves, C. ESMO Virtual Congress 2020. *Lancet Oncol.* **2020**, *21*, 1403–1404. [CrossRef]
119. Pech, O.; Pal, S.; Dash, N.R.; Ahuja, V.; Mohanti, B.K.; Vishnubhatla, S.; Sahni, P.; Chattopadhyay, T.K. Palliative Stenting With or Without Radiotherapy for Inoperable Esophageal Carcinoma: A Randomized Trial. *J. Gastrointest. Cancer* **2010**, *43*, 63–69. [CrossRef]
120. Lai, A.; Lipka, S.; Kumar, A.; Sethi, S.; Bromberg, D.; Li, N.; Shen, H.; Stefaniwsky, L.; Brady, P. Role of Esophageal Metal Stents Placement and Combination Therapy in Inoperable Esophageal Carcinoma: A Systematic Review and Meta-analysis. *Dig. Dis. Sci.* **2018**, *63*, 1025–1034. [CrossRef]

121. Liu, B.; Bo, Y.; Wang, K.; Liu, Y.; Tang, X.; Zhao, Y.; Zhao, E.; Yuan, L. Concurrent neoadjuvant chemoradiotherapy could improve survival outcomes for patients with esophageal cancer: A meta-analysis based on random clinical trials. *Oncotarget* **2017**, *8*, 20410–20417. [CrossRef] [PubMed]
122. Zhao, X.; Ren, Y.; Hu, Y.; Cui, N.; Wang, X.; Cui, Y. Neoadjuvant chemotherapy versus neoadjuvant chemoradiotherapy for cancer of the esophagus or the gastroesophageal junction: A meta-analysis based on clinical trials. *PLOS ONE* **2018**, *13*, e0202185. [CrossRef] [PubMed]
123. Safran, H.; Winter, K.A.; Wigle, D.A.; DiPetrillo, T.A.; Haddock, M.G.; Hong, T.S.; Leichman, L.P.; Rajdev, L.; Resnick, M.B.; Kachnic, L.A.; et al. Trastuzumab with trimodality treatment for esophageal adenocarcinoma with HER2 overexpression: NRG Oncology/RTOG 1010. *J. Clin. Oncol.* **2020**, *38*, 4500. [CrossRef]
124. Colquhoun, A.; Arnold, M.; Ferlay, J.; Goodman, K.J.; Forman, D.; Soerjomataram, I. Global patterns of cardia and non-cardia gastric cancer incidence in 2012. *Gut* **2015**, *64*, 1881–1888. [CrossRef]
125. Rugge, M.; Genta, R.M.; Di Mario, F.; El-Omar, E.M.; El-Serag, H.B.; Fassan, M.; Hunt, R.H.; Kuipers, E.J.; Malfertheiner, P.; Sugano, K.; et al. Gastric Cancer as Preventable Disease. *Clin. Gastroenterol. Hepatol.* **2017**, *15*, 1833–1843. [CrossRef]
126. Hatakeyama, M.; Higashi, H. Helicobacter pylori CagA: A new paradigm for bacterial carcinogenesis. *Cancer Sci.* **2005**, *96*, 835–843. [CrossRef]
127. Capelle, L.G.; Haringsma, J.; De Vries, A.C.; Steyerberg, E.W.; Biermann, K.; Van Dekken, H.; Kuipers, E.J. Narrow Band Imaging for the Detection of Gastric Intestinal Metaplasia and Dysplasia During Surveillance Endoscopy. *Dig. Dis. Sci.* **2010**, *55*, 3442–3448. [CrossRef]
128. Dixon, M.F.; Genta, R.M.; Yardley, J.H.; Correa, P. Classification and Grading of Gastritis. *Am. J. Surg. Pathol.* **1996**, *20*, 1161–1181. [CrossRef]
129. Japanese Gastric Cancer Association Japanese gastric cancer treatment guidelines 2018 (5th edition). *Gastric Cancer* **2021**, *24*, 1–21. [CrossRef]
130. Ono, S.; Fujishiro, M.; Niimi, K.; Goto, O.; Kodashima, S.; Yamamichi, N.; Omata, M. Long-term outcomes of endoscopic submucosal dissection for superficial esophageal squamous cell neoplasms. *Gastrointest. Endosc.* **2009**, *70*, 860–866. [CrossRef]
131. Probst, A.; Schneider, A.; Schaller, T.; Anthuber, M.; Ebigbo, A.; Messmann, H. Endoscopic submucosal dissection for early gastric cancer: are expanded resection criteria safe for Western patients? *Endoscopy* **2017**, *49*, 855–865. [CrossRef] [PubMed]
132. Jin, H.; Pinheiro, P.S.; Callahan, K.E.; Altekruse, S.F. Examining the gastric cancer survival gap between Asians and whites in the United States. *Gastric Cancer* **2016**, *20*, 573–582. [CrossRef] [PubMed]
133. Al-Batran, S.-E.; Homann, N.; Pauligk, C.; O Goetze, T.; Meiler, J.; Kasper, S.; Kopp, H.-G.; Mayer, F.; Haag, G.M.; Luley, K.; et al. Perioperative chemotherapy with fluorouracil plus leucovorin, oxaliplatin, and docetaxel versus fluorouracil or capecitabine plus cisplatin and epirubicin for locally advanced, resectable gastric or gastro-oesophageal junction adenocarcinoma (FLOT4): A randomised, phase 2/3 trial. *Lancet* **2019**, *393*, 1948–1957. [CrossRef] [PubMed]
134. Abe, N.; Watanabe, T.; Sugiyama, M.; Yanagida, O.; Masaki, T.; Mori, T.; Atomi, Y. Endoscopic treatment or surgery for undifferentiated early gastric cancer? *Am. J. Surg.* **2004**, *188*, 181–184. [CrossRef] [PubMed]
135. Hirasawa, T.; Gotoda, T.; Miyata, S.; Kato, Y.; Shimoda, T.; Taniguchi, H.; Fujisaki, J.; Sano, T.; Yamaguchi, T. Incidence of lymph node metastasis and the feasibility of endoscopic resection for undifferentiated-type early gastric cancer. *Gastric Cancer* **2009**, *12*, 148–152. [CrossRef] [PubMed]
136. Spolverato, G.; Ejaz, A.; Kim, Y.; Squires, M.H.; Poultsides, G.A.; Fields, R.C.; Schmidt, C.; Weber, S.M.; Votanopoulos, K.; Maithel, S.K.; et al. Use of Endoscopic Ultrasound in the Preoperative Staging of Gastric Cancer: A Multi-Institutional Study of the US Gastric Cancer Collaborative. *J. Am. Coll. Surg.* **2015**, *220*, 48–56. [CrossRef] [PubMed]
137. Mocellin, S.; Pasquali, S. Diagnostic accuracy of endoscopic ultrasonography (EUS) for the preoperative locoregional staging of primary gastric cancer. *Cochrane Database Syst. Rev.* **2015**, *2015*, CD009944. [CrossRef]
138. Redondo-Cerezo, E.; Martínez-Cara, J.G.; Jiménez-Rosales, R.; Valverde-López, F.; Caballero-Mateos, A.; Jérvez-Puente, P.; Ariza-Fernández, J.L.; Úbeda-Muñoz, M.; López-De-Hierro, M.; De Teresa, J. Endoscopic ultrasound in gastric cancer staging before and after neoadjuvant chemotherapy. A comparison with PET-CT in a clinical series. *United Eur. Gastroenterol. J.* **2017**, *5*, 641–647. [CrossRef]
139. Cunningham, D.; Allum, W.H.; Stenning, S.P.; Thompson, J.N.; Van De Velde, C.J.; Nicolson, M.; Scarffe, J.H.; Lofts, F.J.; Falk, S.J.; Iveson, T.J.; et al. Perioperative Chemotherapy versus Surgery Alone for Resectable Gastroesophageal Cancer. *N. Engl. J. Med.* **2006**, *355*, 11–20. [CrossRef]
140. Rubin, B.P.; Heinrich, M.C.; Corless, C.L. Gastrointestinal stromal tumour. *Lancet* **2007**, *369*, 1731–1741. [CrossRef]
141. Cai, J.-Q.; Yu-Cheng, Z.; Mou, Y.-P.; Pan, Y.; Xu, X.; Zhou, Y.-C.; Huang, C.-J. Laparoscopic versus open wedge resection for gastrointestinal stromal tumors of the stomach: A single-center 8-year retrospective cohort study of 156 patients with long-term follow-up. *BMC Surg.* **2015**, *15*, 1–10. [CrossRef] [PubMed]
142. Kim, H.H.; Uedo, N. Hybrid NOTES. *Gastrointest. Endosc. Clin. North Am.* **2016**, *26*, 335–373. [CrossRef] [PubMed]
143. Fiore, M.; Palassini, E.; Fumagalli, E.; Pilotti, S.; Tamborini, E.; Stacchiotti, S.; Pennacchioli, E.; Casali, P.G.; Gronchi, A. Preoperative imatinib mesylate for unresectable or locally advanced primary gastrointestinal stromal tumors (GIST). *Eur. J. Surg. Oncol. (EJSO)* **2009**, *35*, 739–745. [CrossRef] [PubMed]
144. Etherington, M.S.; DeMatteo, R.P. Tailored management of primary gastrointestinal stromal tumors. *Cancer* **2019**, *125*, 2164–2171. [CrossRef] [PubMed]

145. Joensuu, H.; Eriksson, M.; Hall, K.S.; Hartmann, J.T.; Pink, D.; Schütte, J.; Ramadori, G.; Hohenberger, P.; Duyster, J.; Al-Batran, S.-E.; et al. One vs Three Years of Adjuvant Imatinib for Operable Gastrointestinal Stromal Tumor. *JAMA* **2012**, *307*, 1265–1272. [CrossRef] [PubMed]
146. Corey, B.; Chen, H. Neuroendocrine Tumors of the Stomach. *Surg. Clin. North Am.* **2017**, *97*, 333–343. [CrossRef] [PubMed]
147. Burkitt, M.D.; Pritchard, D.M. Review article: Pathogenesis and management of gastric carcinoid tumours. *Aliment. Pharmacol. Ther.* **2006**, *24*, 1305–1320. [CrossRef]
148. Min, B.-H.; Hong, M.; Lee, J.H.; Rhee, P.-L.; Sohn, T.S.; Kim, S.; Kim, K.-M.; Kim, J.J. Clinicopathological features and outcome of type 3 gastric neuroendocrine tumours. *BJS* **2018**, *105*, 1480–1486. [CrossRef]
149. Sato, Y. Endoscopic diagnosis and management of type I neuroendocrine tumors. *World J. Gastrointest. Endosc.* **2015**, *7*, 346–353. [CrossRef]
150. Kim, M.K. Endoscopic Ultrasound in Gastroenteropancreatic Neuroendocrine Tumors. *Gut Liver* **2012**, *6*, 405–410. [CrossRef]
151. Scherübl, H.; Cadiot, G. Early Gastroenteropancreatic Neuroendocrine Tumors: Endoscopic Therapy and Surveillance. *Visc. Med.* **2017**, *33*, 332–338. [CrossRef] [PubMed]
152. Wang, R.; Zheng-Pywell, R.; Chen, H.A.; A Bibb, J.; Chen, H.; Rose, J. Management of Gastrointestinal Neuroendocrine Tumors. *Clin. Med. Insights: Endocrinol. Diabetes* **2019**, *12*. [CrossRef] [PubMed]
153. Evans, J.A.; Chandrasekhara, V.; Chathadi, K.V.; Decker, G.A.; Early, D.S.; Fisher, D.A.; Foley, K.Q.; Hwang, J.H.; Jue, T.L.; Lightdale, J.R.; et al. The role of endoscopy in the management of premalignant and malignant conditions of the stomach. *Gastrointest. Endosc.* **2015**, *82*, 1–8. [CrossRef] [PubMed]
154. Zullo, A.; Hassan, C.; Cristofari, F.; Andriani, A.; De Francesco, V.; Ierardi, E.; Tomao, S.; Stolte, M.; Morini, S.; Vaira, D. Effects of Helicobacter pylori Eradication on Early Stage Gastric Mucosa–Associated Lymphoid Tissue Lymphoma. *Clin. Gastroenterol. Hepatol.* **2010**, *8*, 105–110. [CrossRef] [PubMed]
155. El-Zahabi, L.M.; Jamali, F.R.; El-Hajj, I.I.; Naja, M.; Salem, Z.; I Shamseddine, A.; El Saghir, N.S.; Zaatari, G.; Geara, F.; Soweid, A.M. The value of EUS in predicting the response of gastric mucosa–associated lymphoid tissue lymphoma to Helicobacter pylori eradication. *Gastrointest. Endosc.* **2007**, *65*, 89–96. [CrossRef] [PubMed]
156. Fukagawa, T. Role of staging laparoscopy for gastric cancer patients. *Ann. Gastroenterol. Surg.* **2019**, *3*, 496–505. [CrossRef]
157. Mezhir, J.J.; Shah, M.A.; Jacks, L.M.; Brennan, M.F.; Coit, D.G.; Strong, V.E. Positive Peritoneal Cytology in Patients with Gastric Cancer: Natural History and Outcome of 291 Patients. *Ann. Surg. Oncol.* **2010**, *17*, 3173–3180. [CrossRef]
158. Marano, L.; Rondelli, F.; Bartoli, A.; Testini, M.; Castagnoli, G.; Ceccarelli, G. Oncologic Effectiveness and Safety of Splenectomy in Total Gastrectomy for Proximal Gastric Carcinoma: Meta-analysis of Randomized Controlled Trials. *Anticancer. Res.* **2018**, *38*, 3609–3617. [CrossRef]
159. Cuschieri, A.; for the Surgical Co-operative Group; Weeden, S.; Fielding, J.; Bancewicz, J.; Craven, J.L.; Joypaul, V.; Sydes, M.R.; Fayers, P.M. Patient survival after D1 and D2 resections for gastric cancer: long-term results of the MRC randomized surgical trial. *Br. J. Cancer* **1999**, *79*, 1522–1530. [CrossRef]
160. Songun, I.; Putter, H.; Kranenbarg, E.M.-K.; Sasako, M.; Van De Velde, C.J.H. Surgical treatment of gastric cancer: 15-year follow-up results of the randomised nationwide Dutch D1D2 trial. *Lancet Oncol.* **2010**, *11*, 439–449. [CrossRef]
161. Kim, H.-H.; Han, S.-U.; Kim, M.-C.; Kim, W.; Lee, H.-J.; Ryu, S.W.; Cho, G.S.; Kim, C.Y.; Yang, H.-K.; Park, D.J.; et al. Effect of Laparoscopic Distal Gastrectomy vs Open Distal Gastrectomy on Long-term Survival Among Patients With Stage I Gastric Cancer. *JAMA Oncol.* **2019**, *5*, 506–513. [CrossRef] [PubMed]
162. Yu, J.; Huang, C.; Sun, Y.; Su, X.; Cao, H.; Hu, J.; Wang, K.; Suo, J.; Tao, K.; He, X.; et al. Effect of Laparoscopic vs Open Distal Gastrectomy on 3-Year Disease-Free Survival in Patients With Locally Advanced Gastric Cancer. *JAMA* **2019**, *321*, 1983–1992. [CrossRef] [PubMed]
163. Wo, J.Y.; Yoon, S.S.; Guimaraes, A.R.; Wolfgang, J.; Mamon, H.J.; Hong, T.S. Gastric lymph node contouring atlas: A tool to aid in clinical target volume definition in 3-dimensional treatment planning for gastric cancer. *Pr. Radiat. Oncol.* **2013**, *3*, e11–e19. [CrossRef] [PubMed]
164. Tepper, J.E.; Gunderson, L.L. Radiation treatment parameters in the adjuvant postoperative therapy of gastric cancer. *Semin. Radiat. Oncol.* **2002**, *12*, 187–195. [CrossRef]
165. Macdonald, J.S.; Smalley, S.R.; Benedetti, J.; Hundahl, S.A.; Estes, N.C.; Stemmermann, G.N.; Haller, D.G.; Ajani, J.A.; Gunderson, L.L.; Jessup, J.M.; et al. Chemoradiotherapy after Surgery Compared with Surgery Alone for Adenocarcinoma of the Stomach or Gastroesophageal Junction. *N. Engl. J. Med.* **2001**, *345*, 725–730. [CrossRef]
166. Ringash, J.; Perkins, G.; Brierley, J.; Lockwood, G.; Islam, M.; Catton, P.; Cummings, B.; Kim, J.; Wong, R.; Dawson, L.A. IMRT for adjuvant radiation in gastric cancer: A preferred plan? *Int. J. Radiat. Oncol.* **2005**, *63*, 732–738. [CrossRef]
167. Wieland, P.; Dobler, B.; Mai, S.; Hermann, B.; Tiefenbacher, U.; Steil, V.; Wenz, F.; Lohr, F. IMRT for postoperative treatment of gastric cancer: covering large target volumes in the upper abdomen: A comparison of a step-and-shoot and an arc therapy approach. *Int. J. Radiat. Oncol.* **2004**, *59*, 1236–1244. [CrossRef]
168. Moningi, S.; Ajani, J.A.; Badgwell, B.D.; Mansfield, P.F.; Murphy, M.A.B.; Ikoma, N.; Ho, J.; Suh, Y.; Holliday, E.B.; Herman, J.M.; et al. The effect of IMRT on acute toxicity in patients with gastric cancer treated with preoperative chemoradiation. *J. Clin. Oncol.* **2019**, *37*, 153. [CrossRef]
169. Badakhshi, H.; Gruen, A.; Graf, R.; Boehmer, D.; Budach, V. Image-guided intensity-modulated radiotherapy for patients with locally advanced gastric cancer: A clinical feasibility study. *Gastric Cancer* **2013**, *17*, 537–541. [CrossRef]

170. Shinde, A.; Novak, J.; Amini, A.; Chen, Y.-J. The evolving role of radiation therapy for resectable and unresectable gastric cancer. *Transl. Gastroenterol. Hepatol.* **2019**, *4*, 64. [CrossRef]
171. Smalley, S.R.; Benedetti, J.K.; Haller, D.G.; Hundahl, S.A.; Estes, N.C.; Ajani, J.A.; Gunderson, L.L.; Goldman, B.; Martenson, J.A.; Jessup, J.M.; et al. Updated Analysis of SWOG-Directed Intergroup Study 0116: A Phase III Trial of Adjuvant Radiochemotherapy Versus Observation After Curative Gastric Cancer Resection. *J. Clin. Oncol.* **2012**, *30*, 2327–2333. [CrossRef] [PubMed]
172. Bonenkamp, J.J.; Hermans, J.; Sasako, M.; Welvaart, K.; Songun, I.; Meyer, S.; Plukker, J.; Van Elk, P.; Obertop, H.; Gouma, D.J.; et al. Extended Lymph-Node Dissection for Gastric Cancer. *N. Engl. J. Med.* **1999**, *340*, 908–914. [CrossRef] [PubMed]
173. Cats, A.; Jansen, E.P.M.; Van Grieken, N.C.T.; Sikorska, K.; Lind, P.A.; Nordsmark, M.; Kranenbarg, E.M.-K.; Boot, H.; Trip, A.K.; Swellengrebel, H.A.M.; et al. Chemotherapy versus chemoradiotherapy after surgery and preoperative chemotherapy for resectable gastric cancer (CRITICS): an international, open-label, randomised phase 3 trial. *Lancet Oncol.* **2018**, *19*, 616–628. [CrossRef]
174. Lee, J.; Lim, D.H.; Kim, S.; Park, S.H.; Park, J.O.; Park, Y.S.; Lim, H.Y.; Choi, M.G.; Sohn, T.S.; Noh, J.H.; et al. Phase III Trial Comparing Capecitabine Plus Cisplatin Versus Capecitabine Plus Cisplatin With Concurrent Capecitabine Radiotherapy in Completely Resected Gastric Cancer With D2 Lymph Node Dissection: The ARTIST Trial. *J. Clin. Oncol.* **2012**, *30*, 268–273. [CrossRef] [PubMed]
175. Park, C.H.; Kim, E.H.; Kim, H.Y.; Roh, Y.H.; Lee, Y.C. Clinical outcomes of endoscopic submucosal dissection for early stage esophagogastric junction cancer: A systematic review and meta-analysis. *Dig. Liver Dis.* **2015**, *47*, 37–44. [CrossRef] [PubMed]
176. Park, S.H.; Zang, D.Y.; Han, B.; Ji, J.H.; Kim, T.G.; Oh, S.Y.; Hwang, I.G.; Kim, J.H.; Shin, D.; Lim, D.H.; et al. ARTIST 2: Interim results of a phase III trial involving adjuvant chemotherapy and/or chemoradiotherapy after D2-gastrectomy in stage II/III gastric cancer (GC). *J. Clin. Oncol.* **2019**, *37*, 4001. [CrossRef]
177. Walsh, T.N.; Noonan, N.; Hollywood, D.; Kelly, A.; Keeling, N.; Hennessy, T.P. A Comparison of Multimodal Therapy and Surgery for Esophageal Adenocarcinoma. *N. Engl. J. Med.* **1996**, *335*, 462–467. [CrossRef]
178. Ajani, J.A.; Winter, K.; Okawara, G.S.; Donohue, J.H.; Pisters, P.W.; Crane, C.H.; Greskovich, J.F.; Anne, P.R.; Bradley, J.D.; Willett, C.; et al. Phase II Trial of Preoperative Chemoradiation in Patients With Localized Gastric Adenocarcinoma (RTOG 9904): Quality of Combined Modality Therapy and Pathologic Response. *J. Clin. Oncol.* **2006**, *24*, 3953–3958. [CrossRef]
179. Slagter, A.E.; Jansen, E.P.M.; Van Laarhoven, H.W.M.; Sandick, J.W.; Van Grieken, N.C.T.; Sikorska, K.; Cats, A.; Muller-Timmermans, P.; Hulshof, M.C.; Boot, H.; et al. CRITICS-II: A multicentre randomised phase II trial of neo-adjuvant chemotherapy followed by surgery versus neo-adjuvant chemotherapy and subsequent chemoradiotherapy followed by surgery versus neo-adjuvant chemoradiotherapy followed by surgery in resectable gastric cancer. *BMC Cancer* **2018**, *18*, 1–12. [CrossRef]
180. Leong, T.; Smithers, B.M.; Haustermans, K.; Michael, M.; Gebski, V.; Miller, D.; Zalcberg, J.; Boussioutas, A.; Findlay, M.; O'Connell, R.L.; et al. TOPGEAR: A Randomized, Phase III Trial of Perioperative ECF Chemotherapy with or Without Preoperative Chemoradiation for Resectable Gastric Cancer: Interim Results from an International, Intergroup Trial of the AGITG, TROG, EORTC and CCTG. *Ann. Surg. Oncol.* **2017**, *24*, 2252–2258. [CrossRef]
181. Schein, P.S. A comparison of combination chemotherapy and combined modality therapy for locally advanced gastric carcinoma. *Cancer* **1982**, *49*, 1771–1777. [CrossRef]
182. Kaya, D.M.; Nogueras-Gonzáles, G.M.; Harada, K.; Amlashi, F.G.; Thomas, I.; Rogers, J.E.; Bhutani, M.S.; Lee, J.H.; Weston, B.; Minsky, B.D.; et al. Potentially curable gastric adenocarcinoma treated without surgery. *Eur. J. Cancer* **2018**, *98*, 23–29. [CrossRef] [PubMed]
183. Li, R.; Hou, W.-H.; Chao, J.; Woo, Y.; Glaser, S.; Amini, A.; Nelson, R.A.; Chen, Y.-J. Chemoradiation Improves Survival Compared With Chemotherapy Alone in Unresected Nonmetastatic Gastric Cancer. *J. Natl. Compr. Cancer Netw.* **2018**, *16*, 950–958. [CrossRef] [PubMed]
184. Koyama, S.; Kawanishi, N.; Fukutomi, H.; Osuga, T.; Iijima, T.; Tsujii, H.; Kitagawa, T. Advanced carcinoma of the stomach treated with definitive proton therapy. *Am. J. Gastroenterol.* **1990**, *85*, 443–447. [PubMed]
185. Shibuya, S.; Takase, Y.; Aoyagi, H.; Orii, K.; Sharma, N.; Tsujii, H.; Tsuji, H.; Iwasaki, Y. Definitive proton beam radiation therapy for inoperable gastric cancer: A report of two cases. *Radiat. Med.* **1991**, *9*, 35–40.
186. Ahmed, K.A.; Caudell, J.J.; El-Haddad, G.; Berglund, A.; Welsh, E.A.; Yue, B.; Hoffe, S.E.; Naghavi, A.O.; Abuodeh, Y.A.; Frakes, J.M.; et al. Radiosensitivity Differences Between Liver Metastases Based on Primary Histology Suggest Implications for Clinical Outcomes After Stereotactic Body Radiation Therapy. *Int. J. Radiat. Oncol.* **2016**, *95*, 1399–1404. [CrossRef]
187. Sandhu, N.; Benson, K.R.K.; Kumar, K.A.; Eyben, R.V.; Chang, D.T.; Gibbs, I.C.; Hancock, S.L.; Meola, A.; Chang, S.D.; Li, G.; et al. Local control and toxicity outcomes of stereotactic radiosurgery for spinal metastases of gastrointestinal origin. *J. Neurosurgery: Spine* **2020**, *33*, 87–94. [CrossRef]
188. Myrehaug, S.; Hallet, J.; Chu, W.; Yong, E.; Law, C.; Assal, A.; Koshkina, O.; Louie, A.V.; Singh, S. Proof of concept for stereo-tactic body radiation therapy in the treatment of functional neuroendocrine neoplasms. *J. Radiosurgery SBRT* **2020**, *6*, 321–324.
189. Qin, Y.; Wu, C.W.; Taylor, W.R.; Sawas, T.; Burger, K.N.; Mahoney, D.W.; Sun, Z.; Yab, T.C.; Lidgard, G.P.; Allawi, H.T.; et al. Discovery, Validation, and Application of Novel Methylated DNA Markers for Detection of Esophageal Cancer in Plasma. *Clin. Cancer Res.* **2019**, *25*, 7396–7404. [CrossRef]
190. Liang, K.; O Ahsen, O.; Murphy, A.; Zhang, J.; Nguyen, T.H.; Potsaid, B.; Figueiredo, M.; Huang, Q.; Mashimo, H.; Fujimoto, J.G. Tethered capsule en face optical coherence tomography for imaging Barrett's oesophagus in unsedated patients. *BMJ Open Gastroenterol.* **2020**, *7*, e000444. [CrossRef]
191. Leggett, C.L.; Gorospe, E.C.; Chan, D.K.; Muppa, P.; Owens, V.; Smyrk, T.C.; A Anderson, M.; Lutzke, L.S.; Tearney, G.J.; Wang, K.K. Comparative diagnostic performance of volumetric laser endomicroscopy and confocal laser endomicroscopy in the detection of dysplasia associated with Barrett's esophagus. *Gastrointest. Endosc.* **2016**, *83*, 880–888.e2. [CrossRef] [PubMed]

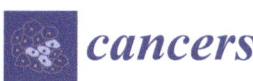

Commentary

Current Trends in Endoscopic Diagnosis and Treatment of Early Esophageal Cancer

Franz Ludwig Dumoulin [1],*, Ralf Hildenbrand [2], Tsuneo Oyama [3] and Ingo Steinbrück [4]

[1] Department of Medicine and Gastroenterology, Gemeinschaftskrankenhaus Bonn, Academic Teaching Hospital, University of Bonn, D-53113 Bonn, Germany
[2] Institute for Pathology Bonn-Duisdorf, D-53123 Bonn, Germany; hildenbrand@patho-bonn.de
[3] Department of Endoscopy, Saku Central Hospital Advanced Care Center, Saku, 3400-28 Nakagomie, Nagano, Japan; oyama@coral.ocn.ne.jp
[4] Department of Medicine, Evangelisches Diakoniekrankenhaus Freiburg, Academic Teaching Hospital, University of Freiburg, D-79110 Freiburg, Germany; ingo.steinbrueck@diak-fr.de
* Correspondence: f.dumoulin@gk-bonn.de; Tel.: +49-228-508-1561

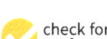

Citation: Dumoulin, F.L.; Hildenbrand, R.; Oyama, T.; Steinbrück, I. Current Trends in Endoscopic Diagnosis and Treatment of Early Esophageal Cancer. *Cancers* **2021**, *13*, 752. https://doi.org/10.3390/cancers13040752

Academic Editor: Ulrich Ronellenfitsch

Received: 30 December 2020
Accepted: 8 February 2021
Published: 11 February 2021

Publisher's Note: MDPI stays neutral with regard to jurisdictional claims in published maps and institutional affiliations.

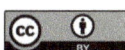

Copyright: © 2021 by the authors. Licensee MDPI, Basel, Switzerland. This article is an open access article distributed under the terms and conditions of the Creative Commons Attribution (CC BY) license (https://creativecommons.org/licenses/by/4.0/).

Simple Summary: Early esophageal cancer is diagnosed in the context of reflux disease, surveillance of Barrett's metaplasia, or during upper gastrointestinal endoscopy for other indications. High definition and virtual or dye chromoendoscopy are mandatory for the screening and evaluation of neoplasia. Endoscopic treatment options include endoscopic mucosal resection (EMR) or endoscopic submucosal dissection (ESD). Resection is considered curative if histopathology confirms low or absent risk of lymph node metastasis. Barrett's high-grade dysplasia or early adenocarcinoma is treated by EMR or ESD, followed by ablation of Barrett's epithelium to avoid metachronous cancer. ESD is the treatment of choice for squamous cell neoplasia. Excellent outcomes have been reported if the ESD of squamous cell cancer with slight submucosal infiltration and thus substantial risk for lymph node metastasis was combined with adjuvant chemo-radiotherapy. In contrast, infiltration of squamous cell cancer exceeding the lamina propria mucosae is not curative. However, despite a substantial risk of lymph node metastasis, excellent outcomes have recently been reported if endoscopic resection of tumors with up to 200 µm submucosal infiltration was combined with adjuvant chemo-radiotherapy.

Abstract: Diagnosis of esophageal adenocarcinoma mostly occurs in the context of reflux disease or surveillance of Barrett's metaplasia. Optimal detection rates are obtained with high definition and virtual or dye chromoendoscopy. Smaller lesions can be treated with endoscopic mucosal resection. Endoscopic submucosal dissection (ESD) is an option for larger lesions. Endoscopic resection is considered curative (i.e., without significant risk of lymph node metastasis) if histopathology confirms en bloc and R0 resection of a well-differentiated (G1/2) tumor without infiltration of lymphatic or blood vessels and the maximal submucosal infiltration depth is 500µm. Ablation of remaining Barrett's metaplasia is important, to reduce the risk of metachronous cancer. Esophageal squamous cell cancer is associated with different risk factors, and most of the detected lesions are diagnosed during upper gastrointestinal endoscopy for other indications. Virtual high definition and dye chromoendoscopy with Lugol's solution are used for screening and evaluation. ESD is the preferred resection technique. The criteria for curative resection are similar to Barrett's cancer, but the maximum infiltration depth must not exceed lamina propria mucosae. Although a submucosal infiltration depth of up to 200 µm carries a substantial risk of lymph node metastasis, ESD combined with adjuvant chemo-radiotherapy gives excellent results. The complication rates of endoscopic resection are low, and the functional outcomes are favorable compared to surgery.

Keywords: squamous cell esophageal cancer; gastro-esophageal reflux disease; Barrett's esophagus; early adenocarcinoma of esophagus; endoscopic submucosal dissection; endoscopic mucosal resection

1. Introduction

According to a recent update from the Globoscan database, esophageal cancer is the seventh most prevalent cancer and the sixth most common cause of cancer-related mortality worldwide [1]. Over 90% of esophageal cancers are due to subtypes of squamous cell cancer or adenocarcinoma. Cancer-related mortality correlates with tumor stage at diagnosis with an overall five year survival rate of less than 20% [2]. While squamous cell cancer is the most prevalent subtype worldwide, dominant in Asia and Africa, there is an increasing prevalence of adenocarcinoma in high-income countries where this subtype today is more prevalent than squamous cell cancer [1,3–5]. This difference is thought to reflect the different distribution of risk factors, i.e., smoking, alcohol consumption, and environmental factors associated with squamous cell cancer versus obesity, gastro-esophageal reflux disease, and Barrett's metaplasia as risk factors for adenocarcinoma. With the advent of high-definition endoscopy and the development of advanced endoscopic resection and ablation techniques, the concept of organ-preserving treatment for early esophageal cancer has been established with excellent survival rates and minimal associated morbidity. This review focuses on the latest trends in the endoscopic diagnosis and treatment of early esophageal neoplasia.

2. Barrett's Esophagus, High-Grade Dysplasia, and Early Adenocarcinoma

2.1. Screening for the Presence of Barrett's Esophagus

The incidences of gastro-esophageal reflux disease, Barrett's esophagus, and esophageal adenocarcinoma are increasing in Western countries. Thus, screening for Barrett's esophagus and surveillance for possible progression to high-grade dysplasia and (early) esophageal adenocarcinoma, including the option of endoscopic treatment, is a desirable concept. However, to date, there is no recommendation for population-based endoscopic screening. Instead, most guidelines suggest selected screening for long standing gastro-esophageal reflux disease with additional risk factors, such as age >50 years, male gender, Caucasian ethnicity, obesity, or family history of Barrett's esophagus or adenocarcinoma [6–9]. A recent evaluation of these guidelines demonstrated poor test characteristics with either low or absent specificity leading to unnecessary endoscopies or unacceptably low sensitivity [10]. To overcome these problems, new technologies are being evaluated. Thus, promising data have been demonstrated for a non-endoscopic cytosponge test to detect the expression of the metaplasia biomarker trefoil factor 3. The method involves swallowing an encapsulated brush attached to a string. The capsule then dissolves in the stomach, and the expanded sponge is withdrawn to obtain the brush cytology [11]. Moreover, a breath test using an artificial intelligence supported sensor system to evaluate patterns of volatile organic compounds was shown to predict the presence of Barrett's esophagus with high sensitivity and specificity [12]. Yet, with current guideline recommendations and pending further optimization of alternative non-endoscopic tests, the detection of Barrett's esophagus still occurs most often in the setting of upper endoscopy performed for other indications than dedicated screening [5]. It is very unfortunate that a recent retrospective study on 123,395 upper gastrointestinal endoscopies calculated a miss rate for esophageal cancer of 6.5% with an associated two year survival rate of only 20% [13]. Thus, it seems to be more than justified to define a neoplasia detection rate as a quality indicator for upper endoscopy in patients with reflux disease [14].

2.2. Detection and Evaluation of High-Grade Dysplasia and Early Adenocarcinoma

Considerable efforts have been made to optimize the detection of dysplasia or early adenocarcinoma during surveillance endoscopy [15]. Important issues are the use of high-definition endoscopes, chromoendoscopy with acetic acid [16,17] and/or virtual chromoendoscopy [18,19], a sufficient inspection time (at least one minute per cm of segment length), and the application of a biopsy protocol with targeted biopsies from any suspicious lesion and four quadrant biopsies every 1–2 cm Barrett's length ("Seattle protocol") [9]. Several classification systems for the detection and evaluation of high-grade dysplasia and early adenocarcinoma in Barrett's esophagus have been proposed. The Barrett's International NBI Group (BING) classification [18] and the Japanese classification [19] both rely on surface and/or vessel irregularities identified with virtual narrow band imaging chromoendoscopy and show good sensitivity (80–87%) and specificity (88–97%) for the detection of dysplasia. The more recent proposed classification relies on surface irregularities and the loss of whitening of the mucosa after the application of acetic acid [16]. Using these descriptive criteria, a high sensitivity and a high negative predictive power for the presence or absence of Barrett's neoplasia could be demonstrated not only for expert, but also for non-expert endoscopists (Table 1; Figure 1 a–d).

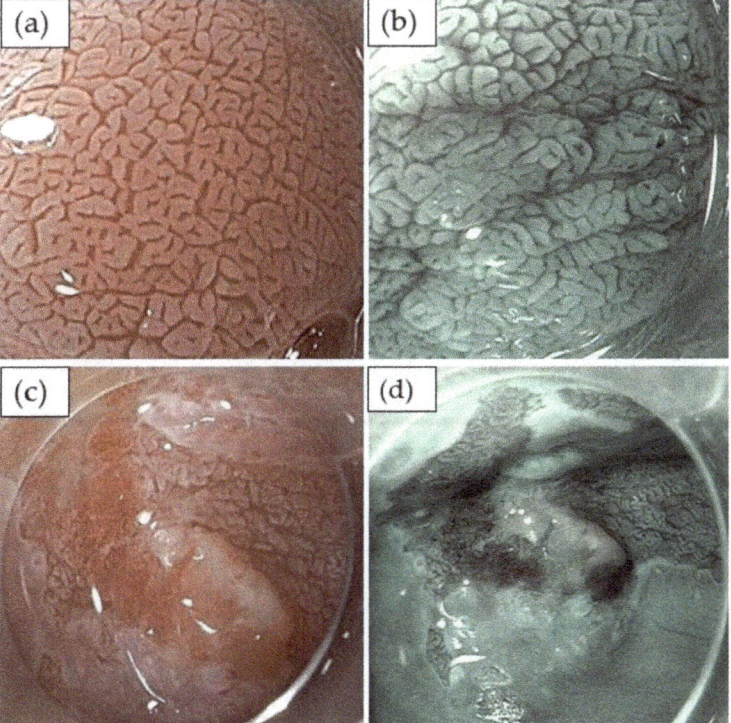

Figure 1. Endoscopic evaluation of Barrett's esophagus and dysplasia with chromoendoscopy using 1.5% acetic acid. Top: non-dysplastic Barrett's with a regular surface structure: (**a**) white light imaging, (**b**) narrow band imaging. Bottom: Barrett's adenocarcinoma with the irregular surface structure and loss of acetowhitening: (**c**) white light imaging, (**d**) narrow band imaging.

Acetic acid staining can also be helpful to evaluate the extent of Barrett's cancer underneath the squamous epithelium [20]. In contrast to endoscopic image analysis (in particular with magnifying endoscopy), endoscopic ultrasound is less accurate in the prediction of infiltration depth [21]. However, endoscopic ultrasound is the most reliable method to detect possible lymph node metastasis and thus can be helpful in selected cases [22]. The additional acquisition of cytology with a specifically designed brush may increase the dysplasia detection rate and is included in the recommendations of the American Society for Gastrointestinal Endoscopy (ASGE) [9,23]. In the near future, artificial intelligence systems will become available to support the detection of dysplasia and early adenocarcinoma [24–26].

Table 1. Classification systems for Barrett's associated neoplasia [16,18,19,27].

Classification System (Barrett's Esophagus)
Paris Classification ('generic" classification of superficial GI neoplasia)
0-Ip (pedunculated), 0-Is (sessile)
0-IIa (slightly elevated), 0-IIb (completely flat) 0-IIc (slightly depressed)
0-III (excavated/ulcerous)
Barrett's International NBI Group (BING) Classification
mucosal pattern regular
• circular, ridged/villous, or tubular patterns
mucosal pattern irregular:
• absent or irregular patterns
vascular pattern regular
• blood vessels situated regularly along or between mucosal ridges and/or showing normal, long, branching patterns
vascular pattern irregular
• focally or diffusely distributed vessels not following the normal architecture of the mucosa
Japan Esophageal Society classification of Barrett's esophagus
mucosal pattern regular
• form/size: similar; arrangement: regular; density: low or same as surrounding area; white zone: clearly visible and/or of homogeneous width.
mucosal pattern irregular:
• form/size: variable; arrangement: irregular; density: high; white zone: obscure/invisible or of heterogeneous width.
vascular pattern regular:
• form: similar or bending and branching gently or regularly; caliber change gradual; location between or in mucosal pattern
vascular pattern irregular:
• form: various or bending and branching steeply or irregularly; caliber change: abrupt; location: beyond or regardless of mucosal patterns
flat pattern (classified as regular)
• completely flat surface without a clear demarcation line; greenish thick and/or long branching vessels
Portsmouth acetic acid (PREDICT) Classification
acetowhitening non-neoplastic:
• no focal loss of acetowhitening
acetowhitening neoplastic:
• focal loss of acetowhitening
surface pattern non-neoplastic:
• uniform evenly spaced pits with normal pit density
surface pattern neoplastic:
• compactly packed small pits with increased pit density; focal irregularity or disorganized pits; absent pit pattern

2.3. Endoscopic Treatment of Dysplasia and Early Adenocarcinoma

Pioneering work from Germany has established the concept of endoscopic mucosal resection (EMR) for high-grade dysplasia and mucosal esophageal adenocarcinoma [28]. This study included endoscopic resections for 1000 consecutive patients with T1a Barrett's mucosal adenocarcinoma. During a follow up period of almost five years, the complete response rate was 96.3%. Surgery was necessary in 3.7% of the patients; metachronous neoplasia was detected in 14.5% and could be re-treated endoscopically in 81.4%, yielding a long-term complete remission rate of 93.8%. The same group also reported a series of 61 patients with endoscopic resection of low-risk T1b Barrett's cancer: 90% of those with lesions ≤2 cm were in remission during a follow up of approximately four years; one patient developed a lymph node metastasis; and there was no tumor-related mortality [29]. Therefore, EMR is the preferred resection technique in Western countries [30] (Figure 2a–d). In contrast, endoscopic submucosal dissection (ESD) is the recommended method in the Japanese guidelines [21]. In fact, ESD is more appropriate for larger lesions, in particular Paris Type 0-Is, and is recommended for suspicious lesions for which en bloc resection is not possible using endoscopic mucosal resection [8,31]. Moreover, ESD compares favorably to EMR with higher en bloc (96% vs. 50%) and R0 resection rates (82% vs. 40%) with less recurrences (2.5% vs. 12.4%) [21]. Complication rates of endoscopic resection are low for both techniques [21,32]. They include perforation, bleeding, and, after resection of

>70–80% of the circumference, also strictures. In cases of early adenocarcinoma, the criteria for curative resection are (i) complete (R0) resection without involvement of lateral and vertical margins, (ii) no invasion of lymphatic or blood vessels, and (iii) tumor grading G1/2. Infiltration depth into the submucosal layer of <500 µm is acceptable, in particular for patients with high perioperative risk [33]. While involved vertical margins are usually an indication for additional surgery, endoscopic controls and secondary resection are recommended in cases of positive lateral margins (Table 2).

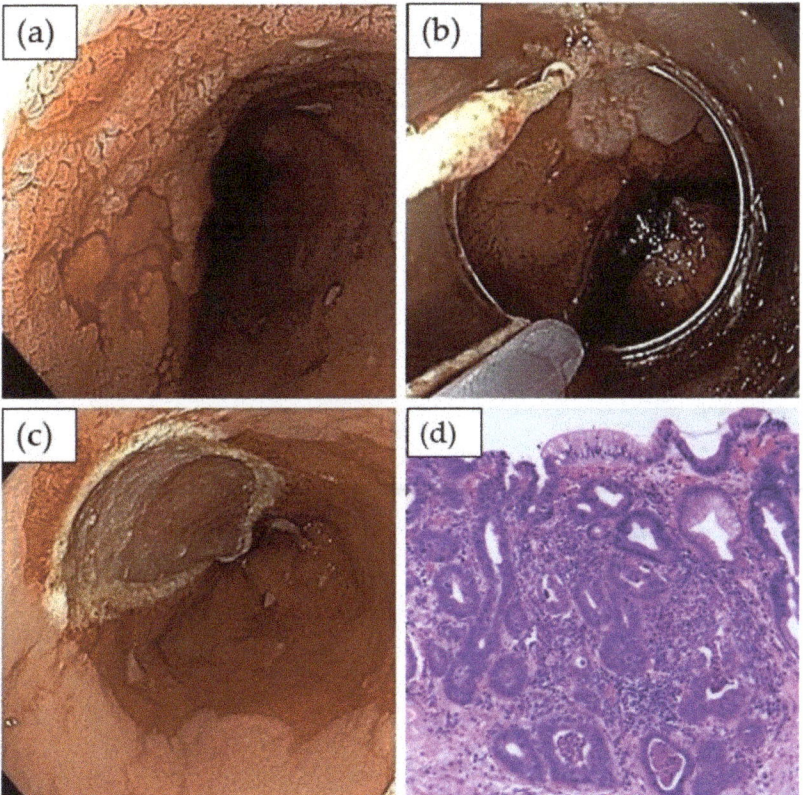

Figure 2. Endoscopic mucosal resection (EMR) of early adenocarcinoma with the suck and cut technique. (**a**) Long segment Barrett's cancer with suspicious lesion to the left (white light imaging, acetic acid 1.5%); (**b**) lesion is band ligated and resected with the snare placed underneath the rubber band; (**c**) resection bed without any associated bleeding; (**d**) histopathology shows well differentiated intramucosal adenocarcinoma without infiltration of lymphatic or blood vessels pT1a m3, ly(-), v(-) G2 (H&E stain, × 400).

Table 2. Criteria for curative endoscopic resection of Barrett's cancer [30].

Criteria for Curative Endoscopic Resection
• Resection en bloc/R0 (vertical margin)
• Grading G1/G21
• No infiltration of lymphatic/blood vessels
• Submucosal infiltration depth ≤500 µm

2.4. Additional Treatment and Follow-Up

The development of metachronous neoplasia from residual Barrett's metaplasia after endoscopic resection of high-grade dysplasia/early adenocarcinoma has been reported in up to 37% of cases during a two year follow up [34]. Thus, current guidelines recommend complete ablation of the remaining Barrett's epithelium [31,33,35] (Figure 3). This is usually performed by radiofrequency ablation starting from ca. 5–10 mm above the squamo-columnar junction to 5–10 mm distal to the "neo Z-line". Tissue ablation can also be achieved by argon plasma coagulation, cryo-ablation, or photodynamic therapy [35,36]. A major complication of ablation therapy is a stricture rate of approximately 5% [33]. A recently published study on 807 patients reported a 4.5% neoplasia recurrence rate after mucosal ablation, which peaked within the first 18 months [37].

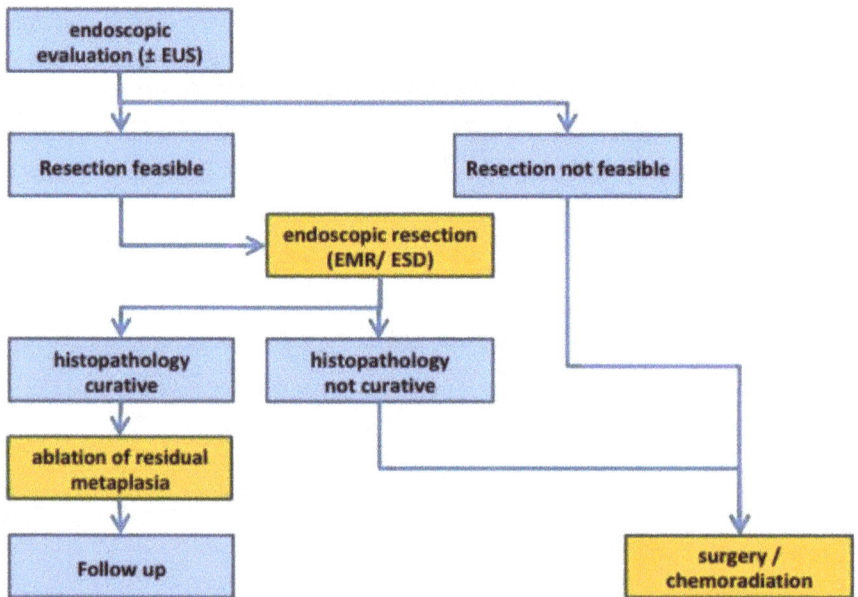

Figure 3. Proposed treatment algorithm according to current guidelines [30]. Evaluation may include endoscopic ultrasound to assess possible lymph node metastasis. Criteria for curative resection are listed in Table 2. EUS, endoscopic ultrasound; EMR, endoscopic mucosal resection; ESD, endoscopic submucosal dissection.

Mucosal ablation can also be considered for confirmed non-visible low-grade dysplasia [38] or high-grade dysplasia and early cancer. However, a recent meta-analysis suggests that visible high-grade dysplasia or early cancer is best treated by a combination of endoscopic resection and additive ablation rather than using just radiofrequency ablation [39]. An endoscopic follow up after 3, 6, and 12 months and yearly thereafter has been suggested after endoscopic resection and/or mucosal ablation [33]. The approach to recurrent or metachronous neoplasia is similar to initial therapy [30] and the vast majority of these lesions can be re-treated endoscopically [28].

3. Squamous Cell High-Grade Dysplasia and Early Cancer

3.1. Screening for Squamous Cell Dysplasia or Early Cancer

As for Barrett's esophagus, there is no established population-based screening for esophageal squamous cell cancer. However, endoscopic screening should be considered in the presence of risk factors, e.g., after diagnosis of head and neck cancer, in cases of long standing achalasia, or for persons with heavy smoking and drinking [40]. Vice versa, there is an increased risk for head and neck cancer in patients treated for superficial esophageal squamous cell cancer [41]. Screening for esophageal cancer is probably best performed by chromoendoscopy, after staining with a low concentration of Lugol's solution or by virtual chromoendoscopy such as narrow band imaging [42,43]. A disadvantage of dye chromoendoscopy with Lugol's solution, in particular at higher concentrations, is the induction of a painful inflammatory reaction. This inflammatory reaction interferes with the delineation of the borders of the lesion for up to several weeks. Thus, dye staining is usually done immediately before the beginning of endoscopic resection.

3.2. Detection and Evaluation of Squamous Cell Dysplasia or Early Cancer

Endoscopic evaluation of a detected lesion to predict the infiltration depth is critical since lymph node metastasis in squamous cell cancer is mainly associated with invasion depth [19]. The simplified classification of the Japan Esophageal Society uses vessel irregularities (loop formation, loss of loop formation, dilated and tortuous vessel) observed with regular or magnification endoscopy to predict infiltration depth [44] (Table 3; Figure 4a–d). The diagnostic accuracy is over 90% for B1 and B3 vessel patterns in predicting either superficial infiltration depth, i.e., epithelial (pT1a-EP) or lamina propria (pT1a-LPM) infiltration, or for the prediction of deep submucosal infiltration (pT1b-pSM2). In contrast, the vessel pattern B2 has an accuracy of only 55.7% for predicting an infiltration depth to the muscularis mucosae (pT1b-MM) or to the upper submucosal layer (pT1b-SM1). Endoscopic ultrasound has a relatively lower diagnostic accuracy for the evaluation of squamous cell cancer infiltration depth, but has its value as the most accurate diagnostic tool to assess possible lymph node metastasis [21,22].

Table 3. Japanese classification for early squamous cell cancer [44].

Japan Esophageal Society (JES) Classification of Early Squamous Cell Cancer to Assess Tumor Infiltration Depth
Vascular pattern regular
Type A vessels
Type B vessels
Abnormal microvessels (severe irregularity/highly dilated abnormal vessels)
• Type B1 with a loop-like formation
• Type B2 without a loop-like formation
• Type B3 highly dilated vessels, the calibers of which appear to be more than three times that of usual B2 vessels

3.3. Endoscopic Treatment

The recommended technique for endoscopic en bloc resection of early esophageal squamous cell cancer is ESD. Compared to EMR, ESD achieves higher en bloc (96% vs. 50%) and R0 resection rates (82% vs. 40%) and lower recurrence rates (2.5% vs. 12.4%) [21]. To facilitate the delineation of the lateral tumor extension, chromoendoscopy with Lugol's solution is performed immediately before the procedure. The use of a traction device, e.g., the clip line technique [45], is useful to facilitate the resection in the narrow lumen of the esophagus. According to the recent Japanese guideline, endoscopic resection should be undertaken for all lesions with the B1 vessel pattern (predicted infiltration depth T1a-EP/LPM), unless the lesion is completely circumferential and has an axial extension of more than 5 cm. In addition, ESD should also be attempted for lesions with B2 vessel patterns (predicted infiltration depth T1a-MM/T1b-SM1) unless completely circumferential since there is a high probability that histopathology may reveal a more superficial infiltration depth and might thus be a curative resection (Figure 5 a–d). Curability is then evaluated by final histopathology: resection is considered curative for R0 resected superficial tumors without infiltration of lymphatic or blood vessels, i.e., pT1a-EP/LPM ly (-), v (-) (Table 4). In cases of vessel infiltration or infiltration of the submucosal layer, additional treatment (either surgery or chemo-radiotherapy) is recommended [21]. Data from observational studies comparing endoscopic resection with surgery for cT1a cancers demonstrate lower complication rates and associated health care costs with similar clinical outcomes for endoscopic treatment [21,46].

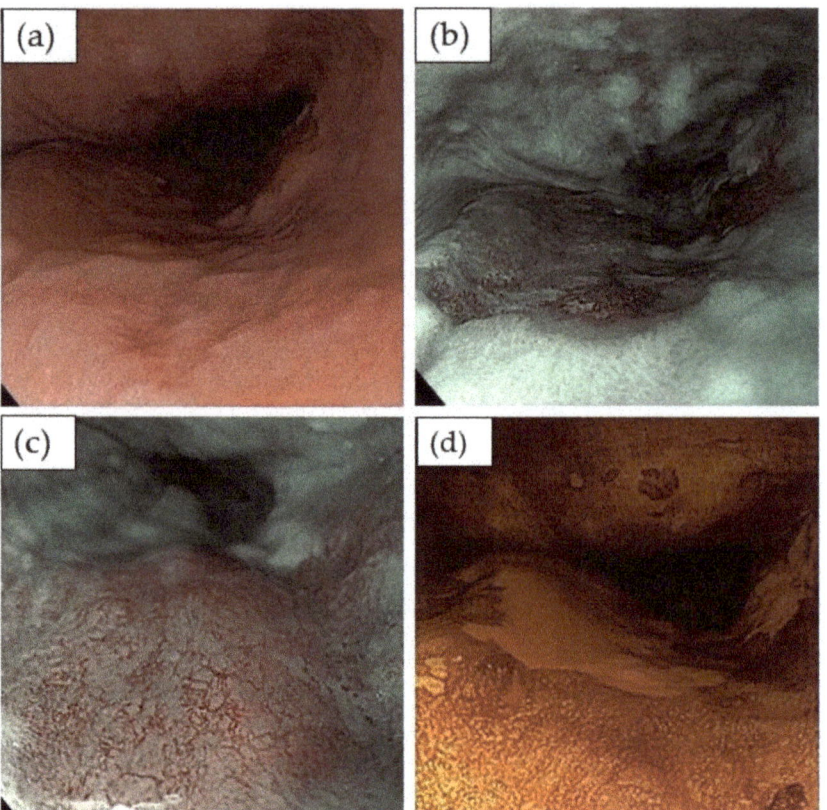

Figure 4. Endoscopic evaluation of early squamous cell cancer by endoscopic submucosal dissection: (**a**) irregular surface structure in the mid esophagus (white light imaging); (**b**) virtual chromoendoscopy of this area shows a brownish are with better definition of the borders (narrow band imaging); (**c**) close view of the lesion showing vessel irregularities (type B2 vessels); (**d**) chromoendoscopy with 0.5% Lugol's solution nicely delineates the borders of the lesions and is ideally used immediately before starting an endoscopic resection.

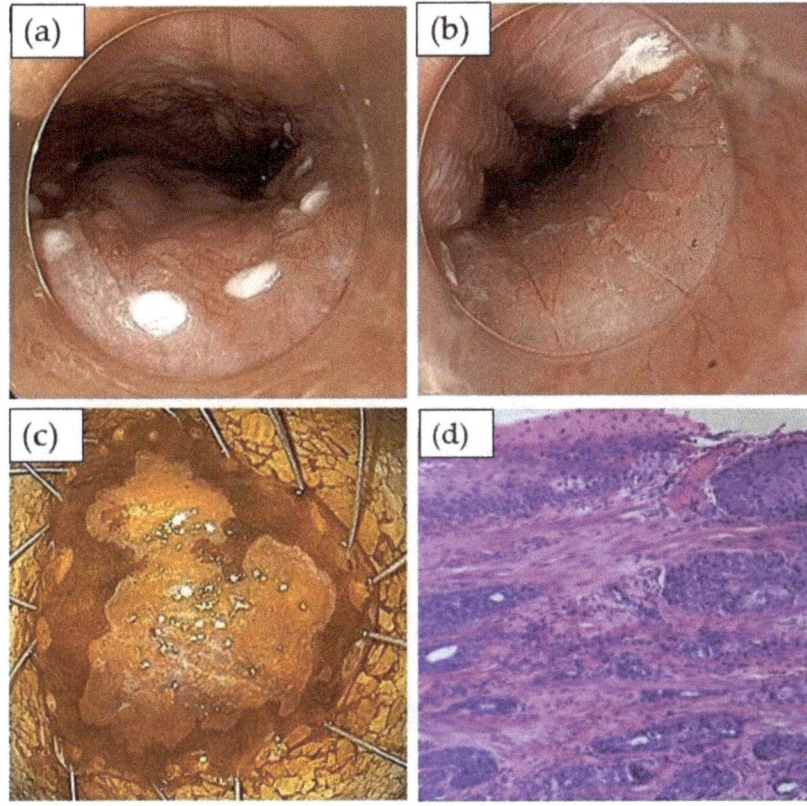

Figure 5. Endoscopic resection of early squamous cell cancer by endoscopic submucosal dissection: (**a**) after chromoendoscopy with Lugol's solution, the borders of the lesion are marked with coagulation points; (**b**) resection bed without any associated bleeding; (**c**) specimen on corkboard (after repeated staining with Lugol's solution); (**d**) histopathology shows poorly differentiated pT1b squamous cell cancer (H&E stain, × 400).

Table 4. Criteria for curative endoscopic resection of early squamous cell cancer.

Criteria for Curative Endoscopic Resection
• Resection en bloc/R0
• Grading G1/G21
• No infiltration of lymphatic/blood vessels
• Infiltration depth pT1a-EP [1] or pT1a-LPM [2]

[1] Abbreviations: EP: epithelial layer; LPM: lamina propria mucosae; MM: muscularis mucosae; sm: submucosal.
[2] The Japanese guideline recommends comprehensive evaluation of the need for additional treatment for pT1a-MM cancers, while additional treatment with surgery or chemoradiotherapy is strongly recommended for pT1b sm1 (≤200 µm) cancers [21].

3.4. Additional Treatment and Follow-Up

Additional surgery or definitive chemo-radiotherapy is recommended after non curative resection [21] (Figure 6). Recently, excellent data have been published for adjuvant chemo-radiotherapy after complete endoscopic resection of T1b (SM1–2) cancers [47]. In this prospective observational study, 176 patients were treated with endoscopic resection of early esophageal squamous cell cancer. After histopathology, eighty-seven patients had either pT1a tumors with lympho-vascular invasion or pT1b tumors. These patients were treated by adjuvant chemo-radiotherapy (41.4 Gy) and had an overall three year survival of 90.7%. This outcome is comparable to published outcome data for surgery, and the rate of local recurrences is less than after primary chemo-radiotherapy [47]. The annual risk for metachronous esophageal is between 2.2 and 9.0%, and most recurrences can be treated endoscopically [19]. Thus, endoscopic follow-up and surveillance are recommended to be done in at least yearly intervals after curative local treatment. In addition, screening for synchronous head and neck, as well as lung cancers is also recommended [21].

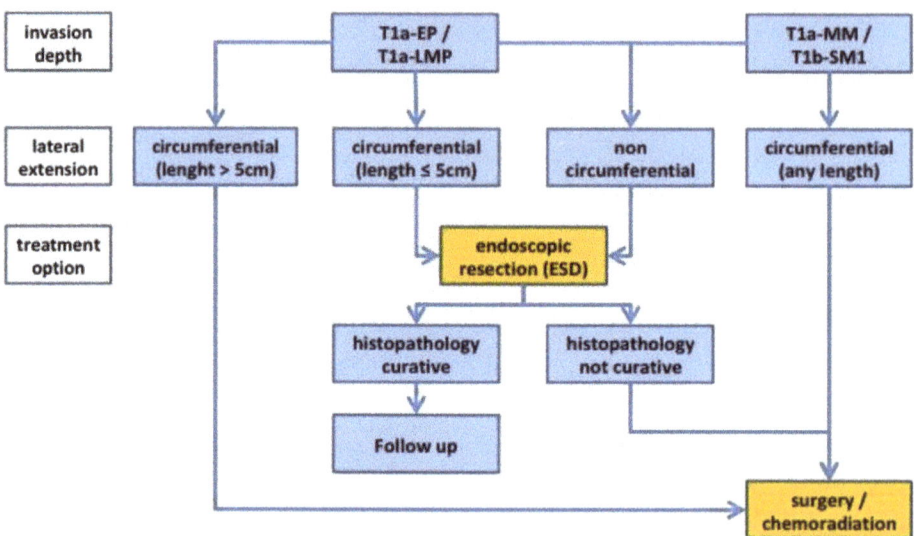

Figure 6. Proposed treatment algorithm of early esophageal squamous cell cancer according to current Japanese guidelines [21]. Evaluation should include endoscopic ultrasound to assess possible lymph node metastasis in selected cases. Invasion depth is diagnosed according to the Japan Esophageal Society (JES) classification (Table 3). Lateral extension is usually visualized by chromoendoscopy with Lugol's solution. Criteria for curative resection are listed in Table 4. ESD, endoscopic submucosal dissection; EP, epithelial layer; LMP, lamina propria mucosae; MM, muscularis mucosae.

4. Conclusions

Endoscopic detection and treatment of high-grade dysplasia and early esophageal cancer are established concepts for neoplasia with low or absent lymph node metastasis risk. Areas of research are (i) indications for endoscopic screening, (ii) optimizing of screening efficiency, and (iii) extending the concept of organ-preserving therapy by adjuvant treatment strategies. Screening may become more efficient with non-endoscopic pretesting, with promising data from cytosponge procedures or the use of an artificial intelligence-based breath test. The optimization of the neoplasia detection rate is important. Here, the widespread availability of high-definition endoscopy with virtual and/or dye-based chromoendoscopy is helpful. Moreover, additional support will soon be available from artificial intelligence image analysis systems. Finally, adjuvant treatment, e.g., chemo-radiotherapy may help to extend the curative ability of minimally invasive endoscopic therapy of early esophageal cancer in cases of high lymph node metastasis risk.

Author Contributions: F.L.D. and I.S. worked out the concept of the paper and wrote the draft. T.O. and R.H. provided additional input and contributed to the figures. All authors read and agreed to the published version of the manuscript.

Funding: This research received no external funding.

Data Availability Statement: No new data were created or analyzed in this study. Data sharing is not applicable to this article.

Conflicts of Interest: The authors declare no conflict of interest.

References

1. Arnold, M.; Abnet, C.C.; Neale, R.E.; Vignat, J.; Giovannucci, E.L.; McGlynn, K.A.; Bray, F. Global Burden of 5 Major Types of Gastrointestinal Cancer. *Gastroenterology* **2020**, *159*, 335–349. [CrossRef]
2. Malhotra, G.K.; Yanala, U.; Ravipati, A.; Follet, M.; Vijayakumar, M.; Are, C. Global trends in esophageal cancer. *J. Surg. Oncol.* **2017**, *115*, 564–579. [CrossRef] [PubMed]
3. Que, J.; Garman, K.S.; Souza, R.F.; Spechler, S.J. Pathogenesis and cells of origin of Barrett's esophagus. *Gastroenterology* **2019**, *157*, 349–364. [CrossRef]
4. Desai, M.; Lieberman, D.A.; Kennedy, K.F.; Hamade, N.; Thota, P.; Parasa, S.; Gorrepati, V.S.; Bansal, A.; Gupta, N.; Gaddam, S.; et al. Increasing prevalence of high-grade dysplasia and adenocarcinoma on index endoscopy in Barrett's esophagus over the past 2 decades: Data from a multicenter U.S. consortium. *Gastrointest. Endosc.* **2019**, *89*, 257–263. [CrossRef]
5. Peters, Y.; Al-Kaabi, A.; Shaheen, N.J.; Chak, A.; Blum, A.; Souza, R.F.; Di Pietro, M.; Iyer, P.G.; Pech, O.; Fitzgerald, R.C.; et al. Barrett oesophagus. *Nat. Rev. Dis. Prim.* **2019**, *5*, 35. [CrossRef]
6. Spechler, S.J.; Sharma, P.; Souza, R.F.; Inadomi, J.M.; Shaheen, N.J. American Gastroenterological Association medical position statement on the management of Barrett's esophagus. *Gastroenterology* **2011**, *140*, 1084–1091. [CrossRef]
7. Fitzgerald, R.C.; Di Pietro, M.; Ragunath, K.; Ang, Y.; Kang, J.Y.; Watson, P.; De Caestecker, J. British Society of Gastroenterology guidelines on the diagnosis and management of Barrett's oesophagus. *Gut* **2014**, *63*, 7–42. [CrossRef] [PubMed]
8. Weusten, B.; Bisschops, R.; Coron, E.; Dinis-Ribeiro, M.; Dumonceau, J.-M.; Esteban, J.-M.; Hassan, C.; Pech, O.; Repici, A.; Bergman, J.; et al. Endoscopic management of Barrett's esophagus: European Society of Gastrointestinal Endoscopy (ESGE) Position Statement. *Eur. Soc. Gastrointest. Endosc. Position Statement* **2017**, *49*, 191–198. [CrossRef]
9. Qumseya, B.; Sultan, S.; Bain, P.; Jamil, L.; Jacobson, B.; Anandasabapathy, S.; Agrawal, D.; Buxbaum, J.L.; Fishman, D.S.; Gurudu, S.R.; et al. ASGE guideline on screening and surveillance of Barrett's esophagus. *Gastrointest. Endosc.* **2019**, *90*, 335–359. [CrossRef] [PubMed]
10. Nguyen, T.H.; Thrift, A.P.; Rugge, M.; El-Serag, H.B. Prevalence of Barrett's esophagus and performance of societal screening guidelines in an unreferred primary care population of U.S. veterans. *Gastrointest. Endosc. e1*. [CrossRef] [PubMed]
11. Fitzgerald, R.C.; di Pietro, M.; O'Donovan, M.; Maroni, R.; Muldrew, B.; Debiram-Beecham, I.; Gaw, M. Cytosponge-trefoil factor 3 versus usual care to identify Barrett's oesophagus in a primary care setting: A multicentre, pragmatic, randomised controlled trial. *Lancet* **2020**, *396*, 333–344. [CrossRef]
12. Peters, Y.; Schrauwen, R.W.M.; Tan, A.C.; Bogers, S.K.; De Jong, B.; Siersema, P.D. Detection of Barrett's oesophagus through exhaled breath using an electronic nose device. *Gut* **2020**, *69*, 1169–1172. [CrossRef]
13. Rodríguez de Santiago, E.; Hernanz, N.; Marcos-Prieto, H.M.; De-Jorge-Turrión M, Á.; Barreiro-Alonso, E.; Rodríguez-Escaja, C.; Albillos, A. Rate of missed oesophageal cancer at routine endoscopy and survival outcomes: A multicentric cohort study. *United Eur. Gastroenterol. J.* **2019**, *7*, 189–198.
14. Parasa, S.; Desai, M.; Vittal, A.; Chandrasekar, V.T.; Pervez, A.; Kennedy, K.F.; Gupta, N.; Shaheen, N.J.; Sharma, P. Estimating neoplasia detection rate (NDR) in patients with Barrett's oesophagus based on index endoscopy: A systematic review and meta-analysis. *Gut* **2019**, *68*, 2122–2128. [CrossRef] [PubMed]
15. Bergman, J.; De Groof, A.J.; Pech, O.; Ragunath, K.; Armstrong, D.; Mostafavi, N.; Lundell, L.; Dent, J.; Vieth, M.; Tytgat, G.; et al. An Interactive Web-Based Educational Tool Improves Detection and Delineation of Barrett's Esophagus–Related Neoplasia. *Gastroenterology* **2019**, *156*, 1299–1308. [CrossRef]
16. Kandiah, K.; Chedgy, F.J.Q.; Subramaniam, S.; Longcroft-Wheaton, G.; Bassett, P.; Repici, A.; Sharma, P.; Pech, O.; Bhandari, P. International development and validation of a classification system for the identification of Barrett's neoplasia using acetic acid chromoendoscopy: The Portsmouth acetic acid classification (PREDICT). *Gut* **2017**, *67*, 2085–2091. [CrossRef] [PubMed]
17. Chedgy, F.J.; Subramaniam, S.; Kandiah, K.; Thayalasekaran, S.; Bhandari, P. Acetic acid chromoendoscopy: Improving neoplasia detection in Barrett's esophagus. *World J. Gastroenterol.* **2016**, *22*, 5753. [CrossRef]
18. Sharma, P.; Bergman, J.J.G.H.M.; Goda, K.; Kato, M.; Messmann, H.; Alsop, B.R.; Gupta, N.; Vennalaganti, P.; Hall, M.; A Konda, V.J.; et al. Development and Validation of a Classification System to Identify High-Grade Dysplasia and Esophageal Adenocarcinoma in Barrett's Esophagus Using Narrow-Band Imaging. *Gastroenterol.* **2016**, *150*, 591–598. [CrossRef] [PubMed]
19. Ishihara, R.; Goda, K.; Oyama, T. Endoscopic diagnosis and treatment of esophageal adenocarcinoma: Introduction of Japan Esophageal Society classification of Barrett's esophagus. *J. Gastroenterol.* **2018**, *54*, 1–9. [CrossRef]

20. Iwaya, Y.; Rowsell, C.; Gupta, V.; Marcon, N. Buried Barrett's Adenocarcinoma Clearly Demonstrated with Acetic Acid Chromoendoscopy. *Am. J. Gastroenterol.* **2018**, *113*, 1580. [CrossRef]
21. Ishihara, R.; Arima, M.; Iizuka, T.; Oyama, T.; Katada, C.; Kato, M.; Goda, K.; Goto, O.; Tanaka, K.; Yano, T.; et al. Endoscopic submucosal dissection/endoscopic mucosal resection guidelines for esophageal cancer. *Dig. Endosc.* **2020**, *32*, 452–493. [CrossRef]
22. Ahmed, O.; A Ajani, J.; Lee, J.H. Endoscopic management of esophageal cancer. *World J. Gastrointest. Oncol.* **2019**, *11*, 830–841. [CrossRef]
23. Raphael, K.L.; Stewart, M.; Sejpal, D.V.; Cheung, M.; Whitson, M.J.; Han, D.; Trindade, A.J. Adjunctive yield of wide-area transepithelial sampling for dysplasia detection after advanced imaging and random biopsies in Barrett's esophagus. *Clin. Transl. Gastroenterol.* **2019**, *10*, 12. [CrossRef] [PubMed]
24. de Groof, A.J.; Struyvenberg, M.R.; Van Der Putten, J.; Van Der Sommen, F.; Fockens, K.N.; Curvers, W.L.; Zinger, S.; Pouw, R.E.; Coron, E.; Baldaque-Silva, F.; et al. Deep-Learning System Detects Neoplasia in Patients With Barrett's Esophagus With Higher Accuracy Than Endoscopists in a Multistep Training and Validation Study With Benchmarking. *Gastroenterologgy* **2020**, *158*, 915–929. [CrossRef] [PubMed]
25. Ebigbo, A.; Mendel, R.; Probst, A.; Manzeneder, J.A.D.S.; Papa, J.P.; Palm, C.; Messmann, H. Computer-aided diagnosis using deep learning in the evaluation of early oesophageal adenocarcinoma. *Gut* **2013**, *68*, 1143. [CrossRef]
26. Hashimoto, R.; Requa, J.; Dao, T.; Ninh, A.; Tran, E.; Mai, D.; Lugo, M.; Chehade, N.E.-H.; Chang, K.J.; Karnes, W.E.; et al. Artificial intelligence using convolutional neural networks for real-time detection of early esophageal neoplasia in Barrett's esophagus (with video). *Gastrointest. Endosc.* **2020**, *91*, 1264–1271. [CrossRef]
27. Endoscopic Classification Review Group. Update on the paris classification of superficial neoplastic lesions in the digestive tract. *Endoscopy* **2005**, *37*, 570–578. [CrossRef] [PubMed]
28. Pech, O.; May, A.; Manner, H.; Behrens, A.; Pohl, J.; Weferling, M.; Hartmann, U.; Manner, N.; Huijsmans, J.; Gossner, L.; et al. Long-term Efficacy and Safety of Endoscopic Resection for Patients With Mucosal Adenocarcinoma of the Esophagus. *Gastroenterol.* **2014**, *146*, 652–660. [CrossRef]
29. Manner, H.; Pech, O.; Heldmann, Y.; May, A.; Pohl, J.; Behrens, A.; Gossner, L.; Stolte, M.; Vieth, M.; Ell, C. Efficacy, Safety, and Long-term Results of Endoscopic Treatment for Early Stage Adenocarcinoma of the Esophagus with Low-risk sm1 Invasion. *Clin. Gastroenterol. Hepatol.* **2013**, *11*, 630–635. [CrossRef] [PubMed]
30. Sharma, P.; Shaheen, N.J.; Katzka, D.; Bergman, J.J. AGA clinical practice update on endoscopic treatment of Barrett's esophagus with dysplasia and/or early cancer: Expert review. *Gastroenterology* **2020**, *158*, 760–769.
31. Noordzij, I.C.; Curvers, W.L.; Schoon, E.J. Endoscopic resection for early esophageal carcinoma. *J. Thorac. Dis.* **2019**, *11*, S713–S722. [CrossRef] [PubMed]
32. Pimentel-Nunes, P.; Dinis-Ribeiro, M.; Ponchon, T.; Repici, A.; Vieth, M.; De Ceglie, A.; Amato, A.; Berr, F.; Bhandari, P.; Bialek, A.; et al. Endoscopic submucosal dissection: European Society of Gastrointestinal Endoscopy (ESGE) Guideline. *Endoscopy* **2015**, *47*, 829–854. [CrossRef] [PubMed]
33. Sharma, P.; Shaheen, N.J.; Katzka, D.; Bergman, J. Clinical Practice Update: Endoscopic Treatment of Barrett's Esophagus With Dysplasia and/or Early Cancer. *Gastroenterology* **2019**. [PubMed]
34. Manner, H.; Rabenstein, T.; Pech, O.; Braun, K.; May, M.A.; Pohl, J.; Behrens, A.; Vieth, M.; Ell, C. Ablation of residual Barrett's epithelium after endoscopic resection: A randomized long-term follow-up study of argon plasma coagulation vs. surveillance (APE study). *Endoscopy* **2013**, *12*. [CrossRef] [PubMed]
35. Lal, P.; Thota, P.N. Cryotherapy in the management of premalignant and malignant conditions of the esophagus. *World J. Gastroenterol.* **2018**, *24*, 4862–4869. [CrossRef] [PubMed]
36. Hamade, N.; Desai, M.; Thoguluva Chandrasekar, V.; Chalhoub, J.; Patel, M.; Duvvuri, A.; Sharma, P. Efficacy of cryotherapy as first line therapy in patients with Barrett's neoplasia: A systematic review and pooled analysis. *Dis. Esophagus* **2019**, *32*, doz040. [CrossRef]
37. Wani, S.; Han, S.; Kushnir, V.; Early, D.; Mullady, D.; Hammad, H.; Brauer, B.; Thaker, A.; Simon, V.; Ezekwe, E.; et al. Recurrence Is Rare Following Complete Eradication of Intestinal Metaplasia in Patients With Barrett's Esophagus and Peaks at 18 Months. *Clin. Gastroenterol. Hepatol.* **2020**. [CrossRef]
38. di Pietro, M.; Fitzgerald, R.C. Revised British Society of Gastroenterology recommendation on the diagnosis and management of Barrett's oesophagus with low-grade dysplasia. *Gut* **2018**, *67*, 392–393. [CrossRef]
39. de Matos, M.V.; da Ponte-Neto, A.M.; de Moura DT, H.; Maahs, E.D.; Chaves, D.M.; Baba, E.R.; de Moura EG, H. Treatment of high-grade dysplasia and intramucosal carcinoma using radiofrequency ablation or endoscopic mucosal resection+ radiofrequency ablation: Meta-analysis and systematic review. *World J. Gastrointest. Endosc.* **2019**, *11*, 239. [CrossRef] [PubMed]
40. van de Ven SE, M.; Bugter, O.; Hardillo, J.A.; Bruno, M.J.; Baatenburg de Jong, R.J.; Koch, A.D. Screening for head and neck second primary tumors in patients with esophageal squamous cell cancer: A systematic review and meta-analysis. *United Eur. Gastroenterol. J.* **2019**, *7*, 1304–1311.
41. Maekawa, A.; Ishihara, R.; Iwatsubo, T.; Nakagawa, K.; Ohmori, M.; Iwagami, H.; Matsuno, K.; Inoue, S.; Arao, M.; Nakahira, H.; et al. High incidence of head and neck cancers after endoscopic resection for esophageal cancer in younger patients. *J. Gastroenterol.* **2019**, *55*, 401–407. [CrossRef] [PubMed]

42. Bugter, O.; van de Ven, S.E.; Hardillo, J.A.; Bruno, M.J.; Koch, A.D.; Baatenburg de Jong, R.J. Early detection of esophageal second primary tumors using Lugol chromoendoscopy in patients with head and neck cancer: A systematic review and meta-analysis. *Head Neck* **2019**, *41*, 1122–1130.
43. Su, H.-A.; Hsiao, S.-W.; Hsu, Y.-C.; Wang, L.-Y.; Yen, H.-H. Superiority of NBI endoscopy to PET/CT scan in detecting esophageal cancer among head and neck cancer patients: A retrospective cohort analysis. *BMC Cancer* **2020**, *20*, 1–9. [CrossRef]
44. Oyama, T.; Inoue, H.; Arima, M.; Momma, K.; Tomori, A.; Ishihara, R.; Hirasawa, D.; Takeuchi, M.; Goda, K. Prediction of the invasion depth of superficial squamous cell carcinoma based on microvessel morphology: Magnifying endoscopic classification of the Japan Esophageal Society. *Esophagus* **2017**, *14*, 105–112. [CrossRef] [PubMed]
45. Oyama, T. Counter Traction Makes Endoscopic Submucosal Dissection Easier. *Clin. Endosc.* **2012**, *45*, 375–378. [CrossRef] [PubMed]
46. Raman, V.; Jawitz, O.K.; Voigt, S.L.; Yang, C.-F.J.; Harpole, D.H.; D'Amico, T.A.; Hartwig, M.G. The effect of age on survival after endoscopic resection versus surgery for T1a esophageal cancer. *J. Thorac. Cardiovasc. Surg.* **2020**, *160*, 295–302. [CrossRef]
47. Minashi, K.; Nihei, K.; Mizusawa, J.; Takizawa, K.; Yano, T.; Ezoe, Y.; Muto, M. Efficacy of endoscopic resection and selective chemoradiotherapy for stage I esophageal squamous cell carcinoma. *Gastroenterology* **2019**, *157*, 382–390. [CrossRef] [PubMed]

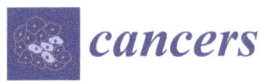

Article

The Role of the Lymph Node Ratio in Advanced Gastric Cancer After Neoadjuvant Chemotherapy

Karol Rawicz-Pruszyński [1,*], Bogumiła Ciseł [1], Radosław Mlak [2], Jerzy Mielko [1], Magdalena Skórzewska [1], Magdalena Kwietniewska [1], Agnieszka Pikuła [1], Katarzyna Gęca [1], Katarzyna Sędłak [1], Andrzej Kurylcio [1] and Wojciech P. Polkowski [1]

1. Department of Surgical Oncology, Medical University of Lublin, 20-080 Lublin, Poland; bogumilacisel@uml.edu.pl (B.C.); jerzymielko@uml.edu.pl (J.M.); magdalenaskorzewska@uml.edu.pl (M.S.); magdalenakwietniewska@uml.edu.pl (M.K.); agnieszkapikula@uml.edu.pl (A.P.); kasiaa.geca@gmail.com (K.G.); sedlak.katarz@gmail.com (K.S.); andrzejkurylcio@uml.edu.pl (A.K.); wojciechpolkowski@uml.edu.pl (W.P.P.)
2. Department of Human Physiology, Medical University of Lublin, 20-080 Lublin, Poland; radoslawmlak@uml.edu.pl
* Correspondence: karolrawiczpruszynski@uml.edu.pl; Tel.: +48-81-531-8137; Fax: +48-81-531-8133

Received: 24 October 2019; Accepted: 28 November 2019; Published: 1 December 2019

Abstract: The ratio of positive lymph nodes (LNs) to the total LN harvest is called the LN ratio (LNR). It is an independent prognostic factor in gastric cancer (GC). The aim of the current study was to evaluate the impact of neoadjuvant chemotherapy (NAC) on the LNR (ypLNR) in patients with advanced GC. We retrospectively analyzed the data of patients with advanced GC, who underwent gastrectomy with N1 and N2 (D2) lymphadenectomy between August 2011 and January 2019 in the Department of Surgical Oncology at the Medical University of Lublin. The exclusion criteria were a lack of preoperative NAC administration, suboptimal lymphadenectomy (<D2 and/or removal of less than 15 lymph nodes), and a lack of data on tumor regression grading (TRG) in the final pathological report. A total of 95 patients were eligible for the analysis. A positive correlation was found between the ypLNR and tumor diameter ($p < 0.001$), post treatment pathological Tumour (ypT) stage ($p < 0.001$), Laurén histological subtype ($p = 0.0001$), and the response to NAC ($p < 0.0001$). A multivariate analysis demonstrated that the ypLNR was an independent prognostic factor in patients with intestinal type GC ($p = 0.0465$) and in patients with no response to NAC ($p = 0.0483$). In the resection specimen, tumor diameter and depth of infiltration, Laurén histological subtype, and TRG may reflect the impact of NAC on LN status, as quantified by ypLNR in advanced GC.

Keywords: gastric cancer; lymph node ratio; neoadjuvant chemotherapy

1. Introduction

In 2018, gastric cancer (GC) was diagnosed in 1,000,000 patients. The cause of an estimated 783,000 deaths, it was the fifth-most frequently diagnosed cancer and the third leading cause of cancer deaths worldwide [1]. Surgery is globally accepted as the only curative treatment option. Radical surgery involves gastrectomy and adequate regional lymph node dissection [2–4]. The latter has been suggested as the most important surgery-dependent prognostic factor in GC [5]. According to the fourth version of the Japanese Gastric Cancer Association guidelines, D1 lymphadenectomy is defined as lymph node (LN) removal from the perigastric area (stations 1–7, N1 tier), whereas N1 and N2 (D2) dissection extends along the lymph nodes at the coeliac axis and its branches (D1 plus no. 8a, 9, 10, 11p, 11d, 12a, and N2 tier) [4]. In contrast to the Far East, in the West it is recommended that surgical treatment be preceded by neoadjuvant (perioperative) chemotherapy [2,3,6,7]. LN metastases are the only independent predictor of survival after chemotherapy and surgery [8], as reported in the analysis of pathologic tumor response and nodal status in the Perioperative Chemotherapy versus Surgery Alone for Resectable Gastroesophageal Cancer (MAGIC) trial [6]. The ratio of positive LNs to the total LN harvest is called the LN ratio (LNR). A recent meta-analysis of 27 studies confirmed that as an independent prognostic factor in GC patients, higher LNR was significantly related to shorter overall survival (OS) [9]. Although several studies investigated the effect of neoadjuvant chemotherapy (NAC) on the nodal status in GC patients [7,8,10–13] and focused on the impact of NAC on the LNR in pancreatic [14], rectal [15], and breast cancer [16] patients, to the best of our knowledge, there are no data available on the influence of NAC on LNR in GC. Therefore, the aim of the current study is to evaluate the impact of NAC on LNR (ypLNR) in patients with advanced GC.

2. Materials and Methods

2.1. Study Subjects

After obtaining institutional review board approval [KE-0254/297/2018], we collected data from a prospectively maintained database of all patients with histologically confirmed and previously untreated primary advanced gastric adenocarcinoma, who were operated on between August 2011 and January 2019 in the Department of Surgical Oncology at the Medical University of Lublin (Poland). The exclusion criteria were a lack of preoperative NAC administration, suboptimal lymphadenectomy (<D2 and/or removal of less than 15 LN), and a lack of data on pathological tumor regression grading (TRG) in the final pathological report. The post treatment clinical M0/post treatment pathological M1 (ycM0/ypM1) patients were included in the study, since these patients were operated on with curative intent. The metastatic setting was revealed only after the final pathological assessment and was available after surgery. A flowchart of the inclusion and exclusion criteria of the study is shown in Figure 1. Since NAC may significantly impact the lymph node status [17], whereas inadequate lymphadenectomy (removal of <15 LNs) causes suboptimal pathological nodal (pN) staging [18], the ypLNR was not calculated in excluded patients. A total of 95 patients were eligible for analysis.

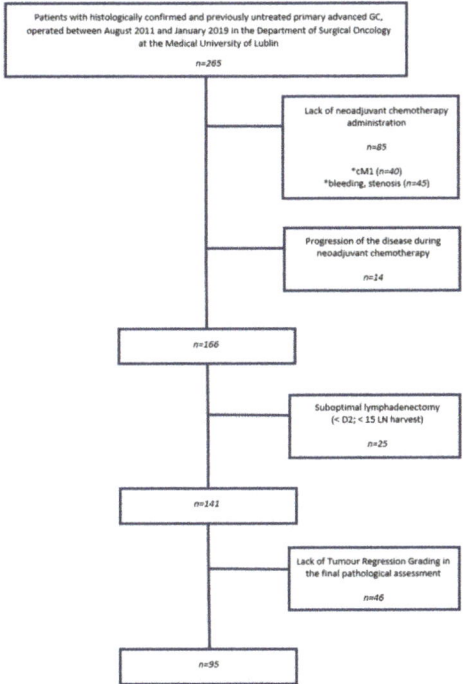

Figure 1. Flow chart of study inclusion and exclusion criteria.

2.2. Preoperative Staging

Between 2011 and 2015, preoperative staging was based on computed tomography (CT) (abdominal and chest CT, and pelvic CT in females) and endoscopic ultrasonography (EUS) if there were suspicions of early GC after initial diagnostic endoscopy. Since 2016, all consecutive patients with locally advanced GC but clinically non-metastatic (cM0) GC (based on CT), have been scheduled for a staging laparoscopy with peritoneal (washings) cytology prior to evaluation of the patient on Multi Disciplinary Team (MDT) meeting.

2.3. Neoadjuvant (Perioperative) Chemotherapy

The perioperative epirubicin, oxaliplatin, and capecitabine (EOX) regimen consisted of 50 mg/m^2 epirubicin and 130 mg/m^2 oxaliplatin on day 1, with 625 mg/m^2 capecitabine administered twice daily on days 1–21. The perioperative regimen was repeated two to three times every three weeks. The docetaxel, oxapliplatin, fluorouracil, and folinic acid (FLOT) chemotherapy consisted of oxaliplatin, 85 mg/m^2; leucovorin, 200 mg/m^2; and docetaxel, 50 mg/m^2. Each was an intravenous infusion followed by fluorouracil, 2600 mg/m^2, as a 24-h continuous intravenous infusion on day 1, repeated every two weeks. The entire cohort was scheduled for adjuvant chemotherapy; however, due to poor performance status, patient preference, and postoperative complications, 16 patients (17%) did not receive postoperative systemic treatment.

2.4. Tumor Regression Grading after NAC

A modified Becker's system was used to assess TRG [19,20]—complete response/no residual tumor (Grade 1), subtotal regression/<10% residual tumor (Grade 2), partial regression/10–50% residual tumor (Grade 3), and no regression/>50% residual tumor (Grade 4). Assessment of TRG with this system is recommended by a panel of gastrointestinal pathology experts [20]. All patients were divided into two cohorts according to the TRG: patients with response to NAC (TRG = 1, 2, 3) and patients who did not respond to NAC (TRG = 4).

2.5. Statistical Analysis

All analyses were performed using MedCalc 15.8 (MedCalc Software, Ostend, Belgium). Data were expressed as a percentage (for categorized variable), mean, standard deviation, median, and range (for continuous variables). We considered p values < 0.05 as statistically significant. Spearman's correlation test was used to calculate correlation coefficients. The comparison of ypLNR values in relation to the selected demographic and clinical variables was carried out with the use of the nonparametric U–Mann–Whitney test (the data had a non-normal distribution) and the Kruskal–Wallis test, if more than two groups were compared. Lymph node stations (LNS) were categorized into three groups: N1 tier (LNS 1–7), N2 tier (LNS 8–12a), and the complete D2 (N1 + N2) tier (LNS 1–12a). In each group, the ypLNR (the ratio of postneoadjuvant, metastatic LNs to the total LN harvest in the postoperative pathological report) was calculated for every patient. Overall survival (OS) time was defined as the length of time from the date of surgery to the patient's death by any cause (complete data) or to the last known observation (censored data). A univariate OS analysis was performed with the use of the Kaplan–Meier estimation method (log-rank), whereas Cox logistic regression models were used in the multivariate OS analysis, with statistically significant factors from the univariate analysis ($\alpha < 0.05$) included as variables. A total of 92 patients (96.8%) were included in the OS analysis. Three patients (3.2%) were lost from follow-up.

2.6. Follow-Up

Initially, patients were seen in the outpatient clinic three weeks after the surgery, then every three months during the first postoperative year, every six months during the second postoperative year, and once a year thereafter. A CT scan and gastroscopy were performed 12 months after surgery, unless patients were symptomatic and/or had signs of recurrence.

3. Results

Among the 95 patients included in the study, 54 were males (56.8%) and 41 were females (43.2%), with the median age being 57 years. The median tumor size tumor upon pathological evaluation was 3.5 cm, and the majority of tumors were poorly differentiated (G3; 82.7%). There were 45 (47.4%) intestinal, 29 (30.5%) diffuse, and 21 (22.1%) mixed tumors. There were 44 patients (46.4%) who did not have tumor regression (TRG 4), 32 patients (33.7%) who presented with partial regression (TRG 3), 9 patients (9.4%) who presented with subtotal regression (TRG 2), and 10 patients (10.5%) who had complete response to NAC (TRG 1). There were 63 tumors (66.6%) that were at least ypT3. Additionally, 53 patients (55.8%) had lymph node metastases (N+) and 19 patients (20%) had distant metastases (ypM1) in the final pathological evaluation. The median LN harvest was 28. The clinicopathological features of selected patients are shown in Table 1.

Table 1. Clinicopathological variables.

Variables	No. of Patients n = 95 (%)
Sex	
Male	54 (56.8%)
Female	41 (43.2%)
Age (years)	
Average	57.37
Standard deviation (±)	10.90
Median (min-max)	57 (31–77)
Tumor maximal diameter (cm)	
Average	4.2
Standard deviation (±)	2.7
Median (min-max)	3.5 (1–15)
Tumor location	
Upper 1/3	29 (31%)
Middle 1/3	27 (28%)
Distal 1/3	39 (41%)
Tumor depth	
Mucosa	2 (2%)
Submucosa	7 (7%)
Muscularis Propria	35 (37%)
Subserosa	14 (15%)
Serosa	37 (39%)
Lauren histological subtype	
Intestinal	45 (47.4%)
Diffuse	29 (30.5%)
Mixed	21 (22.1%)
Grading	
G1	6 (8%)
G2	27 (9.3%)
G3	62 (82.7%)
No. of NAC cycles	
1	2 (2%)
2	8 (8%)
3	56 (60%)
4	20 (21%)
6	6 (6.38%)
8	2 (2.13%)
NAC regimen	
EOX	83 (87.2%)
FLOT	12 (12.8%)
Tumor regression grading (TRG) (Classification of response)	
Complete (Grade 1)	10 (10.5%)
Subtotal (Grade 2)	9 (9.4%)
Partial (Grade 3)	32 (33.7%)
Minimal/No regression (Grade 4)	44 (46.4%)
ypT	
T0	6 (6.3%)
T1	6 (6.3%)
T2	20 (21%)
T3	40 (42%)
T4	23 (24.6%)

Table 1. Cont.

Variables	No. of Patients $n = 95$ (%)
ypN	
N0	42 (44.2%)
N1	7 (7.4%)
N2	14 (14.4%)
N3	32 (34%)
ypM	
M0	76 (80%)
M1	19 (20%)
No. of examined lymph nodes	
Mean	32
Standard deviation (±)	14
Median (min-max)	28 (16–81)

NAC: neoadjuvant chemotherapy. EOX: epirubicin, oxaliplatin and capecitabine. FLOT: docetaxel, oxapliplatin, fluorouracil and folinic acid.

3.1. ypLNR in Selected Subgroups

The median ypLNR for the entire cohort was 0.07. In patients with a tumor diameter of <3.5 cm, the median ypLNR was significantly lower than in the patients with larger (≥3.5 cm) tumors in N1 and N2, as well as in the combined N1 + N2 tiers ($p = 0.0003$, $p = 0.009$, and $p = 0.0005$, respectively). In patients with intestinal-type GC, the median ypLNR was significantly lower than in patients with diffuse- and mixed-type GC in the N1, N2, and N1 + N2 tiers ($p = 0.0005$, $p = 0.001$, and $p = 0.0005$, respectively). In patients with response to NAC, the median ypLNR was significantly lower than in patients without a NAC response in the N1, N2, and N1 + N2 tiers ($p < 0.0001$, $p = 0.001$, and $p < 0.0001$, respectively). In ypT4 patients, the median ypLNR was significantly higher than in ypT0–T3 patients in the N1 and N1 + N2 tiers ($p = 0.001$ and $p = 0.002$, respectively). With respect to nodal status, a significant difference was observed between ypN0 patients (ypLNR = 0) and ypN + patients (ypLNR >0) in the N1, N2, and D2 tiers ($p < 0.0001$). In ypM1 patients, the median ypLNR was significantly higher than in ypM0 patients in the N1, N2, and N1 + N2 tiers ($p < 0.0001$, $p = 0.04$, and $p = 0.001$, respectively). No statistically significant association was found between ypLNR and a patient's sex, age, and tumor location and grading. Differences between ypLNR in the N1, N2, and the N1 + N2 tiers in relation to various clinicopathological features are presented in Table 2.

Table 2. ypLNR in selected clinicopathological variables in the N1, N2, and N1 + N2 (D2) tiers.

Variable:	N1		N2		N1 + N2 (D2)	
	Me	p	Me	p	Me	p
Sex [¥]						
Male	0.08	0.64	0.00	0.56	0.00	0.41
Female	0.00		0.00		0.07	
Age (years) [¥]						
<57	0.08	0.54	0.00	0.83	0.09	0.40
≥57	0.02		0.00		0.04	
Maximal tumor dimension (cm) [¥]						
<3.5	0.00	0.0003	0.00	0.009	0.00	0.0005
≥3.5 cm	0.38		0.00		0.31	
Tumor location [#]						
Upper 1/3	0.00		0.00		0.02	
Middle 1/3	0.30	0.09	0.00	0.28	0.06	0.09
Lower 1/3	0.03		0.00		0.22	

Table 2. Cont.

Variable:	N1		N2		N1 + N2 (D2)	
	Me	p	Me	p	Me	p
Laurén histological subtype [#]						
Intestinal	0.00		0.00		0.00	
Diffuse	0.45	0.0005	0.00	0.001	0.30	0.0005
Mixed	0.30		0.14		0.22	
Grading [#]						
G1	0.01		0.00		0.01	
G2	0.00	0.27	0.00	0.73	0.07	0.46
G3	0.10		0.00		0.09	
Response to NAC (TRG) [¥]						
Response to NAC (TRG 1–3)	0.00	<0.0001	0.00	0.0011	0.00	<0.0001
No response to NAC (TRG 4)	0.40		0.07		0.30	
ypT [¥]						
ypT0-T3	0.00	0.001	0.00	0.06	0.00	0.002
ypT4	0.50		0.08		0.31	
ypN [¥]						
N0	0.00	<0.0001	0.00	<0.0001	0.00	<0.0001
N1-N3b	0.48		0.24		0.36	
ypM [¥]						
M0	0.00	0.0001	0.00	0.04	0.00	0.001
M1	0.53		0.08		0.30	

Me: median. TRG: tumor regression grading; [¥] U–Mann–Whitney test, [#] Kruskal–Wallis test.

3.2. Correlation between ypLNR and Selected Clinicopathological Variables

A significant correlation was shown between the clinical Tumour (cT) stage and ypLNR in the N1 and N1 + N2 tiers ($p = 0.0006$ and $p = 0.0024$, respectively), whereas the correlation between the cT stage and ypLNR in N2 tier was nearly significant ($p = 0.06$). The maximal tumor diameter and ypLNR showed a positive correlation in the N1 and N1 + N2 tiers ($p < 0.0001$ and $p < 0.0001$, respectively). A positive correlation was found between ypLNR and the Laurén histological subtype in the N1 and N1 + N2 tiers (both $p = 0.0001$). There was an upward trend in ypLNR value in intestinal-, mixed-, and diffuse-type GC, respectively. A positive correlation was found between ypLNR and response to NAC in the N1, N2, and N1 + N2 tiers ($p < 0.0001$, $p = 0.0009$, and $p < 0.0001$, respectively). Positive correlation was also observed between ypLNR and ypT in the N1 and N1 + N2 tiers (both $p < 0.0001$) and ypLNR and ypM in the N1, N2, and N1 + N2 tiers ($p < 0.0001$, $p = 0.03$, and $p = 0.001$, respectively). A positive correlation was found between ypLNR and ypN in the N1, N2, and N1 + N2 tiers ($p < 0.0001$, $p < 0.0001$, and $p < 0.000$, respectively). Results of the Spearman's rank correlation coefficient between ypLNR and selected clinicopathological variables are shown in Table 3.

Table 3. Spearman's rank correlation coefficient between ypLNR and selected clinicopathological variables.

Variable (n = 95)	ypLNR					
	N1		N2		N1 + N2 (D2)	
	R (Spearman)	p	R (Spearman)	p	R (Spearman)	p
Age	−0.015	0.88	0.005	0.96	−0.024	0.82
cT	0.344	0.0006	0.192	0.06	0.308	0.002
Tumor max. diameter	0.455	<0.0001	0.246	0.01	0.420	<0.0001
Grading	0.166	0.10	0.068	0.51	0.126	0.22
Laurén histological subtype	0.399	0.0001	0.0179	0.8632	0.387	0.0001
Response to NAC (TRG)	0.528	<0.0001	0.335	0.0009	0.503	<0.0001
No. of NAC cycles	0.120	0.24	0.187	0.07	0.151	0.14
ypT	0.436	<0.0001	0.270	0.008	0.422	<0.0001
ypN	0.903	<0.0001	0.744	<0.0001	0.953	<0.0001
ypM	0.405	<0.0001	0.213	0.03	0.330	0.001

3.3. Tumor Survival Analysis

In the univariate analysis of OS, ypLNR > median showed prognostic significance in patients with intestinal-type GC (11 vs. 37 months, $p = 0.0114$) and diffuse-type GC (15 vs. 39 months, $p = 0.0008$), as well as in patients with response to NAC (14 vs. 39 months; $p = 0.0162$) and in patients with no response to NAC (11 vs. 34 months; $p = 0.0097$). A multivariate analysis demonstrated that ypLNR was an independent prognostic factor in intestinal-type GC ($p = 0.0465$) and in patients with no response to NAC (TRG 4) ($p = 0.0483$). The results of the uni- and multivariate survival analysis are presented in Table 4. The median OS of patients with ypLNR ≤0.07 was 37 months, whereas in patients with ypLNR >0.07, the median OS was 11 months ($p = 0.0002$; log-rank test; HR 2.29; 95% CI: 1.36–3.84). The median follow-up for all patients, ypM0 patients and ypM1 patients was 20, 29 and 9 months, respectively. During follow-up, 71% of patients died. The date of data cut-off was 4 October, 2019.

Table 4. The effect of ypLNR on overall survival (OS) based on the Laurén classification and TRG.

Variable	Univariate		Multivariate
	Months	HR (95%CI) p	HR (95%CI) p
	Intestinal-type GC		
ypLNR > median (0.00)	11	2.69 (1.09–6.64)	2.87 (1.02–8.06) *
ypLNR ≤ median (0.00)	37	0.0114	0.0465
	Diffuse-type GC		
ypLNR > median (0.30)	15	2.99 (1.18–7.60)	2.28 (0.60–8.47)
ypLNR ≤ median (0.30)	39	0.0008	0.3488
	Mixed-type GC		
ypLNR > median (0.22)	10	1.13 (0.41–3.14)	0.48 (0.07–3.17)
ypLNR ≤ median (0.22)	15	0.8150	0.4453
	Response to NAC (TRG 1–3)		
ypLNR > median (0.00)	14	2.18 (0.97–4.91)	2.38 (0.94–6.03)
ypLNR ≤ median (0.00)	39	0.0162	0.0683
	No response to NAC (TRG 4)		
ypLNR > median (0.30)	11	2.29 (1.15–4.55)	2.46 (1.01–5.99) **
ypLNR ≤ median (0.30)	34	0.0097	0.0483

Tumor* grading, tumor maximal diameter, ypM, and ypT were significant variables in univariate analysis. ** grading, tumor location, ypM, and ypT were significant variables in univariate analysis.

4. Discussion

The current study enabled us to distinguish a ypLNR high-risk group among GC patients after NAC. Tumor diameter ≥ 3.5 cm, Laurén intestinal subtype, lack of response to NAC (TRG 4), serosal infiltration, lymph node metastases, and distant metastases were significantly associated with higher ypLNR.

The influence of NAC on nodal status in GC patients has been investigated meticulously [21]. Wu et al. [22] evaluated the influence of clinical, pathological, and treatment variables on the total LN harvest and the number of metastatic LNs after NAC in patients with GC. The study showed that NAC for GC reduced the total LN count and increased the number of patients who had <15 LN harvested. Thus, a decrease in total LN harvest should be expected in patients undergoing resection after neoadjuvant chemotherapy. In a study conducted by Ji et al. [23], the total LN harvest was an independent prognostic factor in ypN0 GC patients, with a minimum LN harvest of 22. Interestingly, in these patients, surgery alone was even more beneficial than neoadjuvant chemotherapy, as reported by Ronellenfitsch et al. [17]. However, in ypN+ patients, survival was longer in those who received NAC [17] and total LN harvest should exceed 30 in order to avoid stage migration after surgery [24].

Recent data from Asian [25,26], North American [27], and European [28,29] populations showed that LNR is considered a more accurate and reliable parameter than TNM classification in terms of GC prognosis. Additionally, LNR could be a better option to compensate for the stage migration effect. The predictive value for prognosis increases with a higher number of retrieved lymph nodes, as shown in a high-volume study from Korea [30]. Moreover, LNR is a prognostic indicator for patients who develop GC liver metastases, as well as nodal and peritoneal recurrences after radical resection [31,32].

The Laurén classification remains an important clinical factor in treatment of GC. A recent study by Wang et al. demonstrated that LNR might be used as an independent predictor of survival in patients with diffuse-type GC [33]. Jimenez et al. [34] studied the chemosensitivity of GC according to Laurén subtypes. Diffuse-type GC was found to be less chemosensitive and was associated with increased mortality. The recent study by Xu et al. [35] focused on the prognostic value of TRG in perioperative treatment of advanced GC. The Laurén classification and the ypT stage were independent factors for TRG, whereas TRG itself was a prognostic variable for ypN+ patients. In the present study, patients with response to NAC had significantly lower ypLNR when compared to nonresponders. Moreover, the Laurén histological subtype analysis revealed an upward trend in ypLNR value—the mean ypLNR was lowest in intestinal-type GC, intermediate in mixed-type GC, and highest in diffuse-type GC. These results show the potential prognostic information of ypLNR in Western patients with advanced GC by means of response to NAC in different histological subtypes.

The accurate prediction of response to neoadjuvant and adjuvant chemotherapy remains a challenge [36–38]. Due to histological heterogeneity, tumor behavior throughout the clinical management of GC remains uncertain. Improved understanding of GC biology will successively favor tailored surgery. Further research could possibly introduce LNR as a new biomarker [39], since it is closely associated with epidermal growth factor receptor (EGFR) expression [40].

In the era of NAC in GC, the potential effect of systemic treatment on lymph node involvement should be investigated. LNR proved to be an important prognostic factor in the adjuvant setting.

This study contains certain limitations. Due to its retrospective nature, it cannot identify causation. Due to the relatively small sample size, a subgroup stratification analysis might be biased. Moreover, our pathological evaluation did not include assessment of molecular subtype, tumor budding, and lymph node regression, which could be of potential prognostic significance in this setting.

5. Conclusions

In resection specimens, tumor diameter and depth of infiltration, Laurén histological subtype, and TRG may reflect the impact of NAC on LN status, as quantified by ypLNR in advanced GC. When validated in prospective studies, ypLNR could serve as a simple and objective parameter in the clinical evaluation of NAC.

Author Contributions: Conceptualization, K.R.-P. and J.M.; Data curation, B.C., R.M., J.M., M.S., M.K., A.P., K.G., K.S. and W.P.P.; Formal analysis, R.M., K.G., K.S. and A.K.; Investigation, K.R.-P., B.C., M.S. and A.P.; Methodology, R.M., J.M., M.K. and A.P.; Resources, M.S.; Software, K.R.-P., R.M., K.G. and K.S.; Supervision, B.C., A.K. and

W.P.P.; Validation, K.R.-P., B.C., J.M., M.S. and W.P.P.; Writing—Original draft, K.R.-P. and M.K.; Writing—Review & editing, A.K. and W.P.P.

Funding: This research received no external funding.

Conflicts of Interest: The authors declare no conflict of interest.

References

1. Bray, F.; Ferlay, J.; Soerjomataram, I.; Siegel, R.L.; Torre, L.A.; Jemal, A. Global cancer statistics 2018: GLOBOCAN estimates of incidence and mortality worldwide for 36 cancers in 185 countries. *CA Cancer J. Clin.* **2018**, *68*, 394–424. [CrossRef]
2. Ajani, J.A.; D'Amico, T.A.; Almhanna, K.; Bentrem, D.J.; Chao, J.; Das, P.; Denlinger, C.S.; Fanta, P.; Farjah, F.; Fuchs, C.S.; et al. Gastric Cancer, Version 3.2016, NCCN Clinical Practice Guidelines in Oncology. *J. Natl. Compr. Canc. Netw.* **2016**, *14*, 1286–1312. [CrossRef]
3. Smyth, E.C.; Verheij, M.; Allum, W.; Cunningham, D.; Cervantes, A.; Arnold, D.; Committee, E.G. Gastric cancer: ESMO Clinical Practice Guidelines for diagnosis, treatment and follow-up. *Ann. Oncol.* **2016**, *27*, v38–v49. [CrossRef]
4. Japanese Gastric Cancer Association. Japanese gastric cancer treatment guidelines 2014 (ver. 4). *Gastric Cancer* **2017**, *20*, 1–19. [CrossRef]
5. Maruyama, K.; Sasako, M.; Kinoshita, T.; Sano, T.; Katai, H. Surgical treatment for gastric cancer: The Japanese approach. *Semin. Oncol.* **1996**, *23*, 360–368.
6. Cunningham, D.; Allum, W.H.; Stenning, S.P.; Thompson, J.N.; Van de Velde, C.J.; Nicolson, M.; Scarffe, J.H.; Lofts, F.J.; Falk, S.J.; Iveson, T.J.; et al. Perioperative chemotherapy versus surgery alone for resectable gastroesophageal cancer. *N. Engl. J. Med.* **2006**, *355*, 11–20. [CrossRef]
7. Al-Batran, S.E.; Homann, N.; Pauligk, C.; Illerhaus, G.; Martens, U.M.; Stoehlmacher, J.; Schmalenberg, H.; Luley, K.B.; Prasnikar, N.; Egger, M.; et al. Effect of Neoadjuvant Chemotherapy Followed by Surgical Resection on Survival in Patients With Limited Metastatic Gastric or Gastroesophageal Junction Cancer: The AIO-FLOT3 Trial. *JAMA Oncol.* **2017**, *3*, 1237–1244. [CrossRef] [PubMed]
8. Smyth, E.C.; Fassan, M.; Cunningham, D.; Allum, W.H.; Okines, A.F.; Lampis, A.; Hahne, J.C.; Rugge, M.; Peckitt, C.; Nankivell, M.; et al. Effect of Pathologic Tumor Response and Nodal Status on Survival in the Medical Research Council Adjuvant Gastric Infusional Chemotherapy Trial. *J. Clin. Oncol.* **2016**, *34*, 2721–2727. [CrossRef] [PubMed]
9. Zhu, J.; Xue, Z.; Zhang, S.; Guo, X.; Zhai, L.; Shang, S.; Zhang, Y.; Lu, H. Integrated analysis of the prognostic role of the lymph node ratio in node-positive gastric cancer: A meta-analysis. *Int. J. Surg.* **2018**, *57*, 76–83. [CrossRef] [PubMed]
10. Davies, A.R.; Myoteri, D.; Zylstra, J.; Baker, C.R.; Wulaningsih, W.; Van Hemelrijck, M.; Maisey, N.; Allum, W.H.; Smyth, E.; Gossage, J.A.; et al. Lymph node regression and survival following neoadjuvant chemotherapy in oesophageal adenocarcinoma. *Br. J. Surg.* **2018**, *105*, 1639–1649. [CrossRef] [PubMed]
11. Kurokawa, Y.; Shibata, T.; Sasako, M.; Sano, T.; Tsuburaya, A.; Iwasaki, Y.; Fukuda, H. Validity of response assessment criteria in neoadjuvant chemotherapy for gastric cancer (JCOG0507-A). *Gastric Cancer* **2014**, *17*, 514–521. [CrossRef] [PubMed]
12. Oyama, K.; Fushida, S.; Kinoshita, J.; Makino, I.; Nakamura, K.; Hayashi, H.; Nakagawara, H.; Tajima, H.; Fujita, H.; Takamura, H.; et al. Efficacy of pre-operative chemotherapy with docetaxel, cisplatin, and S-1 (DCS therapy) and curative resection for gastric cancer with pathologically positive para-aortic lymph nodes. *J. Surg. Oncol.* **2012**, *105*, 535–541. [CrossRef] [PubMed]
13. Fu, T.; Bu, Z.D.; Li, Z.Y.; Zhang, L.H.; Wu, X.J.; Wu, A.W.; Shan, F.; Ji, X.; Dong, Q.S.; Ji, J.F. Neoadjuvant chemoradiation therapy for resectable esophago-gastric adenocarcinoma: A meta-analysis of randomized clinical trials. *BMC Cancer* **2015**, *15*, 322. [CrossRef]

14. Roland, C.L.; Yang, A.D.; Katz, M.H.; Chatterjee, D.; Wang, H.; Lin, H.; Vauthey, J.N.; Pisters, P.W.; Varadhachary, G.R.; Wolff, R.A.; et al. Neoadjuvant therapy is associated with a reduced lymph node ratio in patients with potentially resectable pancreatic cancer. *Ann. Surg. Oncol.* **2015**, *22*, 1168–1175. [CrossRef] [PubMed]
15. Chang, K.H.; Kelly, N.P.; Duff, G.P.; Condon, E.T.; Waldron, D.; Coffey, J.C. Neoadjuvant therapy does not affect lymph node ratio in rectal cancer. *Surgeon* **2016**, *14*, 270–273. [CrossRef]
16. Tsai, J.; Bertoni, D.; Hernandez-Boussard, T.; Telli, M.L.; Wapnir, I.L. Lymph Node Ratio Analysis After Neoadjuvant Chemotherapy is Prognostic in Hormone Receptor-Positive and Triple-Negative Breast Cancer. *Ann. Surg. Oncol.* **2016**, *23*, 3310–3316. [CrossRef]
17. Ronellenfitsch, U.; Schwarzbach, M.; Hofheinz, R.; Kienle, P.; Nowak, K.; Kieser, M.; Slanger, T.E.; Burmeister, B.; Kelsen, D.; Niedzwiecki, D.; et al. Predictors of overall and recurrence-free survival after neoadjuvant chemotherapy for gastroesophageal adenocarcinoma: Pooled analysis of individual patient data (IPD) from randomized controlled trials (RCTs). *Eur. J. Surg. Oncol.* **2017**, *43*, 1550–1558. [CrossRef]
18. Claassen, Y.H.M.; de Steur, W.O.; Hartgrink, H.H.; Dikken, J.L.; van Sandick, J.W.; van Grieken, N.C.T.; Cats, A.; Trip, A.K.; Jansen, E.P.M.; Kranenbarg, W.M.M.; et al. Surgicopathological Quality Control and Protocol Adherence to Lymphadenectomy in the CRITICS Gastric Cancer Trial. *Ann. Surg.* **2018**, *268*, 1008–1013. [CrossRef]
19. Becker, K.; Mueller, J.D.; Schulmacher, C.; Ott, K.; Fink, U.; Busch, R.; Bottcher, K.; Siewert, J.R.; Hofler, H. Histomorphology and grading of regression in gastric carcinoma treated with neoadjuvant chemotherapy. *Cancer* **2003**, *98*, 1521–1530. [CrossRef]
20. Tsekrekos, A.; Detlefsen, S.; Riddell, R.; Conner, J.; Mastracci, L.; Sheahan, K.; Shetye, J.; Lundell, L.; Vieth, M. Histopathologic tumor regression grading in patients with gastric carcinoma submitted to neoadjuvant treatment: Results of a Delphi survey. *Hum. Pathol.* **2019**, *84*, 26–34. [CrossRef]
21. Ott, K.; Blank, S.; Ruspi, L.; Bauer, M.; Sisic, L.; Schmidt, T. Prognostic impact of nodal status and therapeutic implications. *Transl. Gastroenterol. Hepatol.* **2017**, *2*, 15. [CrossRef] [PubMed]
22. Wu, Z.M.; Teng, R.Y.; Shen, J.G.; Xie, S.D.; Xu, C.Y.; Wang, L.B. Reduced lymph node harvest after neoadjuvant chemotherapy in gastric cancer. *J. Int. Med. Res.* **2011**, *39*, 2086–2095. [CrossRef] [PubMed]
23. Ji, X.; Bu, Z.D.; Li, Z.Y.; Wu, A.W.; Zhang, L.H.; Zhang, J.; Wu, X.J.; Zong, X.L.; Li, S.X.; Shan, F.; et al. Prognostic significance of the total number of harvested lymph nodes for lymph node-negative gastric cancer patients. *BMC Cancer* **2017**, *17*, 558. [CrossRef] [PubMed]
24. Deng, J.; Liu, J.; Wang, W.; Sun, Z.; Wang, Z.; Zhou, Z.; Xu, H.; Liang, H. Validation of clinical significance of examined lymph node count for accurate prognostic evaluation of gastric cancer for the eighth edition of the American Joint Committee on Cancer (AJCC) TNM staging system. *Chin. J. Cancer Res.* **2018**, *30*, 477–491. [CrossRef] [PubMed]
25. Lin, D.; Li, Y.; Xu, H.; Chen, J.; Wang, B.; Liu, C.; Lu, P.; Alatengbaolide. Lymph node ratio is an independent prognostic factor in gastric cancer after curative resection (R0) regardless of the examined number of lymph nodes. *Am. J. Clin. Oncol.* **2013**, *36*, 325–330. [CrossRef]
26. Zhou, Y.; Zhang, J.; Cao, S.; Li, Y. The evaluation of metastatic lymph node ratio staging system in gastric cancer. *Gastric Cancer* **2013**, *16*, 309–317. [CrossRef]
27. Kutlu, O.C.; Watchell, M.; Dissanaike, S. Metastatic lymph node ratio successfully predicts prognosis in western gastric cancer patients. *Surg. Oncol.* **2015**, *24*, 84–88. [CrossRef]
28. Marchet, A.; Mocellin, S.; Ambrosi, A.; Morgagni, P.; Garcea, D.; Marrelli, D.; Roviello, F.; de Manzoni, G.; Minicozzi, A.; Natalini, G.; et al. The ratio between metastatic and examined lymph nodes (N ratio) is an independent prognostic factor in gastric cancer regardless of the type of lymphadenectomy: Results from an Italian multicentric study in 1853 patients. *Ann. Surg.* **2007**, *245*, 543–552. [CrossRef]
29. Nelen, S.D.; van Steenbergen, L.N.; Dassen, A.E.; van der Wurff, A.A.; Lemmens, V.E.; Bosscha, K. The lymph node ratio as a prognostic factor for gastric cancer. *Acta Oncol.* **2013**, *52*, 1751–1759. [CrossRef]
30. Kong, S.H.; Lee, H.J.; Ahn, H.S.; Kim, J.W.; Kim, W.H.; Lee, K.U.; Yang, H.K. Stage migration effect on survival in gastric cancer surgery with extended lymphadenectomy: The reappraisal of positive lymph node ratio as a proper N-staging. *Ann. Surg.* **2012**, *255*, 50–58. [CrossRef]
31. Li, M.X.; Jin, Z.X.; Zhou, J.G.; Ying, J.M.; Liang, Z.Y.; Mao, X.X.; Bi, X.Y.; Zhao, J.J.; Li, Z.Y.; Huang, Z.; et al. Prognostic Value of Lymph Node Ratio in Patients Receiving Combined Surgical Resection for Gastric Cancer Liver Metastasis: Results from Two National Centers in China. *Medicine* **2016**, *95*, e3395. [CrossRef]

32. Bilici, A.; Selcukbiricik, F.; Seker, M.; Oven, B.B.; Olmez, O.F.; Yildiz, O.; Olmuscelik, O.; Hamdard, J.; Acikgoz, O.; Cakir, A.; et al. Prognostic Significance of Metastatic Lymph Node Ratio in Patients with pN3 Gastric Cancer Who Underwent Curative Gastrectomy. *Oncol. Res. Treat.* **2019**, *42*, 209–216. [CrossRef] [PubMed]
33. Wang, H.; Xing, X.M.; Ma, L.N.; Liu, L.; Hao, J.; Feng, L.X.; Yu, Z. Metastatic lymph node ratio and Lauren classification are independent prognostic markers for survival rates of patients with gastric cancer. *Oncol. Lett.* **2018**, *15*, 8853–8862. [CrossRef] [PubMed]
34. Jimenez Fonseca, P.; Carmona-Bayonas, A.; Hernandez, R.; Custodio, A.; Cano, J.M.; Lacalle, A.; Echavarria, I.; Macias, I.; Mangas, M.; Visa, L.; et al. Lauren subtypes of advanced gastric cancer influence survival and response to chemotherapy: Real-world data from the AGAMENON National Cancer Registry. *Br. J. Cancer* **2017**, *117*, 775–782. [CrossRef] [PubMed]
35. Xu, X.; Zheng, G.; Zhang, T.; Zhao, Y.; Zheng, Z. Is pathologic tumor regression grade after neo-adjuvant chemotherapy a promising prognostic indicator for patients with locally advanced gastric cancer? A cohort study evaluating tumor regression response. *Cancer Chemother. Pharmacol.* **2019**, *84*, 635–646. [CrossRef]
36. Blackham, A.U.; Greenleaf, E.; Yamamoto, M.; Hollenbeak, C.; Gusani, N.; Coppola, D.; Pimiento, J.M.; Wong, J. Tumor regression grade in gastric cancer: Predictors and impact on outcome. *J. Surg. Oncol.* **2016**, *114*, 434–439. [CrossRef]
37. Mansour, J.C.; Tang, L.; Shah, M.; Bentrem, D.; Klimstra, D.S.; Gonen, M.; Kelsen, D.P.; Brennan, M.F.; Coit, D.G. Does graded histologic response after neoadjuvant chemotherapy predict survival for completely resected gastric cancer? *Ann. Surg. Oncol.* **2007**, *14*, 3412–3418. [CrossRef]
38. Foo, M.; Leong, T. Adjuvant therapy for gastric cancer: Current and future directions. *World J. Gastroenterol.* **2014**, *20*, 13718–13727. [CrossRef]
39. Yamashita, K.; Hosoda, K.; Ema, A.; Watanabe, M. Lymph node ratio as a novel and simple prognostic factor in advanced gastric cancer. *Eur. J. Surg. Oncol.* **2016**, *42*, 1253–1260. [CrossRef]
40. Ema, A.; Waraya, M.; Yamashita, K.; Kokubo, K.; Kobayashi, H.; Hoshi, K.; Shinkai, Y.; Kawamata, H.; Nakamura, K.; Nishimiya, H.; et al. Identification of EGFR expression status association with metastatic lymph node density (ND) by expression microarray analysis of advanced gastric cancer. *Cancer Med.* **2015**, *4*, 90–100. [CrossRef]

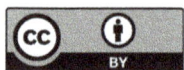

© 2019 by the authors. Licensee MDPI, Basel, Switzerland. This article is an open access article distributed under the terms and conditions of the Creative Commons Attribution (CC BY) license (http://creativecommons.org/licenses/by/4.0/).

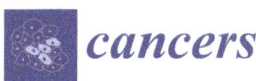

Article

Histopathologic Response Is a Positive Predictor of Overall Survival in Patients Undergoing Neoadjuvant/Perioperative Chemotherapy for Locally Advanced Gastric or Gastroesophageal Junction Cancers—Analysis from a Large Single Center Cohort in Germany

Rebekka Schirren, Alexander Novotny, Helmut Friess and Daniel Reim *

TUM School of Medicine, Department of Surgery, Ismaninger Strasse 22, 81675 Munich, Germany; rebekka.schirren@tum.de (R.S.); alexander.novotny@tum.de (A.N.); helmut.friess@tum.de (H.F.)
* Correspondence: daniel.reim@tum.de; Tel.: +49-89-4140-5019

Received: 1 July 2020; Accepted: 7 August 2020; Published: 11 August 2020

Abstract: There is conflicting evidence regarding the efficacy of neoadjuvant/perioperative chemotherapy (NCT) for gastro-esophageal cancer (GEC) on overall survival. This study aimed to analyze the outcomes of multimodal treatments in a large single center cohort. We performed a retrospective analysis of patients treated with NCT, followed by intended curative oncological surgery for locally advanced gastric cancer. Uni- and multivariate regression analysis were performed to identify the predictors of overall survival. From over 3000 patients, 702 eligible patients were analyzed. In the univariate analysis clinical stage, application of preoperative PLF, requirement of surgical extension, UICC-stage, grading, R-status, Lauren histotype, and HPR were the prognostic survival factors. In multivariate analysis PLF regimen, UICC-stages, R-status, Lauren histotype, and histopathologic regression (HPR) were significant predictors of overall survival. Overall HPR-rate was 26.9%. HPR was highest in the cT2cN0 stage (55.9%), and lowest in the cT3/4 cN+ stage (21.6%). FLOT demonstrated the highest HPR (37.5%). Independent predictors for HPR were the clinical stage and grading. Kaplan Meier analyses demonstrated significant survival benefits for the responding patients ($p < 0.0001$). HPR after NCT was an important prognostic factor to predict overall survival for locally advanced GEC. FLOT should be the preferred regimen in patients undergoing NCT ahead of surgery.

Keywords: gastric/gastroesophageal cancer; perioperative chemotherapy; overall survival; relapse-free survival

1. Introduction

Gastric cancer belongs to the most common malignant diseases worldwide, with the highest incidence in Eastern Asia [1]. Despite decreasing incidence in the West, it remains a therapeutic challenge. In the Western hemisphere, gastric malignancy is often diagnosed at an advanced stage and in contrast to Eastern Asia, it is preferably located in the proximal third of the stomach or the gastro-esophageal junction (GEJ) [2]. Hence, multimodal treatment concepts were introduced, after demonstrating outcome benefits in randomized controlled trials [3–5]. Nevertheless, there is still conflicting evidence, that perioperative chemotherapy might not be effective for all patients, especially those with non-cardia gastric cancer and poorly cohesive type gastro-esophageal cancer [6–8]. New chemotherapeutic regimens were introduced into clinical practice in the last few years, the most promising being the

FLOT regimen (Fluorouracil, Leucovorin, Oxaliplatin, and Docetaxel), which demonstrated higher histopathological regression rates and which was shown to be an independent prognostic factor for overall and disease-free survival [9]. The aim of this analysis was to evaluate oncological outcomes and predictors of perioperative/neoadjuvant chemotherapy in a large German single center cohort.

2. Results

2.1. Patient Data

During the designated period from 1987 to 2014, over 3000 patients were treated for gastric cancer at the Surgical Department of TUM, from which 894 patients underwent intended neoadjuvant/perioperative chemotherapy. Patients undergoing R2 resection ($n = 47$) and the metastatic patients ($n = 145$) were excluded from the analysis. Finally, 702 patients fulfilled the inclusion criteria and were eventually included in this analysis. Most patients were male (75%) and the tumors were predominantly located at the gastro-esophageal junction (68%). The most frequently applied chemotherapeutic regimen was PLF (50%). Two-thirds of the patients required surgical extension for complete tumor removal, mostly extending to the distal esophagus. The overall morbidity rate was 26%. The median number of dissected lymph nodes was 29 [range 5–128]. A total of 72% of all patients demonstrated ypT3/ypT4 tumors and 56% of patients had lymph node metastases. Most patients (73%) had poorly differentiated (G3/G4) histology. Almost half of the cases demonstrated Lauren intestinal-type histology (48%), followed by diffuse-type (25%). R0-resections were achieved in 87%, and almost 27% of patients revealed a histopathological response (Becker 1a/Becker 1b) [10] to preoperative chemotherapy. Moderate response (Becker 2 (10–50% remaining viable tumor cells) was detected in 29% and poor response (Becker 3 (>50% remaining viable tumor cells) was found in 44%. The representative histopathological slides are shown in Figures S1–S3, for each histopathological response grade. The extensive baseline characteristics are depicted in Table 1.

Table 1. Baseline characteristics.

Characteristics	n	%
Gender		
Female	172	24.50
Male	530	75.50
Age (years) *	58.8+/−11.5 (range 3–83 years)	
<70	590	84.05
>70	112	15.95
Localization		
Siewert II/III [#]	477	67.95
Middle	111	15.81
Distal	88	12.54
Total	26	3.70
Clinical Staging [$]		
cT2 cN0	56	7.98
cT1/cT2 cN+	57	8.12
cT3/cT4 cN0	102	14.53
cT3/cT4 cN+	487	69.37
Type of chemotherapy [&]		
PLF	351	50.00
OLF	70	9.97
Taxol+PLF	57	8.12
ECF/ECX	64	9.12
FLOT	56	7.98
Modified platin based CTx	104	14.81

Table 1. Cont.

Characteristics	n	%
Type of Surgery		
Esophagectomy	147	20.94
Transhiatal ext. Gastrectomy	326	46.44
Total gastrectomy	191	27.21
Subtotal gastrectomy	38	5.41
Surgical extension		
None	238	33.90
Luminal/transhiatal	288	41.03
Splenectomy	19	2.71
Colon	5	0.71
Pancreas	18	2.56
Others	134	19.09
Dissected LN [Median]	29 (Range 5–218)	
<=25	232	33.05
>25	470	66.95
Complications ?		
None	515	73.36
CD I/II	84	11.97
CD III-V	103	14.67
pT !		
pT0/is	35	4.99
pT1a	22	3.13
pT1b	50	7.12
pT2	88	12.54
pT3	331	47.15
pT4a	148	21.08
pT4b	28	3.99
pN !		
pN0	306	43.59
pN1	130	18.52
pN2	109	15.53
pN3a	106	15.10
pN3b	51	7.26
UICC !		
UICC 0	32	4.56
UICC IA	58	8.26
UICC IB	69	9.83
UICC IIA	126	17.95
UICC IIB	125	17.81
UICC IIIA	97	13.82
UICC IIIB	134	19.09
UICC IIIC	61	8.69
Grading		
G1/G2	191	27.21
G3/G4	511	72.79
R		
R0	615	87.61
R1	87	12.39
Lauren histotype		
Intestinal	339	48.29
Diffuse	177	25.21
Mixed	92	13.11
Not classified	94	13.39

Table 1. Cont.

Characteristics	n	%
Histopathologic Response		
Becker Ia/Ib	189	26.92
Becker II	202	28.77
Becker III	311	44.30

* Mean ± standard deviation; # GE-Junction cancer according to Siewert classification; $ cT1 = Mucosa/Submucosa; cT2 = Muscularis propria; cT3 = Serosa; cT4 = Adjacent organs; cN0 = no lymph nodemetastasis detected during staging, cN+ = locoregional lymph node metastasis evident during staging; & PLF = 2 cycles preOP; OLF; 2 cycles preOP; Taxol/PLF 2 cycles preOP, ECF/ECX = 3 cycles preOP+3cycles postOP; FLOT = 4 cycles preOP and 4 cycles postOP; ? According to Clavien Dindo classification; ! UICC 8th edition.

Median follow-up was 56 months (range 2–269 months), comprising of 59.5 months [range 12–69 months] for survivors and 18 months (range 1–216) months for deceased patients. During the follow-up period, 346 patients (49.3%) died, the five-year survival rate was 46%, the ten-year survival rate was 32% ($p = 0.003$). Median survival for the histopathologic responders was 216 months and 36 months for non-responders ($p < 0.0001$). The five- and ten-year survival probabilities were 70%/60% for responders and 40%/29% for non-responders, respectively. Kaplan Meier analyses demonstrated a statistically significant survival benefit for responders, compared to non-responders (Figure 1). No survival benefit was detected for the intermediate responders (Becker 2), compared to the non-responding patients ((Becker 3), $p = 0.155$) (Figure 2).

2.2. Predictors of Overall Survival

Univariate regression analysis revealed clinical stage, application of preoperative PLF, requirement of surgical extension, UICC-stage, grading, R-status, Lauren histotype (intestinal and diffuse types), and histopathologic response to be significantly related to postoperative survival (Table 2).

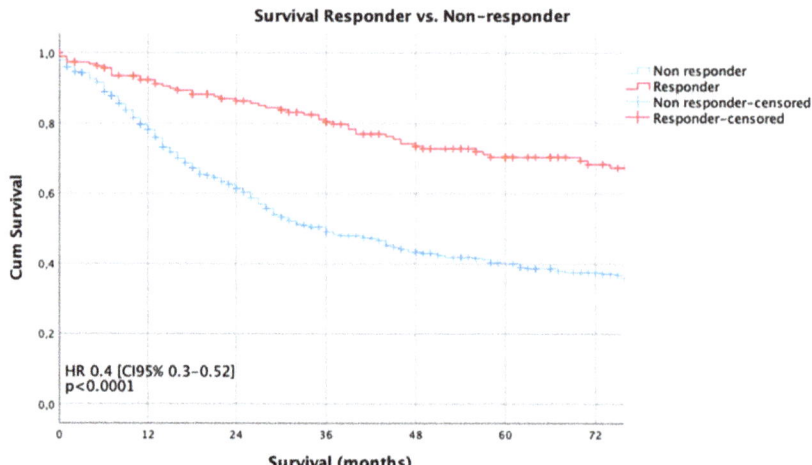

Figure 1. Survival curves according to histopathologic regression (HPR). The Kaplan-Meier method and the log-rank test were used to compare the estimated survival by histopathologic responders and non-responders.

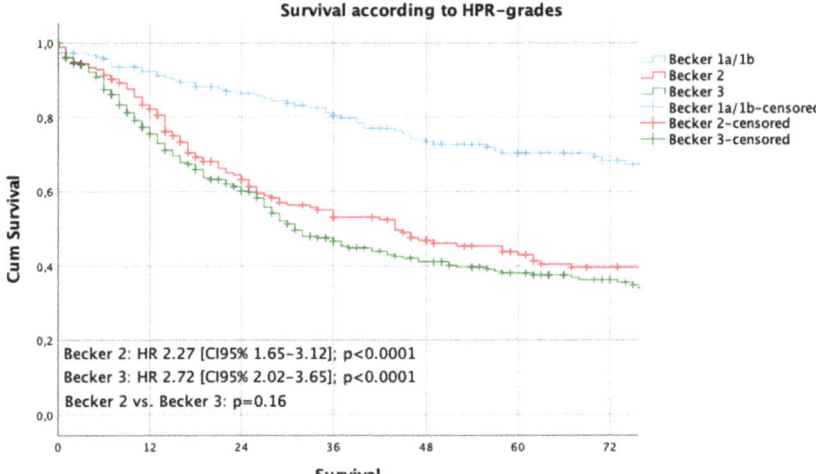

Figure 2. Survival curves according to the Becker grades. The Kaplan-Meier method and the log-rank test were used to compare the estimated survival by each Becker-stage.

Table 2. Univariate analysis of predictors for overall survival.

Univariate	HR	CI95% Lower	CI95% Upper	p
Gender [!]	1.19	0.92	1.53	0.190
Age (>70y)	1.23	0.93	1.64	0.150
Localization [§]	1.26	0.99	1.59	0.060
cT2 cN0 [$]	1.00			0.032
cT3/4 cN0	1.65	0.99	2.74	**0.050**
cT1/2 cN+	1.74	1.00	3.02	**0.050**
cT3/4 cN+	1.90	1.23	2.93	**0.004**
PLF [$]	1.00			**0.007**
OLF	1.20	0.83	1.72	0.335
MAGIC	0.89	0.58	1.37	0.594
FLOT	0.39	0.16	0.96	**0.040**
PLF-Taxol	0.79	0.53	1.17	0.241
Other	1.46	1.10	1.94	**0.008**
Esophagectomy [$]	1.00			0.052
Extended gastrectomy	1.17	0.88	1.56	0.274
Gastrectomy	0.88	0.63	1.22	0.430
Subtotal Gastrectomy	0.67	0.37	1.22	0.192
Surgical Extension	1.37	1.08	1.73	**0.009**
LN dissected (>25/<25)	1.02	0.81	1.28	0.870
Complication (any) [+]	1.21	0.96	1.53	0.110
UICC I [$]	1.00			**0.000**
UICC II	2.74	1.87	4.01	**0.000**
UICC III	5.48	3.80	7.90	**0.000**
G1/2 vs G3/4	1.61	1.24	2.09	**0.000**
R1 vs. R0	2.43	1.84	3.20	**0.000**
Lauren intestinal [$]	1.00			**0.001**

Table 2. Cont.

Univariate	HR	CI95% Lower	CI95% Upper	p
Lauren diffuse	1.51	1.18	1.93	**0.001**
Lauren mixed	0.97	0.68	1.39	0.884
Lauren not classified	0.79	0.56	1.11	0.175
HPR (Y/N)	0.39	0.30	0.52	**0.000**

HR = Hazard Ratio, CI95% lower: 95% Confidence Interval lower boundary, CI95% upper: 95% Confidence Interval upper boundary, p = p-value, HPR=histopathologic response according to Becker; $ cT1 = Mucosa/Submucosa; cT2 = Muscularis propria; cT3 = Serosa; cT4 = Adjacent organs; cN0: no lymph node metastasis detected during staging, cN+: locoregional lymph node metastasis evident during staging; ! male vs. female; § GE-junction vs. distal gastric cancer; $ categorical variable, first value is reference (=1.00); + Any complication vs. no complication. Bold variables are considered statistically significant.

The multivariate analysis demonstrated that PLF regimen, UICC-stages, R-status, Lauren histotype (intestinal and diffuse), and histopathologic response were significantly and independently related to postoperative survival (Table 3).

Table 3. Multivariate analysis of predictors for overall survival.

Multivariate	HR	CI95% Lower	CI95% Upper	p
Gender !	1.22	0.93	1.60	0.154
Age (>70y)	1.08	0.79	1.46	0.635
Localization §	1.20	0.71	2.02	0.492
cT2 cN0 $	1.00			0.550
cT3/4 cN0	1.29	0.76	2.20	0.354
cT1/2 cN+	0.90	0.51	1.61	0.733
cT3/4 cN+	1.05	0.66	1.68	0.830
PLF $				**0.033**
OLF	1.01	0.69	1.47	0.980
MAGIC	0.94	0.61	1.44	0.761
FLOT	0.53	0.21	1.29	0.161
PLF-Taxol	0.74	0.49	1.11	0.140
Other	1.47	1.09	1.99	**0.013**
Esophagectomy $	1.00			0.261
Extended gastrectomy	1.17	0.87	1.57	0.298
Gastrectomy	0.79	0.44	1.43	0.440
Subtotal Gastrectomy	0.61	0.27	1.37	0.228
Surgical Extension	1.00	0.71	1.41	0.992
LN dissected (>25/<25)	0.82	0.64	1.04	0.104
Complication (any) +	1.17	0.91	1.49	0.222
UICC I $	1.00			**0.000**
UICC II	2.07	1.35	3.16	**0.001**
UICC III	3.98	2.58	6.13	**0.000**
G1/2 vs. G3/4	1.21	0.89	1.65	0.234
R1 vs. R0	1.50	1.11	2.02	**0.009**
Lauren intestinal $	1.00			**0.002**
Lauren diffuse	1.40	1.03	1.91	**0.034**
Lauren mixed	0.91	0.62	1.34	0.641
Lauren not classified	0.66	0.45	0.96	**0.031**
HPR (Y/N)	0.71	0.51	0.99	**0.045**

HR = Hazard Ratio, CI95% lower: 95% Confidence Interval lower boundary, CI95% upper: 95% Confidence Interval upper boundary, p = p-value, HPR = histopathologic response according to Becker; $ cT1 = Mucosa/Submucosa; cT2 = Muscularis propria; cT3 = Serosa; cT4 = Adjacent organs; cN0: no lymph node metastasis detected during staging, cN+: locoregional lymph node metastasis evident during staging; ! male vs. female; § GE-junction vs. distal gastric cancer; $ categorical variable, first value is reference (=1.00); + Any complication vs. no complication. Bold variables are considered statistically significant.

2.3. Histopathologic Response

Histopathologic response as defined by grade 1a/1b, according to the Becker classification, was evaluated postoperatively, as described above. The overall histopathologic response rate was 26.9%. Early clinical stages (cT2-4/cN0) revealed higher histopathologic response rates than advanced stages with lymph node involvement (33–55% vs. 21–33%, $p < 0.001$). With regards to the chemotherapeutic regimens, FLOT revealed the highest histopathologic response rate (37.5%), followed by Taxol+PLF (35.1%), PLF (26.1%), ECF (23.4%), and lastly OLF (17.4%). However, this result was not statistically significant ($p = 0.103$). The response rates varied by the UICC stage: In UICC stage I, there were 71.7% responders (114 of 159 patients), in UICC II there were 19.9% (50/251), and in UICC III, there were 8.6% responders (25/265) ($p < 0.0001$). The proportion of histopathologic responders was higher in the AEG-group than in the non-AEG group (29.8% vs. 20.9%, $p < 0.0001$). Results are shown in Table 4.

Table 4. HPR rates according to the clinical factors.

Variable	NR	%	Responder	%	Total	p
cT2 cN– [$]	25	44.6	31	**55.4**	56	**<0.001**
cT3/4 cN–	68	66.7	34	33.3	102	
cT1/2 cN+	38	66.7	19	33.3	57	
cT3/4 cN+	382	78.4	105	21.6	487	
Total	513	73.1	189	26.9	702	
PLF [&]	263	73.9	93	26.1	356	0.103
OLF	58	82.9	12	17.1	70	
MAGIC	49	76.6	15	23.4	64	
FLOT	35	62.5	21	**37.5**	56	
PLF-Taxol	37	64.9	20	35.1	57	
Other	71	71.7	28	28.3	99	
Total	513	73.1	189	26.9	702	
Non-AEG [#]	178	79.11	47	20.89	225	
AEG	335	70.23	142	29.77	477	
Total	513	73.1	189	26.9	702	
UICC I [!]	45	28.30	114	71.70	159	**$p < 0.0001$**
UICC II	201	80.08	50	19.92	251	
UICC III	267	91.44	25	8.56	292	
Total	513	73.1	189	26.9	702	

NR = Non-responder according to Becker classification, Responder = responder according to the Becker classification, p = p-value. [$] cT1 = Mucosa/Submucosa; cT2 = Muscularis propria; cT3 = Serosa; cT4 = Adjacent organs; cN0: no lymph node metastasis detected during staging, cN+: locoregional lymph node metastasis evident during staging; [&] PLF: 2 cycles preOP; OLF; 2 cycles preOP; Taxol/PLF 2 cycles preOP, ECF/ECX: 3 cycles preOP+3cycles postOP; FLOT: 4 cycles preOP and 4 cycles postop; [#] GE-Junction cancer according to Siewert classification; [!] UICC 8th edition. Bold variables are considered statistically significant.

Predictors of HPR

Clinical factors predicting whether patients were more likely to respond to chemotherapy were evaluated by multivariate regression analysis. In the univariate model, tumor location, gender, clinical stage, intestinal Lauren histotype, and grading were the predictors for histopathologic regression. In the multivariate model, only the clinical stage and grading were significantly related to the histopathologic response. The extensive results are shown in Table 5.

Table 5. Uni-/multivariate analysis for the predictors of HPR.

Univariate	OR	CI95% Lower	CI95% Upper	p
Localization §	1.61	1.10	2.34	**0.01**
Gender !	1.53	1.02	2.32	**0.04**
Age (>70y)	0.89	0.56	1.41	0.62
cT2 cN0 $	1.00			**<0.001**
cT3/4 cN0	0.40	0.21	0.79	**0.01**
cT1/2 cN+	0.40	0.19	0.86	**0.02**
cT3/4 cN+	0.22	0.13	0.39	**0.00**
Lauren type (intest. vs. other)	1.77	1.14	2.46	**0.01**
Grading (G1/2 vs. G3/4)	0.34	0.24	0.49	**<0.001**
MULTIVARIATE	OR	CI95% lower	CI95% upper	p
Localization §	1.44	0.83	2.52	0.20
Gender !	1.70	0.92	3.13	0.09
Age (>70y)	0.57	0.29	1.12	0.10
cT2 cN0 $	1.00			**<0.001**
cT3/4 cN0	0.20	0.03	1.18	0.08
cT1/2 cN+	0.58	0.08	4.24	0.59
cT3/4 cN+	0.12	0.02	0.65	**0.01**
Lauren type (intest. vs. other)	1.30	0.75	2.22	0.35
Grading (G1/2 vs. G3/4)	0.47	0.27	0.82	**0.01**

OR = Odds Ratio, CI95% lower: 95% Confidence Interval lower boundary, CI95% upper: 95% Confidence Interval upper boundary, p = p-value, HPR = histopathologic response according to Becker; $ cT1 = Mucosa/Submucosa; cT2=Muscularis propria; cT3 = Serosa; cT4 = Adjacent organs; cN0: no lymph node metastasis detected during staging, cN+: locoregional lymph node metastasis evident during staging; § GE-junction vs. distal gastric cancer; ! male vs. female; $ categorical variable, first value is reference (=1.00). Bold variables are considered statistically significant.

3. Discussion

This analysis of a large single center cohort demonstrated that neoadjuvant/perioperative chemotherapy results in survival benefit only in patients who demonstrate histopathologic response, as demonstrated by Kaplan Meier and multivariate regression analyses. Histopathologic response was defined when there was either no viable or less than 10% viable tumor cells, in relation to the detectable tumor bed. Patients demonstrating intermediate response according to the Becker classification revealed no benefits over those patients not responding to neoadjuvant/perioperative chemotherapy. This analysis found that only a little more than a quarter of patients respond to neoadjuvant/perioperative chemotherapy, which leads to the notion that almost three-quarters of all patients do not benefit from neoadjuvant/perioperative chemotherapy at all. It remains elusive if these patients were not possibly even been harmed by the ineffective treatment ahead of surgery. Interestingly, histopathologic response rates differed, depending on the chemotherapeutic regimen applied. Among these, three substance-based therapies like FLOT and Taxol-PLF were the most effective regarding response rates. However, this effect was not statistically significant, because the case numbers were too small to draw definitive conclusions. The phase III study on FLOT demonstrated promising results, which need to be proven in clinical practice in the near future [9]. Another remarkable result was that the early clinical stages (cT1/cT2) and patients without clinical detection of lymph node involvement (cN0) revealed high HPR rates. The reasons for this fact are difficult to determine. The elusive reasons might be simple understaging of the real situation or favorable tumor biology in earlier stages, when the cancer does not reach its metastatic potential and responsiveness to chemotherapy is higher than that in later stages. Further reasons for reduced histopathologic responsiveness might also be poor or undifferentiated tumor grading, which is a statistically significant predictor for worse response to neoadjuvant chemotherapy [6,11]. Another factor might be Lauren differentiation. In this analysis, almost half of the patients demonstrated intestinal types, which are considered to be more responsive to chemotherapy than Lauren diffuse types. There is an ongoing discussion about chemotherapy responsiveness related to the histopathologic subtype [11,12]. Lauren diffuse types also incorporate signet ring cell cancers, poorly cohesive cancers with signet ring cells, and poorly cohesive cancer without signet ring cell differentiation. Previously, it was found that signet ring cell differentiation might be related to poor responsiveness [8,12]. However, these analyses are difficult to compare because of different "signet ring cell" classifications. A standardized approach was taken by an expert group, however, this was not yet evaluated for patients undergoing neoadjuvant chemotherapy and was not yet validated in an international setting [13]. Nonetheless, in this analysis, the Lauren diffuse type differentiation resulted in a 40% higher risk of death compared to the intestinal type, but the intestinal type was no independent predictor of HPR. Further study on this fact is required to elucidate the influence of Lauren histotype on histopathologic response to neoadjuvant chemotherapy, especially in a standardized and comparable way. In contrast to previously published reports, this analysis could not confirm the influence of tumor localization on histopathologic response [6,14]. Multivariate analyses on both the overall survival and the histopathologic response prediction were not able to demonstrate an effect related to the tumor site (cardia vs. non-cardia).

Several limitations of this analysis were evident, besides its single-center character and retrospective design. The inclusion period covers a long period of time of thirty years. During this period, surgical techniques might not have changed too much (except minimal invasive technologies) but peri-operative care and management of postoperative complications certainly has, which might have influenced oncological outcomes over time. These innovations were not included in this analysis, because the data were not available. Besides this, chemotherapeutic regimens changed over time, influenced by published results from randomized controlled trial [3,5,9,15]. Further, no toxicity data of the chemotherapeutic treatments were available in the database to analyze if dose or cycle reductions were necessary and might have influenced histopathologic response rates. Further, the newest innovation was the introduction of FLOT as a new standard of perioperative chemotherapy, which was underrepresented in this analysis, due to a small number of patients being eligible for analysis [9]. Besides this, comparisons of the regimens might be erroneous as the MAGIC and FLOT protocols consist of additional postoperative (adjuvant) chemotherapy, whereas the other protocols only consist of preoperative (neoadjuvant) treatment [3,9]. Therefore survival outcome comparisons might be biased because the effect of the adjuvant part could not be properly evaluated. Further, recurrence rates and recurrence-free survival data were not analyzed because they were not available from the present database. Lastly, the frequency and quality of comorbidities was not analyzed, because the data were not available in the database. Certainly these comorbidities might have influenced dose adaptions during neoadjuvant chemotherapy and might have influenced not only the oncologic but also surgical outcomes, which represents a substantial limitation of this retrospective analysis.

Certainly, generalizability of the results presented here is limited, due to the fact that neoadjuvant/perioperative chemotherapy is part of clinical practice only in Europe, whereas the concept of primary resection, followed by adjuvant chemotherapy is practiced predominantly in Eastern Asia, and the concept of (neo-)adjuvant chemo-radiation is commonly accepted in the US [3,5,15–17]. Besides this, cardia cancers are often treated by neoadjuvant chemo-radiation, since publication of the CROSS study [4,16]. These practices were not represented in this analysis, which limits the general applicability of the present results.

4. Materials and Methods

4.1. Patients

Data from patients who underwent curative surgery for gastroesophageal cancer at the Surgical Department of TUM School of Medicine from 1987 to 2017 were extracted from a prospectively documented database. Data were obtained from the medical records and transferred to the institutional databases, as soon as the patients were discharged from inpatient hospital care. The inclusion criteria for this analysis were—histologically proven gastroesophageal cancer (Siewert type II/III, all non-cardia cancers) staged cT2-cT4cN$_{any}$ undergoing neoadjuvant/perioperative chemotherapy, after a multidisciplinary team review. Exclusion criteria were—Siewert type I, metastatic disease, hospital mortality within 30 days, loss of follow-up within a 60 months period and macroscopic residual cancer after surgery (R2). Neoadjuvant/perioperative treatment consisted of either preoperative two cycle—cisplatin or oxaliplatin/leucovorin/5-FU (PLF/OLF), only or perioperative three cycles of ECX/ECF (MAGIC) or perioperative four cycles FLOT [3,9]. All surgical procedures were performed according to the Japanese guidelines for GC treatment, including standardized D2-lymphnode dissection [18]. In case of GE junction cancer (Siewert type II and III), the surgical procedure was extended to the distal esophagus. All patients received intraoperative frozen sections for the oral resection margin to confirm R0 resection. Circumferential and aboral resection margins were not determined intraoperatively on a routine basis. All resected specimens were examined by one or two specialized pathologists, classified according to the TNM-classification, and staged according to the UICC-recommendations (8th edition) [19]. Histopathologic response was graded according to the Becker classification. Patients 0–10% remnant viable tumor cells within the tumor area were graded as histopathologic responders (Becker 1a/1b), whereas all other patients (Becker 2 (10–50% remnant viable tumor cells) and Becker 3 (>50% remnant viable tumor cells)) were graded as histopathologic non-responders [10]. Following oncologic surgery, all patients were followed up every six to twelve months, in an outpatient department (Roman Herzog Comprehensive Cancer Center), over the next five years, using EGD and CT scans, according to the institutional protocol.

Only deceased or surviving patients with complete follow-up of at least 60 months were included in this analysis. Survival was computed from the day of surgery. The dataset consisted of patients' gender, age, location (upper, middle, lower third), clinical stages (cT2N0, cT1/cT2cN+, cT3/cT4cN0, cT3/cT4N+), type of chemotherapeutic regimen applied (PLF, OLF, Taxol+PLF, ECF/ECX, FLOT, modified platin-based CTx), type of surgery (esophagectomy, transhiatal gastrectomy, gastrectomy, subtotal gastrectomy), type of required extension (none, luminal/transhiatal, splenectomy, colon, pancreas, others), number of dissected lymph nodes, postoperative complications (none, Clavien–Dindo Grade I/II, and III/IV), pT- (pT0/pT1a/pT1b/pT2/pT3/pT4a/pT4b), pN-(pN0/pN1/pN2/pN3a/pN3b), and UICC-stages (UICC-0/-IA/-IB/-IIA/-IIB/-IIIA/-IIIB/-IIIC), grading (G1/2, G3/4), R-status (R0/R1), Lauren histotype (intestinal, diffuse, mixed, non-classified), and follow-up period with survival status. Institutional Review Board (IRB)-approval for this study was obtained according to the local guidelines (IRB Registration: 364/20 S).

4.2. Statistical Analysis

Wilcoxon and chi-square tests were used to compare the continuous and categorical clinical characteristics. Overall survival (OS) was graphed using empirical Kaplan-Meier curves with differences in 5-year survival rates among the patient groups evaluated using the log-rank test. Associations between prognostic factors, and survival were estimated by uni- and multivariate Cox proportional-hazards regression analysis. Histopathologic response predictors were evaluated by multivariate regression analysis. All variables were included in the multivariate model to rule out possible confounding for both outcomes. All statistical tests were performed at the two-sided 0.05 level of significance. Statistical analyses were performed using SPSS-software (Version 24, IBM Inc., Armonk, NY, USA).

5. Conclusions

In conclusion, histopathologic response after neoadjuvant chemotherapy is an important prognostic factor to predict overall survival for locally advanced gastro-esophageal cancer. FLOT should be the preferred therapeutic regimen in patients undergoing neoadjuvant/perioperative chemotherapy ahead of surgery. Further research should focus on the early detection of patients not responding well to multimodal treatment.

Supplementary Materials: The following are available online at http://www.mdpi.com/2072-6694/12/8/2244/s1, Figure S1a/b: Histopathologic response grade Becker 1a and Becker 1b ((Sub-)total response (0–10% residual tumor cells in relation to tumor bed)); Figure S2: Histopathologic response grade Becker 2 (Partial response (10–50% residual tumor cells in relation to tumor bed)); Figure S3: Histopathologic response grade Becker 3 (Non-response (>50% residual tumor cells in relation to tumor bed)).

Author Contributions: Conceptualization: A.N. and D.R.; methodology D.R.; software, D.R.; validation, R.S., D.R. and A.N.; formal analysis, D.R. and R.S.; investigation; resources; data curation, R.S. and D.R., writing—original draft preparation, R.S. and D.R.; writing—review and editing, D.R. and H.F.; visualization, R.S.; supervision, H.F.; project administration D.R. All authors have read and agreed to the published version of the manuscript.

Funding: This research received no external funding.

Acknowledgments: Slides for demonstrating the histopathologic response grades according to the Becker classification system were provided with kind approval and courtesy of Rupert Langer, Director of the Institute of Pathology, Kepler Universitätsklinikum, Linz, Austria.

Conflicts of Interest: The authors declare no conflict of interest.

References

1. Bray, F.; Ferlay, J.; Soerjomataram, I.; Siegel, R.L.; Torre, L.A.; Jemal, A. Global cancer statistics 2018: GLOBOCAN estimates of incidence and mortality worldwide for 36 cancers in 185 countries. *CA Cancer J. Clin.* **2018**, *68*, 394–424. [CrossRef] [PubMed]
2. Lagarde, S.M.; ten Kate, F.J.; Reitsma, J.B.; Busch, O.R.; van Lanschot, J.J. Prognostic factors in adenocarcinoma of the esophagus or gastroesophageal junction. *J. Clin. Oncol.* **2006**, *24*, 4347–4355. [CrossRef] [PubMed]
3. Cunningham, D.; Allum, W.H.; Stenning, S.P.; Thompson, J.N.; Van de Velde, C.J.; Nicolson, M.; Scarffe, J.H.; Lofts, F.J.; Falk, S.J.; Iveson, T.J.; et al. Perioperative chemotherapy versus surgery alone for resectable gastroesophageal cancer. *N. Engl. J. Med.* **2006**, *355*, 11–20. [CrossRef] [PubMed]
4. Van Hagen, P.; Hulshof, M.C.; van Lanschot, J.J.; Steyerberg, E.W.; van Berge Henegouwen, M.I.; Wijnhoven, B.P.; Richel, D.J.; Nieuwenhuijzen, G.A.; Hospers, G.A.; Bonenkamp, J.J.; et al. Preoperative chemoradiotherapy for esophageal or junctional cancer. *N. Engl. J. Med.* **2012**, *366*, 2074–2084. [CrossRef] [PubMed]
5. Ychou, M.; Boige, V.; Pignon, J.P.; Conroy, T.; Bouche, O.; Lebreton, G.; Ducourtieux, M.; Bedenne, L.; Fabre, J.M.; Saint-Aubert, B.; et al. Perioperative chemotherapy compared with surgery alone for resectable gastroesophageal adenocarcinoma: An FNCLCC and FFCD multicenter phase III trial. *J. Clin. Oncol.* **2011**, *29*, 1715–1721. [CrossRef] [PubMed]
6. Reim, D.; Gertler, R.; Novotny, A.; Becker, K.; zum Büschenfelde, C.M.; Ebert, M.; Dobritz, M.; Langer, R.; Hoefler, H.; Friess, H.; et al. Adenocarcinomas of the esophagogastric junction are more likely to respond to preoperative chemotherapy than distal gastric cancer. *Ann. Surg. Oncol.* **2012**, *19*, 2108–2118. [CrossRef] [PubMed]
7. Ronellenfitsch, U.; Schwarzbach, M.; Hofheinz, R.; Kienle, P.; Kieser, M.; Slanger, T.E.; Burmeister, B.; Kelsen, D.; Niedzwiecki, D.; Schuhmacher, C.; et al. Preoperative chemo(radio)therapy versus primary surgery for gastroesophageal adenocarcinoma: Systematic review with meta-analysis combining individual patient and aggregate data. *Eur. J. Cancer* **2013**, *49*, 3149–3158. [CrossRef]
8. Piessen, G.; Messager, M.; Leteurtre, E.; Jean-Pierre, T.; Mariette, C. Signet ring cell histology is an independent predictor of poor prognosis in gastric adenocarcinoma regardless of tumoral clinical presentation. *Ann. Surg.* **2009**, *250*, 878–887. [CrossRef]
9. Al-Batran, S.E.; Homann, N.; Pauligk, C.; Goetze, T.O.; Meiler, J.; Kasper, S.; Kopp, H.G.; Mayer, F.; Haag, G.M.; Luley, K.; et al. Perioperative chemotherapy with fluorouracil plus leucovorin, oxaliplatin, and docetaxel versus fluorouracil or capecitabine plus cisplatin and epirubicin for locally advanced, resectable gastric or gastro-oesophageal junction adenocarcinoma (FLOT4): A randomised, phase 2/3 trial. *Lancet* **2019**, *393*, 1948–1957. [CrossRef]
10. Becker, K.; Mueller, J.D.; Schulmacher, C.; Ott, K.; Fink, U.; Busch, R.; Böttcher, K.; Siewert, J.R.; Höfler, H. Histomorphology and grading of regression in gastric carcinoma treated with neoadjuvant chemotherapy. *Cancer* **2003**, *98*, 1521–1530. [CrossRef] [PubMed]

11. Xu, X.; Zheng, G.; Zhang, T.; Zhao, Y.; Zheng, Z. Is pathologic tumor regression grade after neo-adjuvant chemotherapy a promising prognostic indicator for patients with locally advanced gastric cancer? A cohort study evaluating tumor regression response. *Cancer Chemother. Pharmacol.* **2019**, *84*, 635–646. [CrossRef] [PubMed]
12. Hass, H.G.; Smith, U.; Jäger, C.; Schäffer, M.; Wellhäuber, U.; Hehr, T.; Markmann, H.U.; Nehls, O.; Denzlinger, C. Signet ring cell carcinoma of the stomach is significantly associated with poor prognosis and diffuse gastric cancer (Lauren's): Single-center experience of 160 cases. *Onkologie* **2011**, *34*, 682–686. [CrossRef] [PubMed]
13. Mariette, C.; Carneiro, F.; Grabsch, H.I.; van der Post, R.S.; Allum, W.; de Manzoni, G. Correction to: Consensus on the pathological definition and classification of poorly cohesive gastric carcinoma. *Gastric Cancer* **2019**, *22*, 421. [CrossRef] [PubMed]
14. Becker, K.; Langer, R.; Reim, D.; Novotny, A.; Meyer zum Buschenfelde, C.; Engel, J.; Friess, H.; Hofler, H. Significance of histopathological tumor regression after neoadjuvant chemotherapy in gastric adenocarcinomas: A summary of 480 cases. *Ann. Surg.* **2011**, *253*, 934–939. [CrossRef] [PubMed]
15. Schuhmacher, C.; Gretschel, S.; Lordick, F.; Reichardt, P.; Hohenberger, W.; Eisenberger, C.F.; Haag, C.; Mauer, M.E.; Hasan, B.; Welch, J.; et al. Neoadjuvant chemotherapy compared with surgery alone for locally advanced cancer of the stomach and cardia: European Organisation for Research and Treatment of Cancer randomized trial 40954. *J. Clin. Oncol.* **2010**, *28*, 5210–5218. [CrossRef] [PubMed]
16. Shapiro, J.; van Lanschot, J.J.B.; Hulshof, M.; van Hagen, P.; van Berge Henegouwen, M.I.; Wijnhoven, B.P.L.; van Laarhoven, H.W.M.; Nieuwenhuijzen, G.A.P.; Hospers, G.A.P.; Bonenkamp, J.J.; et al. Neoadjuvant chemoradiotherapy plus surgery versus surgery alone for oesophageal or junctional cancer (CROSS): Long-term results of a randomised controlled trial. *Lancet Oncol.* **2015**, *16*, 1090–1098. [CrossRef]
17. Bang, Y.J.; Kim, Y.W.; Yang, H.K.; Chung, H.C.; Park, Y.K.; Lee, K.H.; Lee, K.W.; Kim, Y.H.; Noh, S.I.; Cho, J.Y.; et al. Adjuvant capecitabine and oxaliplatin for gastric cancer after D2 gastrectomy (CLASSIC): A phase 3 open-label, randomised controlled trial. *Lancet* **2012**, *379*, 315–321. [CrossRef]
18. Japanese gastric cancer treatment guidelines 2014 (ver. 4). *Gastric Cancer* **2017**, *20*, 1–19. [CrossRef] [PubMed]
19. Sano, T.; Coit, D.G.; Kim, H.H.; Roviello, F.; Kassab, P.; Wittekind, C.; Yamamoto, Y.; Ohashi, Y. Proposal of a new stage grouping of gastric cancer for TNM classification: International Gastric Cancer Association staging project. *Gastric Cancer* **2017**, *20*, 217–225. [CrossRef] [PubMed]

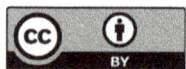

© 2020 by the authors. Licensee MDPI, Basel, Switzerland. This article is an open access article distributed under the terms and conditions of the Creative Commons Attribution (CC BY) license (http://creativecommons.org/licenses/by/4.0/).

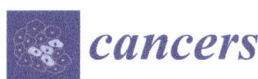

Article

Long-Term Outcomes of Induction Chemotherapy Followed by Chemo-Radiotherapy as Intensive Neoadjuvant Protocol in Patients with Esophageal Cancer

Nicola Simoni [1,*,†], Michele Pavarana [2,†], Renato Micera [1], Jacopo Weindelmayer [3], Valentina Mengardo [3], Gabriella Rossi [1], Daniela Cenzi [4], Anna Tomezzoli [5], Paola Del Bianco [6], Simone Giacopuzzi [3], Giovanni De Manzoni [3,‡] and Renzo Mazzarotto [1,‡]

1. Department of Radiotherapy, Ospedale Civile Maggiore, Azienda Ospedaliera Universitaria Integrata Verona, 37126 Verona, Italy; renato.micera@aovr.veneto.it (R.M.); gabriella.rossi@aovr.veneto.it (G.R.); renzo.mazzarotto@aovr.veneto.it (R.M.)
2. Department of Oncology, Ospedale G.B. Rossi, Azienda Ospedaliera Universitaria Integrata Verona, 37126 Verona, Italy; michele.pavarana@aovr.veneto.it
3. Department of General and Upper G.I. Surgery, Ospedale Civile Maggiore, Azienda Ospedaliera Universitaria Integrata Verona, 37126 Verona, Italy; jacopo.weindelmayer@aovr.veneto.it (J.W.); valentina.mengardo@gmail.com (V.M.); simone.giacopuzzi@univr.it (S.G.); giovanni.demanzoni@univr.it (G.D.M.)
4. Department of Radiology, Ospedale Civile Maggiore, Azienda Ospedaliera Universitaria Integrata Verona, 37126 Verona, Italy; daniela.cenzi@aovr.veneto.it
5. Department of Pathology, Ospedale G.B. Rossi, Azienda Ospedaliera Universitaria Integrata Verona, 37126 Verona, Italy; anna.tomezzoli@aovr.veneto.it
6. Clinical Research Unit, Istituto Oncologico Veneto IOV-IRCCS, 35100 Padova, Italy; paola.delbianco@iov.veneto.it
* Correspondence: nicola.simoni@aovr.veneto.it or nicolasimoni81@gmail.com; Tel.: +39-0-458-122-478
† Nicola Simoni and Michele Pavarana contributed equally to this work.
‡ Giovanni De Manzoni and Renzo Mazzarotto contributed equally to this work as senior authors.

Received: 20 October 2020; Accepted: 30 November 2020; Published: 3 December 2020

Simple Summary: Neoadjuvant chemo-radiotherapy (nCRT) represents a standard approach for both Squamous Cell Carcinoma (SCC) and Adenocarcinoma (ADC) of the esophagus, leading to a 10–15% improvement in survival rate as compared with surgery alone in clinical trials. In this observational study, we report the efficacy and safety of an intensive nCRT protocol in the daily clinical practice, including 122 patients treated with induction chemotherapy, followed by concomitant chemo-radiotherapy, and surgery. Our findings showed good long-term survival and high pathological complete response (pCR) rates, with acceptable side-effects. Notably, the oncological outcome was the same in ADC and SCC responder patients. Although the nCRT protocol here reported represents a distinctive single-center experience, our results contribute to better define the role of an intensive neoadjuvant approach as a reliable therapy for the treatment of locally advanced esophageal cancer, and enrich the current literature on this challenging context.

Abstract: Background: A phase II intensive neoadjuvant chemo-radiotherapy (nCRT) protocol for esophageal cancer (EC) was previously tested at our Center with promising results. We here present an observational study to evaluate the efficacy of the protocol also in "real life" patients. Methods: We retrospectively reviewed 122 ECs (45.1% squamous cell (SCC) and 54.9% adenocarcinoma (ADC)) treated with induction docetaxel, cisplatin, and 5-fluorouracil (TCF), followed by concomitant TCF and radiotherapy (50–50.4 Gy/25–28 fractions), between 2008 and 2017. Primary endpoints were overall survival (OS), event-free survival (EFS) and pathological complete response (pCR). Results: With a median follow-up of 62.1 months (95% CI 50–67.6 months), 5-year OS and EFS rates were

54.8% (95% CI 44.7–63.9) and 42.7% (95% CI 33.1–51.9), respectively. A pCR was observed in 71.1% of SCC and 37.1% of ADC patients ($p = 0.001$). At multivariate analysis, ypN+ was a significant prognostic factor for OS (Hazard Ratios (HR) 4.39 [95% CI 2.36–8.18]; $p < 0.0001$), while pCR was a strong predictor of EFS (HR 0.38 [95% CI 0.22–0.67]; $p < 0.0001$). Conclusions: The nCRT protocol achieved considerable long-term survival and pCR rates also in "real life" patients. Further research is necessary to evaluate this protocol in a watch-and-wait approach.

Keywords: induction chemotherapy; chemo-radiotherapy; neoadjuvant treatment; esophageal cancer

1. Introduction

Esophageal Cancer (EC) represents a major health problem worldwide, ranking seventh among leading causes of cancer-related death [1]. Multimodal treatment, including chemotherapy, radiotherapy, and surgery, is currently accepted as standard of care for locally advanced stage disease [2,3]. Several randomized trials demonstrated a survival benefit with neoadjuvant chemo-radiotherapy (nCRT) followed by surgery, compared to surgery alone, both in patients with Squamous Cell Carcinoma (SCC) and Adenocarcinoma (ADC) of the esophagus and gastroesophageal junction (EGJ) [4–9]. Notably, responders to nCRT have a better prognosis than non-responders [10], and an intensification of the preoperative approach is often advocated to improve oncological outcomes [11].

In our previous experience, an intensive nCRT protocol was tested in a phase II trial, with encouraging results [12]. The nCRT protocol schedule consisted of an induction phase of weekly administered docetaxel, cisplatin, and 5-fluorouracil (TCF) for 3 weeks, followed by concomitant TCF administered weekly for 5 weeks along with radiotherapy (50–50.4 Gy in 25–28 fractions). Remarkably, a pathological complete response (pCR) was obtained in 47% of patients with a 5-year overall survival (OS) rate of 43% (77% for pCR group). These results could be explained by the use of a more intensive chemotherapy schedule and an increased radiotherapy dose compared to other preoperative approaches reported in the literature [6]. Based on these results, this protocol was considered the standard nCRT for both advanced esophageal SCCs and ADCs treated in our center.

However, since trial participants do not represent the population as a whole, applying this protocol in the daily practice could have led to poorer results. [13]. Based on this consideration, we performed a novel analysis of the efficacy and safety of this nCRT protocol in the daily clinical practice.

2. Results

2.1. Baseline Characteristics

A total of 122 consecutive patients were included in the analysis: 55 (45.1%) with SCC and 67 (54.9%) with ADC. Baseline characteristics are outlined in Table 1.

Table 1. Clinical and tumor characteristics of 122 patients.

		N	%
Age, years	Median (IQR)	63 (57–79)	
	<60	42	34.4
	60–69	51	41.8
	≥70	29	23.8
Gender	Female	46	37.7
	Male	76	62.3
Histology	SCC	55	45.1
	ADC	67	54.9

Table 1. Cont.

		N	%
BMI	Median (IQR)	22.9 (19.6–27.5)	
ASA score °	I	5	4.7
	II	75	70
	III	27	25.3
Tumor location	Upper third	18	14.8
	Middle third	28	22.9
	Distal third	36	29.5
	EGJ	40	32.8
Tumor length, cm	Median (IQR)	5.5 (4.1–7.0)	
Clinical T stage	1	2	1.6
	2	12	9.8
	3	98	80.3
	4	9	7.4
	X *	1	0.8
Clinical N stage	N0	19	15.6
	N+	103	84.4
Clinical stage group	IIA	17	13.9
	IIB	12	9.8
	III	92	75.5
	X §	1	0.8

IQR: interquartile range; SCC: squamous cell carcinoma; ADC: adenocarcinoma; BMI: body mass index; EGJ: gastroesophageal junction; * clinical T stage not evaluable because of incomplete endoscopic ultrasound (EUS); § clinical stage TxN1; ° only patients who underwent surgery.

2.2. Treatment Completion

One hundred and nineteen (97.5%) patients underwent concurrent chemo-radiotherapy after the first induction phase, while three (2.5%) were excluded: two due to disease progression during induction chemotherapy, and one due to acute intestinal occlusion requiring surgery. One hundred and sixteen (97.5%) patients received the full prescribed radiation dose, while 3 (2.5%) did not complete the treatment schedule due to toxicity. In five (4.2%) patients the prescription dose was reduced to 45 Gy due to patient's frailty or to large field nodal volume. The median relative dose intensity (RDI) for the chemotherapy schedule was 0.86 (0.74–0.95). During the induction phase, no reduction in the administered chemotherapy doses was needed, and the average relative dose intensity (RDI) was 0.96 (0.88–1). Instead, during the concomitant phase, the average RDI was reduced to 0.77 (0.61–0.90), with a similar reduction for all drugs (average RDI 0.75 [0.57–0.88], 0.79 [0.60–0.91] and 0.75 [0.65–0.98] for docetaxel, cisplatin, and 5-fluorouracil, respectively). Table S1 (Supplementary Material) describes relative dose intensity (RDI), dose density, as well as nCRT protocol treatment details.

One hundred and seven (87.7%) patients underwent surgery. Radical resection (R0) was achieved in 105 patients (98.1% of resected patients). Table 2 reports details on surgery and pathological assessment.

Table 2. Details on surgery and pathological assessment.

		N	%
Total		119 §	
Surgery	No	12	10.1
	W&W *	5	41.7
	Death before surgery °	5	41.7
	PD during nCRT	1	8.3
	Patient unfit for surgery	1	8.3

Table 2. *Cont.*

		N	%
	Yes	107	89.9
	McKeown [+]	36	33.7
	Ivor-Lewis [#]	65	60.7
	Total Gastrectomy ^	6	5.6
Months between nCRT and surgery	Median (IQR)	1.97 (1.63–2.30)	
pT	0	63	58.9
	1	14	13.1
	2	14	13.1
	3	13	12.1
	4	3	2.8
pN	N0	79	73.8
	N1	19	17.8
	N2	5	4.7
	N3	4	3.7
pM	M0	105	98.1
	M1	2	1.9
Pathological complete response	T0N0M0	55	51.4
Radicality	R0	105	98.1
	R1	2	1.9
Positive Nodes	Median (IQR)	0 (0–1)	
Retrieved Nodes	Median (IQR)	26.5 (19–35)	
LN ratio	Median (IQR)	0 (0–0.03)	
TRG [§]	1	58	54.2
	2	17	15.9
	3	6	5.6
	4	8	7.5

PD: progression disease; nCRT: neoadjuvant chemoradiotherapy; IQR: interquartile range; LN: lymph node; TRG: tumor regression grade. [§] Patients evaluated for surgery after chemo-radiotherapy; * watch-and-wait strategy following evidence of a complete response to nCRT protocol (bite-on-bite biopsies proven); ° 4 (4.1%) patients due to presumable nCRT toxicity and 1 (0.8%) patient for causes not tumor related; [§] information on TRG was missing in 19 patients (the sum of patients for this column does not match the total due to missing data); [+] McKeown procedure: Tri-incisional subtotal esophagectomy with cervical esophago-gastric anastomosis; [#] Ivor-Lewis procedure: partial esophagectomy with right intrathoracic esophago-gastrostomy; ^ total gastrectomy and distal esophagectomy with intramediastinal anastomosis.

2.3. Treatment Outcomes

The estimated median follow-up time was 62.1 months (95% CI 49.0–67.6 months). Median OS and EFS of the entire cohort were 78.5 months (95% CI 42.3-NE [not estimable]) and 39.5 months (95% CI 27.3–82.6), respectively (Figure 1A,B), and increased in resected patients to 97.4 months (Hazard Ratios (HR) 0.24 95% CI 0.12–0.47, $p < 0.0001$) and 46.2 months (HR 0.28 95% CI 0.15–0.52, $p < 0.0001$), respectively. The OS rates at 1, 2, 3, and 5 years were 89.3% (95% CI 82.4–93.7), 77.8% (95% CI 69.4–84.2), 64.2% (95% CI 54.7–72.2), and 54.8% (95% CI 44.7–63.9), and the comparable EFS rates were 77.0% (95% CI 68.5–83.5), 60.7% (95% CI 51.4–68.7), 51.1% (95% CI 41.8–59.6), and 42.7% (95% CI 33.1–51.9), respectively. Median OS and EFS did not significantly differ between SCC versus ADC patients (Figure 1C,D).

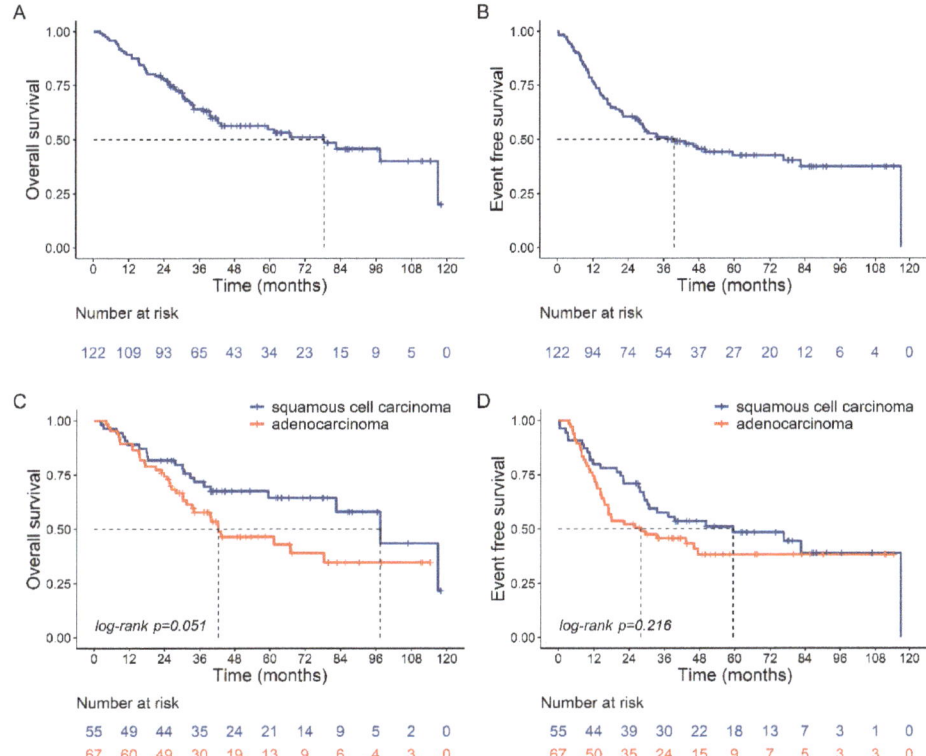

Figure 1. Overall Survival (OS) and Event-Free Survival (EFS) estimated by Kaplan–Meier method. (**A**) OS and (**B**) EFS of the entire cohort; (**C**) OS and (**D**) EFS as a function of histotype (squamous cell carcinoma vs. adenocarcinoma).

2.4. Pathological Complete Response

Among resected patients, pCR was achieved in 51.4% (55/107) of patients, including 71.1% (32/45) of SCC and 37.1% (23/62) of ADC patients ($p < 0.001$). Median OS and EFS were particularly high in pCR cases, being 117 months (HR 0.30 95% CI 0.16–0.56, $p < 0.0001$) and 117 months (HR 0.35 95% CI 0.20–0.61, $p < 0.0001$), respectively (Figure 2A,B), with a similar trend for SCC and ADC patients (Figure 2C,D). The 3- and 5-year OS rates were 82.8% (95% CI 69.5–90.7) and 70.5% (95% CI 56.4–80.8), and the comparable EFS rates were 78.2% (95% CI 63.9–87.4) and 63.5% (95% CI 48.6–75.1), respectively, in pCR patients, as compared with 53.8% (95% CI 38.9–66.6) and 37.6% (95% CI 24.5–50.7), and 40.4% (95% CI 25.9–54.6) and 29.1% (95% CI 16.6–42.8) in non-pCR patients, respectively ($p < 0.001$). Tumor relapse occurred in 48 resected patients (44.9%), with a loco-regional pattern in 7 (6.5%) (Table S2, Supplementary Material).

In the univariate analysis, gender, pCR, pTstage, pNstage and Tumor Regression Grade (TRG) were significantly associated with OS and EFS (Table 3). In the multivariate analysis, pNstage remained a significant predictor for OS (the HR of pN1 cases with respect to pN0 cases was 4.39 (95% CI 2.36–8.18; $p < 0.0001$)), while pCR remained significant for EFS (the HR of pCR cases with respect to non-pCR cases was 0.38 (95% CI 0.22–0.67; $p < 0.0001$) (Table 3)).

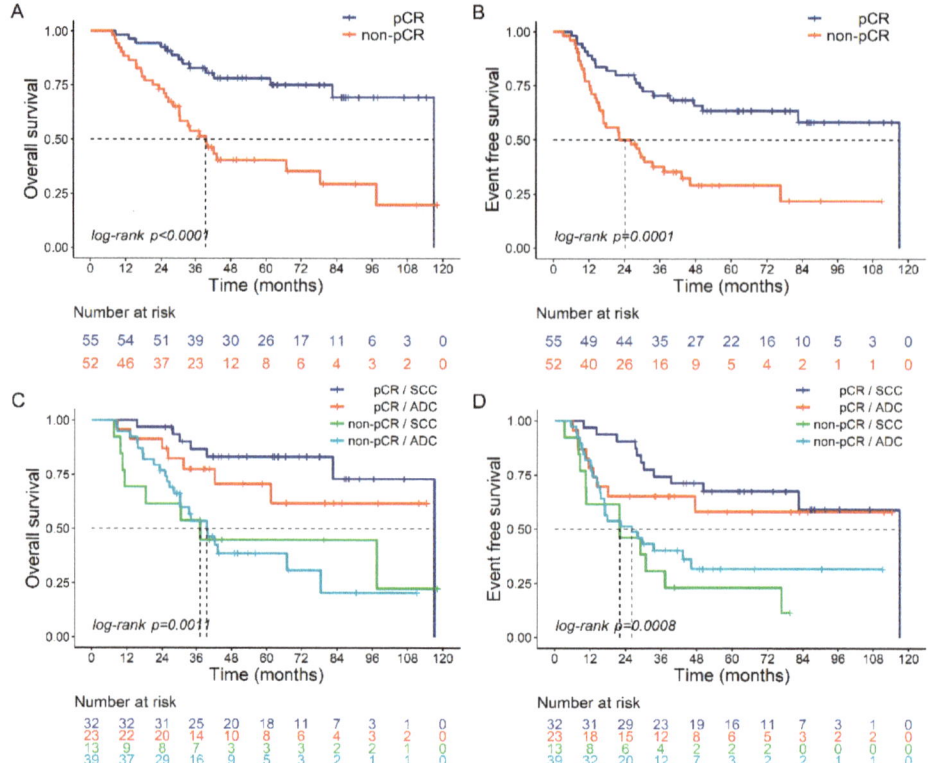

Figure 2. (**A**) Overall Survival (OS) and (**B**) Event-Free Survival (EFS) estimated by Kaplan–Meier method as a function of pathological complete response (pCR vs. non-pCR) in resected patients. (**C**) OS and (**D**) EFS as a function of pCR and histotype (squamous cell carcinoma vs. adenocarcinoma). pCR: pathological complete response; SCC: squamous cell carcinoma; ADC: adenocarcinoma.

Table 3. Univariate and Multivariate Hazard Ratios (HR) and 95% CIs of factors associated with OS and EFS in resected patients.

OS Variable		Univariable Analysis HR (95% CI)	p Value	Multivariable Analysis HR (95% CI)	p Value
Age	<60	1			
	60–69	0.91 (0.50–1.65)	0.7582		
	≥70	0.73 (0.35–1.53)	0.4066		
Gender	Male	1		1	
	Female	0.44 (0.24–0.83)	0.01	0.37 (0.16–0.84)	0.017
Histology	SCC	1			
	ADC	1.72 (0.99–2.99)	0.051		
pCR	No	1			
	Yes	0.30 (0.16–0.56)	<0.0001		
pT stage	T0	1			
	T1–4	2.06 (1.14–3.71)	0.0162		
pN stage	N0	1		1	
	N1	5.11 (2.76–9.47)	<0.0001	4.39 (2.36–8.18)	<0.0001

Table 3. Cont.

OS Variable		Univariable Analysis HR (95% CI)	p Value	Multivariable Analysis HR (95% CI)	p Value
TRG	1	1			
	2–4	2.71 (1.29–5.67)	0.008		
EFS Variable		Univariable Analysis HR (95% CI)	p Value	Multivariable Analysis HR (95% CI)	p Value
Age	<60	1			
	60–69	0.8 (0.5–1.4)	0.4614		
	≥70	0.7 (0.4–1.3)	0.3014		
Gender	Male	1		1	
	Female	0.43 (0.25–0.75)	0.0029	0.44 (0.22–0.87)	0.0184
Histology	SCC	1			
	ADC	1.36 (0.84–2.20)	0.22		
pCR	No	1		1	
	Yes	0.35 (0.20–0.61)	<0.0001	0.38 (0.22–0.67)	<0.0001
pT stage	T0	1			
	T1–4	1.99 (1.17–3.38)	0.0109		
pN stage	N0	1			
	N1	3.73 (2.14–6.49)	<0.0001		
TRG	1	1			
	2–4	2.09 (1.09–3.99)	0.03		

OS: overall survival; EFS: event-free survival; HR: hazard ratio; CI: confidence interval; SCC: squamous cell carcinoma; ADC: adenocarcinoma; pCR: pathological complete response; TRG: tumor regression grade.

2.5. Protocol Toxicity and Postoperative Complications

Of the 119 (97.5%) patients who completed the nCRT protocol, 92 (77.3%) experienced at least one adverse event. Details of toxic effects are shown in Table 4. Thirty-two (26.9%) patients had grade ≥3 acute hematological toxicity, while 23 (19.3%) had acute grade ≥3 non hematological events. Overall, a potentially treatment-related death occurred in 4 (3.4%) patients.

Table 4. Neoadjuvant chemoradiotherapy protocol-related toxicity.

At Least One Adverse Event	92/119 (77.3%)		
	Grade 1/2	Grade 3/4	Grade 5
Nausea, n (%)	57 (47.9)	6 (5.0)	0 (0.0)
Vomiting, n (%)	16 (13.4)	3 (2.5)	0 (0.0)
Esophagitis *, n (%)	42 (35.3)	12 (10.1)	0 (0.0)
Diarrhea, n (%)	30 (25.2)	0 (0.0)	0 (0.0)
Fatigue, n (%)	49 (41.2)	7 (5.9)	0 (0.0)
Skin toxicity, n (%)	15 (12.6)	2 ° (1.7)	0 (0.0)
Neutropenia, n (%)	36 (30.3)	25 (21.0)	2 § (1.7)
Thrombocytopenia, n (%)	14 (11.8)	2 (1.7)	0 (0.0)
Anemia, n (%)	4 (3.4)	4 (3.4)	0 (0.0)
Cardiac toxicity, n (%)	0 (0.0)	0 (0.0)	2 ˆ (1.7)
Radiation pneumonia, n (%)	0 (0.0)	1 (0.8)	0 (0.0)
Aorto-esophageal fistula, n (%)	0 (0.0)	1 ⁿ (0.8)	0 (0.0)

* appearance or worsening; § neutropenic fever and sepsis; ° taxane-related skin reaction; ˆ heart failure; ⁿ requiring an intravascular stent implantation.

None of the patients who underwent surgery died within 30 days after resection or in-hospital. Fifty-nine (55.1%) patients had at least one post-operative complication (Table 5), most of which were mild [14]. Considering severe complications alone (Clavien Dindo ≥3b according to the Esophagectomy Complications Consensus Group [15]), 8 (7.3%) cases required reoperation or ICU. Of these, surgical serious events occurred in 5 (4.6%) patients while medical severe complications were reported in 3 (2.8%).

Table 5. Postoperative complications.

Complications	Clavien Dindo Classification	Events, n (%)
Global, n patients (%)		59 (55.1)
	Grade I	8 (7.4)
	Grade II	22 (20.6)
	Grade III a	21 (19.6)
	Grade III b	5 (4.6)
	Grade IV a	3 (2.8)
	Grade IV b	0 (0.0)
	Grade V	0 (0.0)
Surgical, n events (%)		39 (36.4)
	Grade I	11 (10.3)
	Grade II	8 (7.5)
	Grade III a	15 (14.0)
	Grade III b	5 (4.6)
	Grade IV a	0 (0.0)
	Grade IV b	0 (0.0)
	Grade V	0 (0.0)
Medical, n events (%)		30 (28.0)
	Grade I	1 (0.9)
	Grade II	19 (17.8)
	Grade III a	7 (6.5)
	Grade III b	0 (0.0)
	Grade IV a	3 (2.8)
	Grade IV b	0 (0.0)
	Grade V	0 (0.0)
Frequent complication, n events (%)	Anastomotic leak	9 (8.4)
	Pulmonary/Pleuric Complication	21 (19.6)
	Cardiac Complication	17 (15.8)
Median LOS, days (range)		10 (6–41)
Mortality (30 days or In-Hospital)		0 (0.0)

LOS: Length of Hospital Stay.

3. Discussion

Over the last 15 years, neoadjuvant chemo-radiotherapy and peri-operative chemotherapy have become the standard approaches for locally advanced EC, leading to a 10–15% improvement in long-term survival rates as compared with surgery alone in clinical trials [7–9,16]. However, which is the optimal strategy is still under debate. This observational study reports the efficacy and safety of an intensive nCRT protocol in the daily clinical practice for locally advanced EC. To the best of our knowledge, this study includes one of the largest cohorts of patients treated with induction chemotherapy, followed by chemo-radiotherapy, as the preoperative approach in EC. This nCRT protocol has previously been tested at our institution in a phase II trial, with good long-term survival (median OS 55 months) and pCR (47% of patients) [12]. The results of the present study, with an estimated median follow-up of 62.1 months, confirm the high OS and EFS rate (median 78.5 and 39.5 months, respectively) also in "real life" patients. This finding is relevant, and emphasizes the efficacy, in terms of survival benefit, for neoadjuvant chemo-radiotherapy when added to surgery in patients with EC.

Noteworthy, pCR was achieved in 51.4% of resected patients, one of the highest percentages reported so far [17]. Indeed, a pCR is considered one of the best available predictors of outcome for EC patients who undergo chemo-radiation therapy followed by esophagectomy [18,19]. A recent MDACC cohort study showed that pCR was associated with an improved survival (median OS 71.28 months for pCR versus 35.87 for non-pCR cases, $p = 0.002$) [10]. Of the 911 treated patients, 218 (23.9%) achieved a pCR, with a rate of 32.2% for SCC and of 23.1% for ADC ($p = 0.06$). In our study, pCR patients achieved a 5-year OS rate of 70.5% (versus 37.6% in non-pCR patients), with a similar survival trend for SCC and ADC responder patients (Figure 2C,D). This result supports the role of pCR as a trustworthy surrogate predictor marker of survival advantage.

In the ChemoRadiotherapy for Oesophageal cancer followed by Surgery Study (CROSS) trial, pCR rate was 29%, with a significantly larger number of SCC patients (49% versus 23% for ADC, $p = 0.008$) [7]. In our study, 32 of 45 (71.1%) SCC patients had a pCR in the surgical specimen. This percentage is remarkable and confirms the greater sensitivity of SCC to full-dose chemo-radiotherapy as previously reported by other authors [20]. Another issue is whether surgery on demand is advisable in selected clinical complete responder patients. In a subgroup analysis of our study, we found that the percentage of pCR was significantly higher for SCC vs. ADC tumors (17/21, 81% vs. 4/16, 25%, $p = 0.002$) in females, while no significant difference was observed in males (15/24, 63% for SCC vs. 19/46, 41% for ADC, $p = 0.15$). Moreover, in patients with a pCR, median OS and EFS were particularly high in females (not achievable versus 82.6 months in males, $p = 0.01$, and not achievable versus 33.6 months in males, $p = 0.002$, respectively). Based on these results, the female population with SCC seems to be the ideal candidate for a watch-and-wait approach. The ongoing randomized SANO trial, comparing salvage surgery with immediate surgery in clinical complete responders after nCRT, will provide results over the next few years [21,22].

Controversy exists over the optimal neoadjuvant approach for gastroesophageal junction (EGJ) adenocarcinomas [23]. Neoadjuvant chemo-radiation is associated with an increased local control of the tumor compared with perioperative chemotherapy alone, but this does not translate into an increased survival [24]. Furthermore, the pCR rates in ADCs treated with chemo-radiotherapy are significantly worse than SCCs, being less than 20–25% [6,7,20]. An increase in pCR rate, correlated with the use of higher doses of radiotherapy, compared to 41.4 Gy used in the CROSS trial [7], has been described in the literature. In detail, the use of doses between 45 and 50.4 Gy, in combination with carboplatin-paclitaxel, produced a pCR in 29–36% of treated patients, with acceptable toxicity [25–27]. In our series the pCR rate for ADCs was noticeably high, being 37.1%, and in this subset of patients both median OS and EFS were 117 months. This may be due to the use of an intensive schedule with docetaxel, cisplatin plus 5-fluorouracil (5-FU) during the induction phase and concomitant with radiotherapy (RT), as well as to the 50–50.4 Gy dose administered in this protocol that could have helped maximize local response. This finding further supports the potential effectiveness and generalizability of the use of nCRT in ADC of the esophagus, as a reliable or even better alternative to perioperative chemotherapy in selected patients, although the design of the study does not permit to draw definitive conclusions, due to the lack of a control group [28]. However, many ADCs are extremely resistant to chemo-radiotherapy: these ADC patients may not benefit from this treatment but are exposed to its negative consequences such as toxicity and delayed surgical therapy. To this regard, a multicenter, randomized phase II study on BIRC3-expression driven therapy (nCRT versus upfront surgery), in patients with resectable ADC of the esophagus and EGJ, is currently ongoing (BoRgES trial, NCT04269083) at the authors' institution.

According to the literature [29], this study confirms that nodal downstaging (ypN0) is a strong predictor for OS. We can assume that nodal response might be as important as downstaging on the primary tumor, and that a poor nodal response cannot be compensated even by radical surgery, thus representing a reliable biological marker for poorer survival. Instead, pCR remains the predominant prognostic factor for EFS, presumably indicating that complete response to nCRT corresponds to a particularly favorable tumor biology or treatment efficacy or both. This latter finding is particularly intriguing for the squamous histology. As mentioned above, if the pCR rate is extremely high in this subgroup, and the consequent EFS markedly prolonged, close observation with salvage surgery might be an embraceable option to improve patients' quality of life (QoL) [30].

One potential criticism regarding the use of this intensive nCRT protocol is toxicity, leading to death in about 3% of treated patients. Thus, its use should be recommended only in specialized centers. However, the vast majority of patients were able to complete the planned preoperative treatment, and, notably, the subsequent surgery was not jeopardized by the nCRT protocol. The R0 surgical rate is also remarkable, amounting to 98.1% of resected patients (86.1% for the entire cohort). Hence, considering that tumor shrinkage after nCRT can significantly increase the R0 resection rate that 73.8% of patients achieved a ypN0 and 51.4% a pCR, and that nCRT adverse events did not represent a contraindication for surgery, we can assert that the protocol survival benefit was not counteracted by an excessive toxicity.

Our study presents some limitations. Indeed, it is an observational study, with a 10-year enrollment period, during which some variations in diagnostic accuracy, management of patients and post-operative surveillance occurred. Moreover, the indication to the nCRT protocol was defined on the basis of our previous experience and as a distinctive practice of our multidisciplinary team, thus our results could be biased by the patient selection process. Finally, this analysis included different histologies (SCC and ADC), which could have added heterogeneity to the outcomes measured.

4. Materials and Methods

4.1. Study Design

This study is an Institutional Review Board (IRB)-approved (Number DBCES001) observational single-center analysis of prospectively collected data, designed to assess the real-life effectiveness and safety of our nCRT protocol in patients with SCC and ADC of the esophagus and gastroesophageal junction. We considered all consecutive patients treated at our Institution from January 2008 to December 2017. The following perioperative data were collected: baseline demographics, diagnostic work-up, neoadjuvant protocol details, intra-operative findings, and post-operative data. According to the main international guidelines [2], patients with Siewert III type tumors were treated as gastric cancers, while patients with SC cervical tumors were assigned to definitive chemo-radiotherapy and therefore excluded from the analysis.

4.2. Staging

The pre-treatment staging consisted of clinical examination, blood chemistries including tumor markers, contrast-enhanced total body CT scan, fluorodeoxyglucose positron-emission tomography (^{18}FDG-PET/CT), esophagogastroduodenoscopy with biopsies, and endoscopic ultrasound (EUS). In SCC patients, tracheobronchoscopy, esophageal magnetic resonance (MR), and cervical ultrasound were also performed. Patients were staged according to the Union for International Cancer Control [UICC] TNM cancer staging [31] and the therapeutic approach was defined by the institutional multidisciplinary tumor board.

4.3. Chemo-Radiotherapy Schedule

Treatment schedule consisted of a first phase of induction chemotherapy for 3 weeks (days 1–22), followed by a second phase of concurrent chemotherapy and radiotherapy for 5 weeks (days 29–63), as previously described [12]. Briefly, the chemotherapy treatment plan was as follows: docetaxel 35 mg/m^2 and cisplatin 25 mg/m^2 on days 1, 8, 15, 29, 36, 43, 50 and 57 plus 5 fluorouracil (5-FU) 180 mg/m^2 as protracted venous infusion (c.i.) on days 1 to 21 and 150 mg/m^2 c.i. on days 29 to 63. The detailed treatment schedule is represented in Table S3 (Supplementary Material).

Radiation therapy (RT) was delivered concurrently with chemotherapy starting on day 29. The prescribed dose was 50–50.4 Gy delivered in 25–28 fractions. The gross tumor volume (GTV) included the primary lesion and any regionally involved lymph nodes. The GTV was contoured using data from CT scan, EUS, and PET/CT fusion scans. The clinical target volume (CTV) was generated by expanding the GTV tumor by 3 cm cranially and caudally and 1 cm radially, while positive lymph nodes were uniformly expanded by 1 cm. The CTV was usually completed with the addition of the elective nodal irradiation (ENI) volume [32]. A CTV-to-PTV margin of 8–10 mm was applied. Until 2013, RT was delivered using three-dimensional conformal radiotherapy (3D-CRT). From 2014, 3D-CRT was replaced by intensity-modulated radiotherapy (IMRT) and volumetric modulated arc radiotherapy (VMAT). Image-guided radiation therapy (IGRT) was routinely used.

4.4. Restaging, Surgery and Pathological Analysis

Patients were restaged with pretreatment work-up procedures between the fourth and fifth week after treatment completion. Response evaluation was performed using response evaluation criteria in solid tumors (RECIST and PERCIST Criteria) [33,34]. Surgery with radical intent was performed 6 to 8 weeks after nCRT completion. A Two- or 3-field lymph node dissection was performed based on tumor site and clinical nodal status at diagnosis. Abdominal D2 and standard mediastinal lymphadenectomy was the standard approach for ADC. Extension to the recurrent nerve chain nodes or a complete 3-field lymphadenectomy was performed for SCC based on node involvement. Peritoneal lavage cytology was evaluated in all ADC patients. Positive cytology was considered to be metastatic. Surgical complications were registered according to Clavien Dindo Classification [15]. A positive resection margin (R1) was defined as vital tumor cells within 1 mm of the proximal and distal resection margins, while a circumferential margin was considered involved if neoplastic cells were found at the cut margin. Pathological complete response (pCR) was defined as no vital tumor cells in the resection specimen (ypT0N0M0), and Tumor Regression Grade (TRG) was scored according to a modified Mandard score system [35].

4.5. Follow-Up

Follow-up examination was performed every 6 months after surgery for resected cases and every 3 months after nCRT protocol completion for non-resected patients. The follow-up schedule included: total body contrast-enhanced CT scan, esophagogastroscopy, tumor markers, neck endoscopic ultrasound in SCC and a clinical assessment. Toxicity data were collected during follow-up according to common terminology criteria for adverse events (CTCAE) version 4.0 [36].

4.6. Statistical Analysis

Quantitative variables were described as median and interquartile range (IQR) or mean and standard deviation (SD), categorical variables were summarized as counts and percentages. The median follow-up time was based on the reverse Kaplan-Meier estimator. Primary endpoints considered were OS, event-free survival (EFS) and pCR. Secondary endpoint was toxicity.

OS was the time from the start of induction chemotherapy to death, and EFS was calculated from the start of induction chemotherapy to the date of a documented disease progression, relapse, or death. Patients who did not develop an event during the study period were censored at the date of last observation. The survival probabilities were estimated using the Kaplan-Meier method and reported with their 95% confidence interval (CI). Comparisons among strata were performed using the log-rank test. Hazard ratios (HR) and 95% CI for each group were estimated using univariate Cox proportional hazards models. No deviation from the proportional hazards assumption were found by the numerical methods of Lin et al. [37]. The independent role of each covariate in predicting survival was verified in a multivariable model considering all characteristics significantly associated with the outcome in the univariate analyses. Associations were assessed using the χ^2 or Fisher exact test as appropriate. All statistical tests were two-sided and a p value <0.05 was considered statistically significant. Statistical analyses were performed using the RStudio (RStudio: Integrated Development for R. RStudio Inc., Boston, MA, USA).

5. Conclusions

In conclusion, this intensive neoadjuvant schedule with induction chemotherapy followed by chemo-radiotherapy, based on docetaxel, cisplatin, 5-fluorouracil, and 50–50.4 Gy radiotherapy, achieves considerable results in terms of survival and pCR rate also in "real life" patients, largely counterbalancing the risk of not negligible adverse events. Noteworthy, the protocol does not jeopardize the achievement of radical resection and does not increase the rate of postoperative complications. Further studies are necessary to evaluate the use of this protocol also in a watch-and-wait approach.

Supplementary Materials: The following are available online at http://www.mdpi.com/2072-6694/12/12/3614/s1. Table S1. Neoadjuvant chemo-radiotherapy protocol details. Table S2. Incidence and pattern of failure distribution among resected patients (first site of recurrence). Table S3. Neoadjuvant chemo-radiotherapy protocol schedule.

Author Contributions: Conceptualization, N.S.; methodology, N.S. and M.P.; software, P.D.B.; validation, S.G., G.D.M. and R.M. (Renzo Mazzarotto); formal analysis, N.S., J.W. and P.D.B.; data curation, M.P., R.M. (Renato Micera), V.M., and G.R.; writing—original draft preparation, N.S., R.M. (Renato Micera) and J.W.; writing—review and editing, V.M., D.C., A.T., P.D.B., and S.G.; supervision, G.D.M. and R.M. (Renzo Mazzarotto). All authors have read and agreed to the published version of the manuscript.

Funding: This research received no external funding.

Conflicts of Interest: The authors declare no conflict of interest

References

1. Siegel, R.; Ma, J.; Zou, Z.; Jemal, A. Cancer statistics, 2014. *CA Cancer J. Clin.* **2014**, *64*, 9–29. [CrossRef] [PubMed]
2. NCCN. NCCN Guidelines—Esophageal and Esophagogastric Junction Cancers. Version 1. 2020. Available online: https://www.nccn.org/professionals/physician_gls/pdf/esophageal.pdf (accessed on 1 October 2020).
3. Lordick, F.; Mariette, C.; Haustermans, K.; Obermannová, R.; Arnold, D.; ESMO Guidelines Committee. Oesophageal cancer: ESMO Clinical Practice Guidelines for diagnosis, treatment and follow-up. *Ann. Oncol.* **2016**, *27*, v50–v57. [CrossRef] [PubMed]
4. Walsh, T.N.; Noonan, N.; Hollywood, D.; Kelly, A.; Keeling, N.; Hennessy, T.P. A comparison of multimodal therapy and surgery for esophageal adenocarcinoma. *N. Engl. J. Med.* **1996**, *335*, 462–467. [CrossRef] [PubMed]
5. Bosset, J.F.; Gignoux, M.; Triboulet, J.P.; Tiret, E.; Mantion, G.; Elias, D.; Lozach, P.; Ollier, J.C.; Pavy, J.J.; Mercier, M.; et al. Chemoradiotherapy followed by surgery compared with surgery alone in squamous-cell cancer of the esophagus. *N. Engl. J. Med.* **1997**, *337*, 161–167. [CrossRef] [PubMed]
6. Tepper, J.; Krasna, M.J.; Niedzwiecki, D.; Hollis, D.; Reed, C.E.; Goldberg, R.; Kiel, K.; Willett, C.; Sugarbaker, D.; Mayer, R. Phase III trial of trimodality therapy with cisplatin, fluorouracil, radiotherapy, and surgery compared with surgery alone for esophageal cancer: CALGB 9781. *J. Clin. Oncol.* **2008**, *26*, 1086–1092. [CrossRef] [PubMed]
7. Van Hagen, P.; Hulshof, M.C.; van Lanschot, J.J.; Steyerberg, E.W.; van Berge Henegouwen, M.I.; Wijnhoven, B.P.; Richel, D.J.; Nieuwenhuijzen, G.A.P.; Hospers, G.A.P.; Bonenkamp, J.J.; et al. Preoperative chemoradiotherapy for esophageal or junctional cancer. *N. Engl. J. Med.* **2012**, *366*, 2074–2084. [CrossRef] [PubMed]
8. Shapiro, J.; van Lanschot, J.J.B.; Hulshof, M.C.C.M.; van Hagen, P.; van Berge Henegouwen, M.I.; Wijnhoven, B.P.L.; van Laarhoven, H.W.M.; Nieuwenhuijzen, G.A.P.; Hospers, G.A.P.; Bonenkamp, J.J.; et al. Neoadjuvant chemoradiotherapy plus surgery versus surgery alone for oesophageal or junctional cancer (CROSS): Long-Term results of a randomised controlled trial. *Lancet Oncol.* **2015**, *16*, 1090–1098. [CrossRef]
9. Yang, H.; Liu, H.; Chen, Y.; Zhu, C.; Fang, W.; Yu, Z.; Mao, W.; Xiang, J.; Han, Y.; Chen, Z.; et al. Neoadjuvant chemoradiotherapy followed by surgery versus surgery alone for locally advanced squamous cell carcinoma of the esophagus (NEOCRTEC5010): A phase III multicenter, randomized, open-label clinical trial. *J. Clin. Oncol.* **2018**, *36*, 2796–2803. [CrossRef] [PubMed]

10. Blum Murphy, M.; Xiao, L.; Patel, V.R.; Maru, D.M.; Correa, A.M.; Amlashi, F.G.; Liao, Z.; Komaki, R.; Lin, S.H.; Skinner, H.D.; et al. Pathological complete response in patients with esophageal cancer after the trimodality approach: The association with baseline variables and survival-The University of Texas MD Anderson Cancer Center experience. *Cancer* **2017**, *123*, 4106–4113. [CrossRef] [PubMed]
11. Iams, W.T.; Villaflor, V.M. Neoadjuvant treatment for locally invasive esophageal cancer. *World J. Surg.* **2017**, *41*, 1719–1725. [CrossRef] [PubMed]
12. Pasini, F.; de Manzoni, G.; Zanoni, A.; Grandinetti, A.; Capirci, C.; Pavarana, M.; Tomezzoli, A.; Rubello, D.; Cordiano, C. Neoadjuvant therapy with weekly docetaxel and cisplatin, 5-fluorouracil continuous infusion, and concurrent radiotherapy in patients with locally advanced esophageal cancer produced a high percentage of long-lasting pathological complete response: A phase 2 study. *Cancer* **2013**, *119*, 939–945. [CrossRef] [PubMed]
13. Zarbin, M. Real life outcomes vs. clinical trial results. *J. Ophthalmic Vis. Res.* **2019**, *14*, 88–92. [CrossRef] [PubMed]
14. Low, D.E.; Alderson, D.; Cecconello, I.; Chang, A.C.; Darling, G.E.; D'Journo, X.B.; Griffin, S.M.; Hölscher, A.H.; Hofstetter, W.L.; Jobe, B.A.; et al. International consensus on standardization of data collection for complications associated with esophagectomy: Esophagectomy Complications Consensus Group (ECCG). *Ann. Surg.* **2015**, *262*, 286–294. [CrossRef]
15. Clavien, P.A.; Barkun, J.; de Oliveira, M.L.; Vauthey, J.N.; Dindo, D.; Schulick, R.D.; de Santibañes, E.; Pekolj, J.; Slankamenac, K.; Bassi, C.; et al. The Clavien-Dindo classification of surgical complications: Five-year experience. *Ann. Surg.* **2009**, *250*, 187–196. [CrossRef] [PubMed]
16. Ronellenfitsch, U.; Schwarzbach, M.; Hofheinz, R.; Kienle, P.; Kieser, M.; Slanger, T.E.; Jensen, K.; GE Adenocarcinoma Meta-analysis Group. Perioperative chemo(radio)therapy versus primary surgery for resectable adenocarcinoma of the stomach, gastroesophageal junction, and lower esophagus. *Cochrane Database Syst. Rev.* **2013**, *5*, CD008107. [CrossRef] [PubMed]
17. De Gouw, D.J.J.M.; Klarenbeek, B.R.; Driessen, M.; Bouwense, S.A.W.; van Workum, F.; Fütterer, J.J.; Rovers, M.M.; Ten Broek, R.P.G.; Rosman, C. Detecting pathological complete response in esophageal cancer after neoadjuvant therapy based on imaging techniques: A diagnostic systematic review and meta-analysis. *J. Thorac. Oncol.* **2019**, *14*, 1156–1171. [CrossRef] [PubMed]
18. Chirieac, L.R.; Swisher, S.G.; Ajani, J.A.; Komaki, R.R.; Correa, A.M.; Morris, J.S.; Roth, J.A.; Rashid, A.; Hamilton, S.R.; Wu, T.T. Posttherapy pathologic stage predicts survival in patients with esophageal carcinoma receiving preoperative chemoradiation. *Cancer* **2005**, *103*, 1347–1355. [CrossRef]
19. Meredith, K.L.; Weber, J.M.; Turaga, K.K.; Siegel, E.M.; McLoughlin, J.; Hoffe, S.; Marcovalerio, M.; Shah, N.; Kelley, S.; Karl, R. Pathologic response after neoadjuvant therapy is the major determinant of survival in patients with esophageal cancer. *Ann. Surg. Oncol.* **2010**, *17*, 1159–1167. [CrossRef]
20. Bollschweiler, E.; Metzger, R.; Drebber, U.; Baldus, S.; Vallböhmer, D.; Kocher, M.; Hölscher, A.H. Histological type of esophageal cancer might affect response to neo-adjuvant radiochemotherapy and subsequent prognosis. *Ann. Oncol.* **2009**, *20*, 231–238. [CrossRef]
21. Noordman, B.J.; Spaander, M.C.W.; Valkema, R.; Wijnhoven, B.P.L.; van Berge Henegouwen, M.I.; Shapiro, J.; Biermann, K.; van der Gaast, A.; van Hillegersberg, R.; Hulshof, M.C.C.M.; et al. Detection of residual disease after neoadjuvant chemoradiotherapy for oesophageal cancer (preSANO): A prospective multicentre, diagnostic cohort study. *Lancet Oncol.* **2018**, *19*, 965–974. [CrossRef]
22. Noordman, B.J.; Wijnhoven, B.P.L.; Lagarde, S.M.; Boonstra, J.J.; Coene, P.P.L.O.; Dekker, J.W.T.; Doukas, M.; van der Gaast, A.; Heisterkamp, J.; Kouwenhoven, E.A.; et al. Neoadjuvant chemoradiotherapy plus surgery versus active surveillance for oesophageal cancer: A stepped-wedge cluster randomised trial. *BMC Cancer* **2018**, *18*, 142. [CrossRef] [PubMed]
23. Petrelli, F.; Ghidini, M.; Barni, S.; Sgroi, G.; Passalacqua, R.; Tomasello, G. Neoadjuvant chemoradiotherapy or chemotherapy for gastroesophageal junction adenocarcinoma: A systematic review and meta-analysis. *Gastric Cancer* **2019**, *22*, 245–254. [CrossRef] [PubMed]
24. Al-Batran, S.E.; Homann, N.; Pauligk, C.; Goetze, T.O.; Meiler, J.; Kasper, S.; Kopp, H.G.; Mayer, F.; Haag, G.M.; Luley, K.; et al. Perioperative chemotherapy with fluorouracil plus leucovorin, oxaliplatin, and docetaxel versus fluorouracil or capecitabine plus cisplatin and epirubicin for locally advanced, resectable gastric or gastro-oesophageal junction adenocarcinoma (FLOT4): A randomised, phase 2/3 trial. *Lancet* **2019**, *393*, 1948–1957. [CrossRef] [PubMed]

25. Mukherjee, S.; Hurt, C.N.; Gwynne, S.; Sebag-Montefiore, D.; Radhakrishna, G.; Gollins, S.; Hawkins, M.; Grabsch, H.I.; Jones, G.; Falk, S.; et al. NEOSCOPE: A randomised phase II study of induction chemotherapy followed by oxaliplatin/capecitabine or carboplatin/paclitaxel based pre-operative chemoradiation for resectable oesophageal adenocarcinoma. *Eur. J. Cancer* **2017**, *74*, 38–46. [CrossRef] [PubMed]
26. Nabavizadeh, N.; Shukla, R.; Elliott, D.A.; Mitin, T.; Vaccaro, G.M.; Dolan, J.P.; Maggiore, R.J.; Schipper, P.H.; Hunter, J.G.; Thomas, C.R., Jr.; et al. Preoperative carboplatin and paclitaxel-based chemoradiotherapy for esophageal carcinoma: Results of a modified CROSS regimen utilizing radiation doses greater than 41.4 Gy. *Dis. Esophagus* **2016**, *29*, 614–620. [CrossRef] [PubMed]
27. Paireder, M.; Jomrich, G.; Kristo, I.; Asari, R.; Rieder, E.; Beer, A.; Ilhan-Mutlu, A.; Preusser, M.; Schmid, R.; Schoppmann, S.F. Modification of preoperative radiochemotherapy for esophageal cancer (CROSS protocol) is safe and efficient with no impact on surgical morbidity. *Strahlenther. Onkol.* **2020**, *196*, 779–786. [CrossRef]
28. Zhou, H.Y.; Zheng, S.P.; Li, A.L.; Gao, Q.L.; Ou, Q.Y.; Chen, Y.J.; Wu, S.T.; Lin, D.G.; Liu, S.B.; Huang, L.Y.; et al. Clinical evidence for association of neoadjuvant chemotherapy or chemoradiotherapy with efficacy and safety in patients with resectable esophageal carcinoma (NewEC study). *EClinicalMedicine* **2020**, *24*, 100422. [CrossRef]
29. Zanoni, A. Nodal downstaging in esophageal and esophagogastric junction cancer: More important than ever. *J. Thorac. Dis.* **2017**, *9*, 1839–1842. [CrossRef]
30. Park, S.R.; Yoon, D.H.; Kim, J.H.; Kim, Y.H.; Kim, H.R.; Lee, H.J.; Jung, H.Y.; Lee, G.H.; Song, H.J.; Kim, D.H.; et al. A randomized phase III trial on the role of esophagectomy in complete responders to Preoperative chemoradiotherapy for esophageal Squamous cell Carcinoma (ESOPRESSO). *Anticancer Res.* **2019**, *39*, 5123–5133. [CrossRef]
31. Sobin, L.H.; Gospodarowicz, M.K.; Wittekind, C. *TNM Classification of Malignant Tumors*, 7th ed.; Wiley-Liss: New York, NY, USA, 2009.
32. Wu, A.J.; Bosch, W.R.; Chang, D.T.; Hong, T.S.; Jabbour, S.K.; Kleinberg, L.R.; Mamon, H.J.; Thomas, C.R., Jr.; Goodman, K.A. Expert consensus contouring guidelines for intensity modulated radiation therapy in esophageal and gastroesophageal junction cancer. *Int. J. Radiat. Oncol. Biol. Phys.* **2015**, *92*, 911–920. [CrossRef]
33. Eisenhauer, E.A.; Therasse, P.; Bogaerts, J.; Schwartz, L.H.; Sargent, D.; Ford, R.; Dancey, J.; Arbuck, S.; Gwyther, S.; Mooney, M.; et al. New response evaluation criteria in solid tumours: Revised RECIST guideline (version 1.1). *Eur. J. Cancer* **2009**, *45*, 228–247. [CrossRef] [PubMed]
34. Wahl, R.L.; Jacene, H.; Kasamon, Y.; Lodge, M.A. From RECIST to PERCIST: Evolving Considerations for PET response criteria in solid tumors. *J. Nucl. Med.* **2009**, *50*, 122S–150S. [CrossRef] [PubMed]
35. Mandard, A.M.; Dalibard, F.; Mandard, J.C.; Marnay, J.; Henry-Amar, M.; Petiot, J.F.; Roussel, A.; Jacob, J.H.; Segol, P.; Samama, G.; et al. Pathologic assessment of tumor regression after preoperative chemoradiotherapy of esophageal carcinoma. Clinicopathologic correlations. *Cancer* **1994**, *73*, 2680–2686. [CrossRef]
36. National Cancer Institute. *Common Terminology Criteria for Adverse Events (CTCAE) v.4.03*; National Cancer Institute: Bethesda, MD, USA; NIH: Bethesda, MD, USA, 2010.
37. Lin, D.Y.; Wei, L.J.; Ying, Z. Checking the cox model with cumulative sums of martingale-based residuals. *Biometrika* **1993**, *80*, 557–572. [CrossRef]

Publisher's Note: MDPI stays neutral with regard to jurisdictional claims in published maps and institutional affiliations.

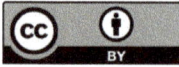

© 2020 by the authors. Licensee MDPI, Basel, Switzerland. This article is an open access article distributed under the terms and conditions of the Creative Commons Attribution (CC BY) license (http://creativecommons.org/licenses/by/4.0/).

Article

Significance of Lauren Classification in Patients Undergoing Neoadjuvant/Perioperative Chemotherapy for Locally Advanced Gastric or Gastroesophageal Junction Cancers—Analysis from a Large Single Center Cohort in Germany

Rebekka Schirren [1], Alexander Novotny [1], Christian Oesterlin [1], Julia Slotta-Huspenina [2], Helmut Friess [1] and Daniel Reim [1,*]

[1] Department of Surgery, TUM School of Medicine, Technical University Munich, 81675 Munich, Germany; rebekka.schirren@tum.de (R.S.); alexander.novotny@tum.de (A.N.); christian.oesterlin@mri.tum.de (C.O.); helmut.friess@tum.de (H.F.)
[2] Institute of Pathology, TUM School of Medicine, Technical University Munich, 81675 Munich, Germany; julia.slotta-huspenina@tum.de
* Correspondence: daniel.reim@tum.de

Citation: Schirren, R.; Novotny, A.; Oesterlin, C.; Slotta-Huspenina, J.; Friess, H.; Reim, D. Significance of Lauren Classification in Patients Undergoing Neoadjuvant/Perioperative Chemotherapy for Locally Advanced Gastric or Gastroesophageal Junction Cancers—Analysis from a Large Single Center Cohort in Germany. *Cancers* **2021**, *13*, 290. https://doi.org/10.3390/cancers13020290

Received: 1 December 2020
Accepted: 31 December 2020
Published: 14 January 2021

Publisher's Note: MDPI stays neutral with regard to jurisdictional claims in published maps and institutional affiliations.

Copyright: © 2021 by the authors. Licensee MDPI, Basel, Switzerland. This article is an open access article distributed under the terms and conditions of the Creative Commons Attribution (CC BY) license (https://creativecommons.org/licenses/by/4.0/).

Simple Summary: Chemotherapy ahead of surgery is standard of care for locally advanced stomach cancer or cancer at the junction between esophagus and stomach in Europe. However, response to chemotherapy may depend on microscopic features of the tumor. Three types were defined before: intestinal, diffuse and mixed types. The authors aimed to investigate if these characteristics influence survival after end of treatment (chemotherapy+surgery) in a large cohort treated in a University hospital. It was found that intestinal type patients demonstrate longer survival after chemotherapy+surgery than those with diffuse types. In the mixed type group no clear conclusion regarding the effect of chemotherapy ahead of surgery may be taken. Conclusively, patients with diffuse type tumors do not benefit from chemotherapy ahead of surgery.

Abstract: Background: the purpose of this analysis was to analyze the outcomes of multimodal treatment that are related to Lauren histotypes in gastro-esophageal cancer (GEC). Methods: patients with GEC between 1986 and 2013 were analyzed. Uni- and multivariate regression analysis were performed to identify predictors for overall survival. Lauren histotype stratified overall survival (OS)-rates were analyzed by the Kaplan–Meier method. Further, propensity score matching (PSM) was performed to balance for confounders. Results: 1290 patients were analyzed. After PSM, the median survival was 32 months for patients undergoing primary surgery (PS) and 43 months for patients undergoing neoadjuvant chemotherapy (nCTx) ahead of surgery. For intestinal types, median survival time was 34 months (PS) vs. 52 months (nCTx+surgery) $p = 0.07$, 36 months (PS) vs. (31) months (nCTx+surgery) in diffuse types ($p = 0.44$) and 31 months (PS) vs. 62 months (nCTx+surgery) for mixed types ($p = 0.28$). Five-/Ten-year survival rates for intestinal, diffuse, and mixed types were 44/29%, 36/17%, and 43/33%, respectively. After PSM, Kaplan–Meier showed a survival benefit for patients undergoing nCTx+surgery in intestinal and mixed types. Conclusion: the Lauren histotype might be predictive for survival outcome in GEC-patients after neoadjuvant/perioperative chemotherapy.

Keywords: gastric/gastroesophageal cancer; perioperative chemotherapy; Lauren histotype

1. Introduction

Gastric cancer belongs to the most common malignant diseases worldwide with the highest incidence in Eastern Asia [1]. Despite decreasing incidence in the West, it remains a therapeutic challenge. In the Western hemisphere gastric malignancy is often diagnosed at an advanced stage and, in contrast to Eastern Asia, it is preferably located in the proximal third of the stomach or the gastro-esophageal junction (GEJ) [2]. Hence, multimodal treatment concepts have been introduced after demonstrating outcome benefits in randomized controlled trials [3–5]. Nevertheless, not all patients are benefitting from neoadjuvant or perioperative chemotherapy, depending on localization, regimen, and also on the histological subtype. In the past, a signet ring cell, like gastric cancer, was identified to be non-responsive to neoadjuvant chemotherapy [6,7]. However, the data published so far have been difficult to interpret, as there were numerous definitions on the histology of signet ring cell or signet ring cell, like gastric cancer [8]. A pragmatic and feasible sub-classification was only recently published [9]. However, none of the prospective trials investigating the value of neoadjuvant chemotherapy applied this classification system before. Therefore, it is of special interest if already established histopathological classifications may stratify and identify patients to benefit from neoadjuvant/perioperative chemotherapy. This may be accomplished by the widely accepted Lauren classification, because all of the relevant histopathological subtypes (signet ring cell type, poorly-cohesive signet ring cell type, poorly cohesive non-signet-ring cell type, mucinous, papillary, and tubular) are summarized here [10]. Therefore, it was hypothesized that the Lauren histotype dependent histopathologic response may influence survival outcomes after neoadjuvant/perioperative chemotherapy and the aim of this analysis was to evaluate the oncologic outcomes of perioperative/neoadjuvant chemotherapy in a large German single center cohort, depending on the Lauren histotype.

2. Results

For this retrospective analysis, the institutional database for gastric cancer patients was screened and identified 2782 patients having been treated by either surgery or chemotherapy followed by surgery. After removing all cases not fulfilling the defined inclusion criteria (n = 1573), 1209 patients were included in this analysis. 730 patients underwent primary surgery and 479 underwent neoadjuvant/perioperative chemotherapy ahead of surgery. Overall, 663 were diagnosed with Lauren intestinal (398 surgery, 265 nCTx), 359 Lauren diffuse (216 surgery, 143 nCTx), and 187 Lauren mixed type (116 surgery, 71 nCTx). In the entire patient cohort, 247 patients received PLF (20.4%), 41 patients PLF+Taxol (3.4%), 53 (4.4%) OLF, 47 (3.9%) MAGIC, 17 (1.4%) FLOT, and 63 patients received modified regimens (5.2%). The analysis of the baseline characteristics showed significant differences between the primary surgery and neoadjuvant/perioperative chemotherapy group regarding gender distribution (more female patients for intestinal and diffuse. but not mixed Laurentype), older age for patients undergoing primary surgery (all Lauren subtypes), higher proportion of distal cancer locations in primary surgery patients (all groups, especially intestinal type), less advanced cT-stages in the surgery only group (cT2 vs. cT3/4 over all Lauren subtypes), earlier clinical stages, higher proportion of patients requiring extension to the distal esophagus in the chemotherapy group (all Lauren subtypes), higher D2 rates and higher median number of dissected lymph-nodes (LN) in patients undergoing direct surgery (especially in intestinal and mixed Lauren histotype, not so in diffuse type), more pT4a cancers in the primary resection group for all of the Lauren subtypes, earlier UICC stages in those patients undergoing neoadjuvant/perioperative chemotherapy. The proportion of Lauren subtypes, histiopathologic grading, R0-status, and complication rates were balanced between the groups. The histopathologic response rates (Becker Ia/Ib) were 22% in Lauren intestinal type, 9% in Lauren diffuse type, and 21% in Lauren mixed type tumors. Tables 1–3 depict the complete baseline characteristics.

Table 1. Baseline characteristics for patients with intestinal Lauren subtype before and after propensity score matching (PSM).

	Intestinal Subtype (n = 663), Unmatched					Intestinal Subtype (n = 340) PS-Matched				
	Surgery Only (n = 398)		CTX + Surgery (n = 265)		p-Value	Surgery Only (n = 170)		CTX + Surgery (n = 170)		p-Value
	n	%	n	%		n	%	n	%	
Gender					<0.001					0.14
Female	132	33.17	42	15.85		30	17.65	42	24.71	
Male	266	66.83	223	84.15		140	82.35	128	75.29	
Age	68.7 ± 10.8		60.1 ± 10.5		<0.001	65.8 ±10.3		61.6 ±11.1		<0.001
<70	188	47.24	206	77.74	<0.001	112	65.88	114	67.06	0.91
>70	210	52.76	59	22.26		58	34.12	56	32.94	
Localization					<0.001					0.24
Proximal	238	59.80	219	82.64		129	75.88	134	78.82	
Middle	63	15.83	21	7.92		15	8.82	16	9.41	
Distal	90	22.61	25	9.43		22	12.94	20	11.76	
Total	7	1.76	0	0.00		4	2.35	0	0.00	
Clinical Staging					<0.001					0.21
cT2 cN+/cNx	161	40.45	31	11.70	<0.001	30	17.65	31	18.24	0.99
cT3/cT4 cN0	23	5.78	26	9.81		15	8.82	15	8.82	
cT3/cT4 cN+/cNx	213	53.52	208	78.49		125	73.53	124	72.94	
Dissected LN (Median)	33 (1–105)		29 (5–71)		0.002	33 (7–105)		30 (12–71)		0.10
≤25	101	25.38	97	36.60		44	25.88	51	30.00	0.47
>25	297	74.62	168	63.40		126	74.12	119	70.00	
Complications					0.25					0.58
None	298	74.87	187	70.57		123	72.35	125	73.53	
CD I/II	67	16.83	46	17.36		30	17.65	24	14.12	
CD III-V	33	8.29	32	12.08		17	10.00	21	12.35	
pT					<0.001					0.11
pT0/is	0	0.00	14	5.28		0	0.00	6	3.53	
pT1a	10	2.51	5	1.89		1	0.59	2	1.18	
pT1b	35	8.79	21	7.92		5	2.94	7	4.12	
pT2	66	16.58	42	15.85		24	14.12	24	14.12	
pT3	183	45.98	139	52.5		92	54.12	99	58.24	
pT4a	84.00	21.11	38	14.3		40.00	23.53	28	16.47	
pT4b	14	3.52	6	2.26		8	4.71	4	2.35	
pN					0.65					0.27
pN0	141	35.43	104	39.25		55	32.35	53	31.18	
pN1	85	21.36	54	20.4		34	20.00	36	21.18	
pN2	74	18.59	51	19.2		33	19.41	38	22.35	
pN3a	70	17.59	44	16.6		28	16.47	34	20.00	
pN3b	28	7.04	12	4.53		20	11.76	9	5.29	
UICC					0.001					0.19
UICC 0	0	0.00	14	5.28		0	0.00	6	3.53	
UICC IA	34	8.54	18	6.79		5	2.94	4	2.35	
UICC IB	37	9.30	32	12.1		15	8.82	13	7.65	
UICC IIA	77	19.35	44	16.6		33	19.41	33	19.41	
UICC IIB	71	17.84	49	18.5		28	16.47	32	18.82	
UICC IIIA	83	20.85	50	18.9		38	22.35	38	22.35	
UICC IIIB	68	17.09	45	17		31	18.24	34	20.00	
UICC IIIC	28	7.04	13	4.91		20	11.76	10	5.88	

Table 1. Cont.

	Intestinal Subtype (n = 663), Unmatched					Intestinal Subtype (n = 340) PS-Matched				
	Surgery Only (n = 398)		CTX + Surgery (n = 265)		p-Value	Surgery Only (n = 170)		CTX + Surgery (n = 170)		p-Value
	n	%	n	%		n	%	n	%	
Grading					0.17					0.66
G1/G2	164	41.21	124	46.79		72	42.35	77	45.29	
G3/G4	234	58.79	141	53.21		98	57.65	93	54.71	
R					0.08					0.86
R0	373	93.72	238	89.81		152	89.41	154	90.59	
R1	25	6.28	27	10.19		18	10.59	16	9.41	
Tumor regression grade										
Becker Ia/Ib			70	26.42				37	21.76	
Becker II			66	24.91				43	25.29	
Becker III			129	48.68				90	52.94	

Legend: cT1 = Mucosa/Submucosa; cT2 = Muscularis propria; cT3 = Serosa; cT4 = Adjacent organs; cN0 = no lymph nodemetastasis detected during staging, cN+ = locoregional lymph node metastasis evident during staging; CD = Clavien Dindo Classification; Staging according to UICC 8th edition; p-values printed in bold are considered statistically significant.

Table 2. Baseline characteristics for patients with diffuse Lauren subtype before and after PSM.

	Diffuse Subtype (n = 359), Unmatched					Diffuse Subtype (n = 210) PS-Matched				
	Surgery Only (n = 216)		CTX + Surgery (n = 143)		p-Value	Surgery Only (n = 105)		CTX + Surgery (n = 105)		p-Value
	n	%	n	%		n	%	n	%	
Gender					0.004					1.00
Female	114	52.78	53	37.06		41	39.05	42	40.00	
Male	102	47.22	90	62.94		64	60.95	63	60.00	
Age	63.9 ±12.3		56.2 ±11.9		<0.001	60.8 ±12.1		57.1 ±12.4		0.03
<70	138	63.89	123	86.01	<0.001	84	80.00	85	80.95	1.00
>70	78	36.11	20	13.99		21	20.00	20	19.05	
Localization					0.03					0.14
Proximal	74	34.26	63	44.06		40	38.10	49	46.67	
Middle	63	29.17	35	24.48		30	28.57	24	22.86	
Distal	63	29.17	27	18.88		30	28.57	21	20.00	
Total	16	7.41	18	12.59		5	4.76	11	10.48	
Clinical Staging					<0.001					0.40
cT2 cN+/cNx	75	34.72	14	9.79	<0.001	15	14.29	14	13.33	
cT3/cT4 cN0	19	8.80	21	14.69		12	11.43	12	11.43	
cT3/cT4 cN+/cNx	122	56.48	108	75.52		78	74.29	79	75.24	
Dissected LN (Median)	34 (1–104)		30 (9–89)		0.01	35 (1–102)		31 (9–70)		0.13
≤25	55	25.46	36	25.17	1.00	26	24.76	23	21.90	0.74
>25	161	74.54	107	74.83		79	75.24	82	78.10	
Complications					0.77					0.4
None	160	74.07	107	74.83		81	77.14	76	72.38	
CD I/II	30	13.89	22	15.38		13	12.38	20	19.05	
CD III-V	26	12.04	14	9.79		11	10.48	9	8.57	

Table 2. Cont.

	Diffuse Subtype (n = 359), Unmatched					Diffuse Subtype (n = 210) PS-Matched				
	Surgery Only (n = 216)		CTX + Surgery (n = 143)		p-Value	Surgery Only (n = 105)		CTX + Surgery (n = 105)		p-Value
	n	%	n	%		n	%	n	%	
pT					<0.001					0.002
pT0/is	0	0.00	3	2.10		0	0.00	1	0.95	
pT1a	18	8.33	1	0.70		6	5.71	0	0.00	
pT1b	18	8.33	6	4.20		8	7.62	2	1.90	
pT2	16	7.41	8	5.59		4	3.81	4	3.81	
pT3	48	22.22	65	45.5		22	20.95	46	43.81	
pT4a	104.00	48.15	54	37.8		57	54.29	46	43.81	
pT4b	12	5.56	6	4.20		8	7.62	6	5.71	
pN					0.05	35	33.33	29	27.62	0.03
pN0	76	35.19	61	42.66		8	7.62	17	16.19	
pN1	23	10.65	21	14.7		23	21.90	20	19.05	
pN2	42	19.44	22	15.4		18	17.14	29	27.62	
pN3a	39	18.06	29	20.3		21	20.00	10	9.52	
pN3b	36	16.67	10	6.99						
UICC					<0.001					0.006
UICC 0	0	0.00	3	2.1		0	0.00	1	0.95	
UICC IA	29	13.43	6	4.2		12	11.43	1	0.95	
UICC IB	11	5.09	4	2.8		3	2.86	1	0.95	
UICC IIA	22	10.19	33	23.1		9	8.57	17	16.19	
UICC IIB	30	13.89	26	18.2		14	13.33	15	14.29	
UICC IIIA	48	22.22	33	23.1		28	26.67	32	30.48	
UICC IIIB	39	18.06	26	18.2		16	15.24	26	24.76	
UICC IIIC	37	17.13	12	8.39		23	21.90	12	11.43	
Grading					0.65					1.00
G1/G2	4	1.85	1	0.70		2	1.90	1	0.95	
G3/G4	212	98.15	142	99.30		103	98.10	104	99.05	
R					0.59					1.00
R0	173	80.09	118	82.52		81	77.14	82	78.10	
R1	43	19.91	25	17.48		24	22.86	23	21.90	
Tumor regression grade										
Becker Ia/Ib			22	15.38				9	8.57	
Becker II			37	25.87				25	23.81	
Becker III			84	58.74				71	67.62	

Legend: cT1 = Mucosa/Submucosa; cT2 = Muscularis propria; cT3 = Serosa; cT4 = Adjacent organs; cN0 = no lymph nodemetastasis detected during staging, cN+ = locoregional lymph node metastasis evident during staging; CD = Clavien Dindo Classification; Staging according to UICC 8th edition; p-values printed in bold are considered statistically significant.

Table 3. Baseline characteristics for patients with mixed Lauren subtype before and after PSM.

	Mixed Subtype (n = 187), Unmatched					Mixed Subtype (n = 112) PS-Matched				
	Surgery Only (n = 116)		CTX + Surgery (n = 71)		p-Value	Surgery Only (n = 56)		CTX + Surgery (n = 56)		p-Value
	n	%	n	%		n	%	n	%	
Gender					0.87					0.84
Female	40	34.48	23	32.39		19	33.93	17	30.36	
Male	76	65.52	48	67.61		37	66.07	39	69.64	
Age					<0.0001					0.79
<70	69	59.48	62	87.32		49	87.50	47	83.93	
>70	47	40.52	9	12.68		7	12.50	9	16.07	
Localization					0.04					0.21
Proximal	55	47.41	40	56.34		28	50.00	26	46.43	
Middle	23	19.83	20	28.17		12	21.43	20	35.71	
Distal	36	31.03	9	12.68		15	26.79	8	14.29	
Total	2	1.72	2	2.82		1	1.79	2	3.57	
Clinical Staging					<0.0001					0.93
cT2 cN+/cNx	39	33.62	10	14.08		11	19.64	10	17.86	
cT3/cT4 cN0	10	8.62	8	11.27		5	8.93	6	10.71	
cT3/cT4 cN+/cNx	67	57.76	53	74.65		40	71.43	40	71.43	
Dissected LN (Median)	34 (7–83)		30 (11–68)		0.02	33 (7–83)		30 (11–60)		0.19
≤25	24	20.69	24	33.80	0.06	13	23.21	20	35.71	0.21
>25	92	79.31	47	66.20		43	76.79	36	64.29	
Complications					0.89					0.81
None	84	72.41	51	71.83		43	76.79	40	71.43	
CD I/II	17	14.66	12	16.90		8	14.29	10	17.86	
CD III-V	15	12.93	8	11.27		5	8.93	6	10.71	
pT					0.17					0.41
pT0/is	0	0.00	3	4.23		0	0.00	3	5.36	
pT1a	2	1.72	0	0.00		0	0.00	0	0.00	
pT1b	11	9.48	7	9.86		5	8.93	6	10.71	
pT2	15	12.93	12	16.90		6	10.71	9	16.07	
pT3	43	37.07	30	42.25		24	42.86	24	42.86	
pT4a	40.00	34.48	16	22.54		18	32.14	12	21.43	
pT4b	5	4.31	3	4.23		3	5.36	2	3.57	
pN					0.02					0.03
pN0	27	23.28	29	40.85		10	17.86	23	41.07	
pN1	16	13.79	14	19.72		10	17.86	13	23.21	
pN2	23	19.83	5	7.04		11	19.64	5	8.93	
pN3a	35	30.17	17	23.94		17	30.36	12	21.43	
pN3b	15	12.93	6	8.45		8	14.29	3	5.36	
UICC					0.15					0.19
UICC 0	0	0.00	3	4.23		0	0.00	3	5.36	
UICC IA	8	6.90	7	9.86		2	3.57	6	10.71	
UICC IB	8	6.90	7	9.86		2	3.57	5	8.93	
UICC IIA	9	7.76	10	14.08		6	10.71	8	14.29	
UICC IIB	16	13.79	12	16.90		9	16.07	10	17.86	
UICC IIIA	26	22.41	11	15.49		13	23.21	10	17.86	
UICC IIIB	34	29.31	15	21.13		17	30.36	11	19.64	
UICC IIIC	15	12.93	6	8.45		7	12.50	3	5.36	

Table 3. Cont.

	Mixed Subtype (n = 187), Unmatched					Mixed Subtype (n = 112) PS-Matched				
	Surgery Only (n = 116)		CTX + Surgery (n = 71)		p-Value	Surgery Only (n = 56)		CTX + Surgery (n = 56)		p-Value
	n	%	n	%		n	%	n	%	
Grading					0.32					1
G1/G2	8	6.90	2	2.82		3	5.36	2	3.57	
G3/G4	108	93.10	69	97.18		53	94.64	54	96.43	
R										0.78
R0	100	86.21	61	85.92	1.00	48	85.71	50	89.29	
R1	16	13.79	10	14.08		8	14.29	6	10.71	
Tumor regression grade										
Becker Ia/Ib			14	19.72				12	21.43	
Becker II			21	29.58				18	32.14	
Becker III			36	50.70				26	46.43	

Legend: cT1 = Mucosa/Submucosa; cT2 = Muscularis propria; cT3 = Serosa; cT4 = Adjacent organs; cN0 = no lymph nodemetastasis detected during staging, cN+ = locoregional lymph node metastasis evident during staging; CD = Clavien Dindo Classification; Staging according to UICC 8th edition; p-values printed in bold are considered statistically significant.

The median follow-up was 30 months (range 1–242 months), comprising of 61 months (range 1–242 months) for survivors and 19 months (range 1–183) months for deceased patients. During the follow-up period 658 patients (54.4%) died, the five-year survival rate was 42%, the ten-year survival rate was 32%. Median survival was 38 months for patients undergoing primary surgery and 46 months for patients undergoing chemotherapy ahead of surgery ($p = 0.06$). Five-year survival rates (FYSR)/ten-year survival rates (TYSR) after primary surgery and after neoadjuvant/perioperative chemotherapy followed by surgery were identical (44/33%). The UICC stage dependent analysis revealed that this effect was only reproducible in UICC stage III (19 vs. 24 months median survival, $p = 0.03$), but not in the other UICC stages (UICC I: median survival not met, $p = 0.58$; UICC II: median survival 72 (surgery) vs. 57 (nCTx+surgery) months, $p = 0.7$). In patients with Lauren intestinal subtype, the median survival time was 51 months (45 months for primary surgery vs. 57 months for neoadjuvant/perioperative chemotherapy + surgery, $p = 0.025$), in the diffuse type group 33 months (35 months for primary surgery vs. 28 months for neoadjuvant/perioperative chemotherapy + surgery, $p = 0.16$) and 40 months (26 months for primary surgery vs. 62 months for neoadjuvant/perioperative chemotherapy + surgery, $p = 0.05$) in the Lauren mixed type group. FYSR and TYSR for patients with Lauren intestinal, diffuse, and mixed subtype were 48/35%, 39/31%, and 42/32%, respectively.

The following variables were included in the cox regression analysis: age, gender, localization, neoadjuvant/perioperative chemotherapy, UICC-stage, Lauren subtype, number of dissected LN, R-stage, grading, and postoperative complications, because these are the most relevant factors in predicting survival. The pT- and pN-stages were not included, as these factors are summarized in the UICC-stage. All of the factors were entered in the multivariate model without selection. Univariate regression analysis revealed age, tumor location (all locations), all UICC-stages, Lauren intestinal and diffuse subtypes, R-status, grading, and the occurrence of postoperative complications to be significantly associated with post-therapeutic survival (Table 4). The multivariate analysis demonstrated that age, localization (proximal, middle, distal), application of neoadjuvant/chemotherapy, all UICC-stages, all Lauren subtypes, R-stage, and occurrence of postoperative complications were significantly and independently related to postoperative survival. Because of the imbalanced baseline characteristics, propensity score matching (PSM) was performed, and further analysis was performed on the PS-matched cohorts.

Table 4. Univariate and Multivariate regression analysis for overall survival (OS).

Univariate	HR	CI 95%	p	Multivariate	HR	CI 95%	p
Age > 70	1.36	1.16–1.60	<0.001	Age > 70	1.46	1.24–1.73	<0.001
Gender [!]	1.06	0.90–1.25	0.48	Gender [!]	1.06	0.89–1.26	0.50
Proximal [$]	1.00		<0.001	Proximal [$]	1.00		<0.001
Middle [$]	0.59	0.47–0.74	<0.001	Middle [$]	0.56	0.44–0.72	<0.001
Distal [$]	0.67	0.54–0.82	<0.001	Distal [$]	0.79	0.63–0.98	0.03
Whole [$]	1.59	1.11–2.27	0.01	Whole [$]	1.03	0.72–1.48	0.88
nCTx	0.88	0.75–1.03	0.11	nCTx	0.84	0.71–1.00	0.05
UICC I [$]	1.00		<0.001	UICC I [$]	1.00		<0.001
UICC II [$]	2.39	1.77–3.23	<0.001	UICC II [$]	2.26	1.67–3.07	<0.001
UICC III [$]	5.23	3.93–6.92	<0.001	UICC III [$]	4.82	3.59–6.47	<0.001
Lauren intestinal [$]	1.00		0.016	Lauren intestinal	1.00		<0.001
Lauren diffuse [$]	1.27	1.08–1.51	0.005	Lauren diffuse [$]	1.40	1.15–1.72	<0.001
Lauren mixed [$]	1.19	0.94–1.49	0.143	Lauren mixed [$]	1.29	1.01–1.65	0.04
Number of LN dissected	1.06	0.89–1.27	0.51	Number of LN dissected	0.91	0.76–1.09	0.31
pR0	1.00						
pR1	2.49	2.01–3.09	<0.001	pR	1.55	1.23–1.94	<0.001
Grading (G1/2 vs. G3/4)	1.23	1.03–1.47	0.03	Grading (G1/2 vs. G3/4)	0.98	0.80–1.21	0.85
Clavien Dindo 0 [$]	1.00		<0.001	Clavien Dindo 0 [$]	1.00		<0.001
Grade I/II [$]	1.29	1.04–1.59	0.02	Clavien Dindo I/II [$]	1.27	1.03–1.56	0.03
Grade III/IV [$]	1.66	1.32–2.09	<0.001	Clavien Dindo III/IV [$]	1.47	1.16–1.86	<0.001

Legend: HR = Hazard Ratio, CI95% lower: 95% Confidence Interval lower boundary, CI95% upper: 95% Confidence Interval upper boundary, p = p-value, [!] male vs. female; [$] categorical variable, first value is reference (=1.00): Localization, UICC-stage, Lauren subtype, Clavien Dindo grade; p-values printed in bold are considered statistically significant.

Results after PSM

Those variables demonstrating clinically meaningful baseline differences within the respective Lauren subgroups were matched through PSM (age, gender, location, clinical stage, UICC stage) in order to balance possible confounders (Supplementary Figure S1). The matching algorithm matched 170 patients each (surgery/nCTx+surgery) in the Lauren intestinal, 105 patients each in the Lauren diffuse, and 56 patients each in the Lauren mixed subtype groups. Analysis of the baseline characteristics demonstrated that the following variables were then well balanced in all of the groups: Gender, age distribution, tumor localization, clinical stages, D2 dissection rate, number of dissected LN, postop complications, pT-stages (in the Lauren intestinal and mixed, not in the diffuse subtype), UICC (intestinal and mixed subtypes, not diffuse), and grading and R0 status. Tables 1–3 show the results.

Median follow-up was 26 months (range 1–242 months), comprising of 55 months (range 1–242 months for survivors and 16 months (range 1–144) months for deceased patients. During the follow-up period, 367 patients (55.4%) died, the five-year survival rate was 41%, and the ten-year survival rate was 25%. The median survival was 32 months for patients undergoing primary surgery and 43 months for patients undergoing chemotherapy ahead of surgery ($p = 0.16$). FYSR/TYSR after primary surgery and after neoadjuvant/perioperative chemotherapy, followed by surgery were 42/31% and 44/32%. The UICC stage dependent analysis revealed no significant survival differences for UICC stages I and II (UICC I: median survival not met, $p = 0.33$; UICC II: median survival 91 (surgery) vs. 80 (nCTx+surgery) months, $p = 0.72$). In UICC III, there was a statistically significant survival difference in favor of those patients undergoing neoadjuvant/perioperative chemotherapy (median survival 18 (surgery) vs. 26 (nCTx+surgery) months (*p* = 0.02), Figures S2–S4. In patients with Lauren intestinal subtype, the median survival time was 46 months (34 months for primary surgery vs. 52 months for neoadjuvant/perioperative chemotherapy + surgery, *p* = 0.07), in patients with diffuse subtype group 35 months (36 months for primary surgery vs. 31 months for neoadjuvant/perioperative chemotherapy + surgery, *p* = 0.44) and 57 months (31 months for primary surgery vs. 62 months for neoadjuvant/perioperative chemotherapy + surgery, *p* = 0.28) in patients with the Lauren mixed subtype. FYSR/TYSR for Lauren intestinal, diffuse, and mixed subtypes were 44/29%, 36/17%, and 43/33%, respectively. Kaplan–Meier analysis revealed that survival benefit for those patients undergoing neoadjuvant/perioperative chemotherapy was detectable for Lauren intestinal (*p* = 0.07) and mixed types (0.28) without statistical significance (Figures 1 and 2). The overall survival was (statistically not significantly) worse for Lauren diffuse type gastric cancer patients when undergoing neoadjuvant/perioperative chemotherapy (*p* = 0.44), (Figure 3). A survival benefit was detectable for Lauren intestinal type patients revealing histopathologic response (HPR) (median survival unmet vs. 43 months in non-responders and 34 months in patients undergoing primary surgery, *p* = 0.01) (Figure 4). There was no significant survival difference between patients undergoing primary surgery and non-responders to nCTx (*p* = 0.65) (Figure 4). This was not reproducible in Lauren diffuse type patients: The median survival was 21 months in responders vs. 33 months in non-responders (*p* = 0.52) and 36 months in patients undergoing primary surgery (*p* = 0.49). There was no survival difference in patients undergoing primary surgery and non-responders to nCTx (*p* = 0.5) (Figure 5). In the Lauren mixed type patients, there was a trend towards improved survival for responders without statistical significance: the median survival was 103 months in responders vs. 57 months in non-responders (*p* = 0.12) and 31 months in patients undergoing primary surgery (*p* = 0.13). There was no survival difference in patients undergoing primary surgery and non-responders to nCTx (*p* = 0.5) (Figure 6).

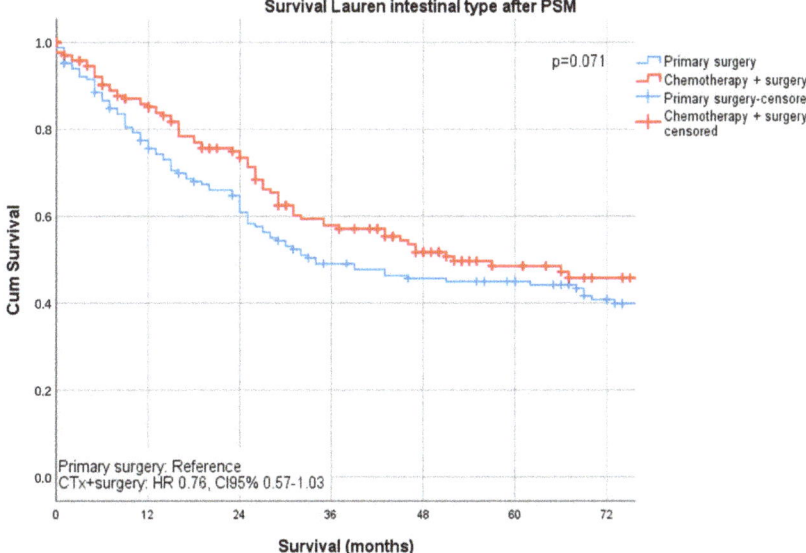

Figure 1. Survival curves for Lauren intestinal subtype after PSM stratified by surgery only vs. chemotherapy plus surgery.

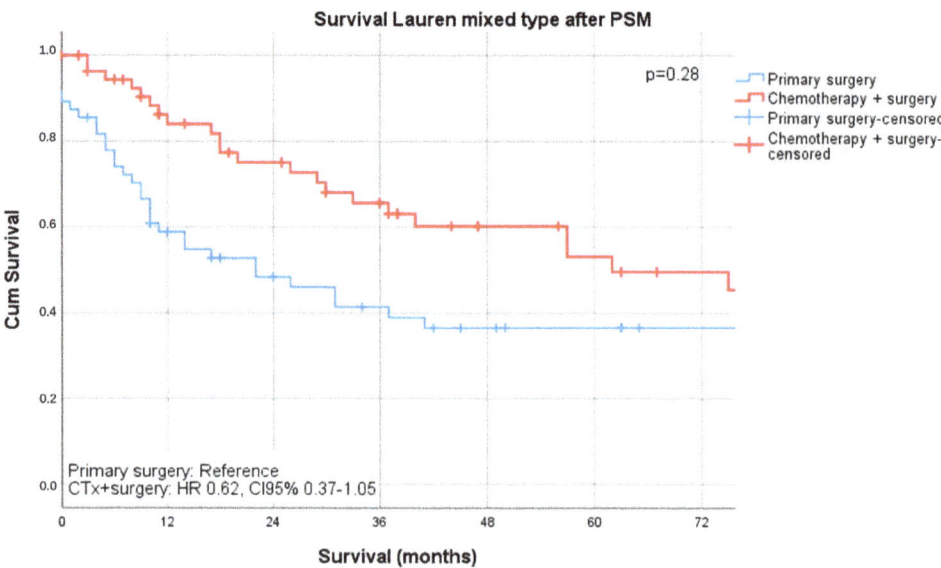

Figure 2. Survival curves for Lauren mixed subtype after PSM stratified by surgery only vs. chemotherapy plus surgery.

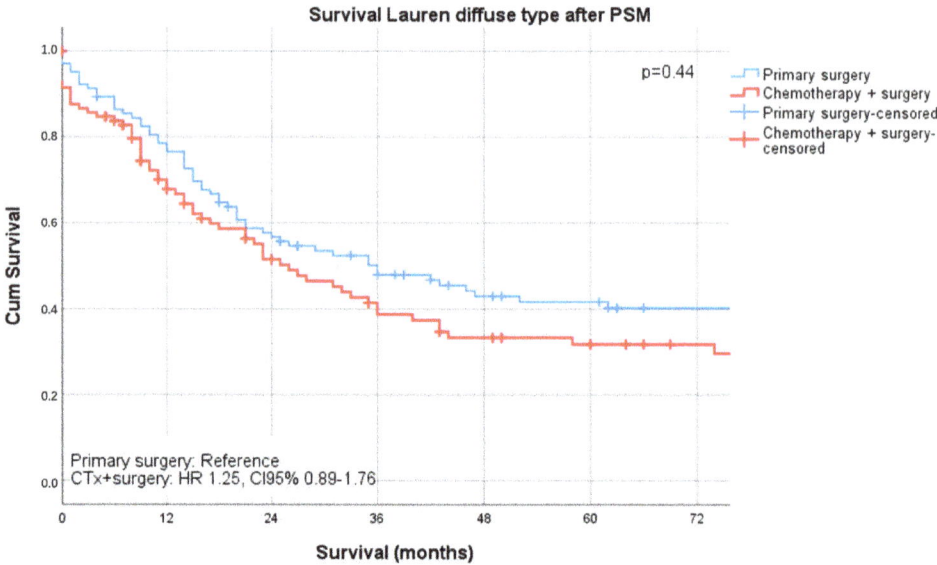

Figure 3. Survival curves for Lauren diffuse subtype after PSM stratified by surgery only vs. chemotherapy plus surgery.

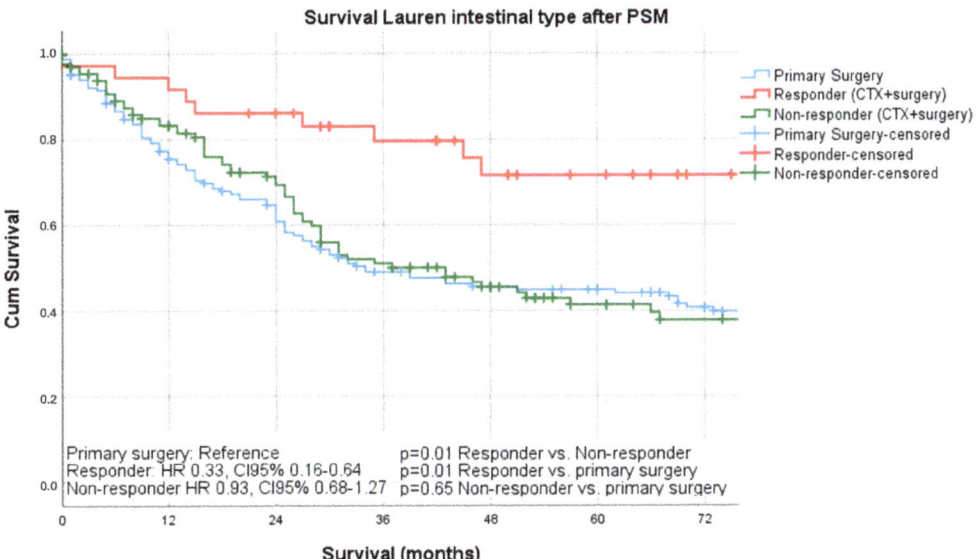

Figure 4. Survival curves for intestinal subtype after PSM differentiated by responders, non-responders, and surgery only.

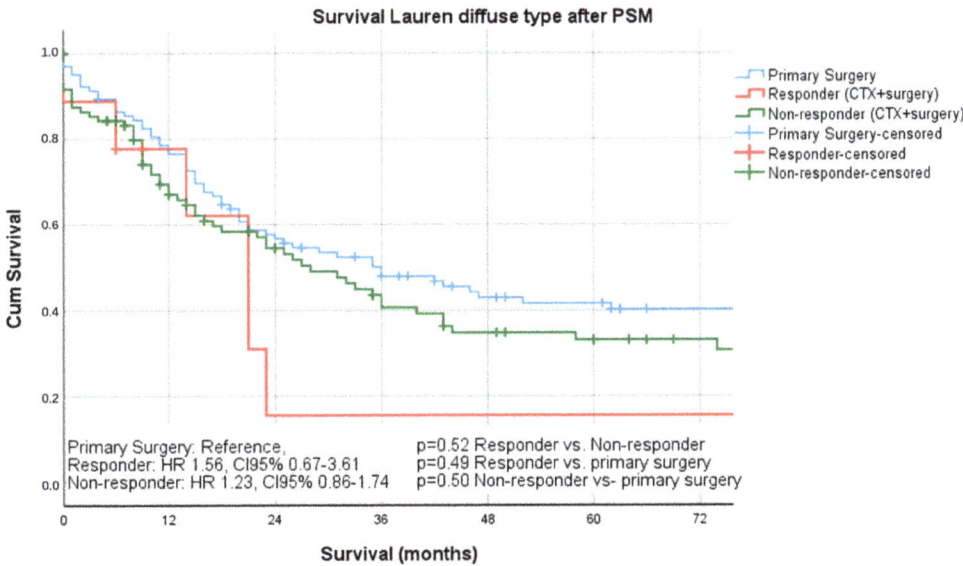

Figure 5. Survival curves for diffuse subtype after PSM differentiated by responders, non-responders and surgery only.

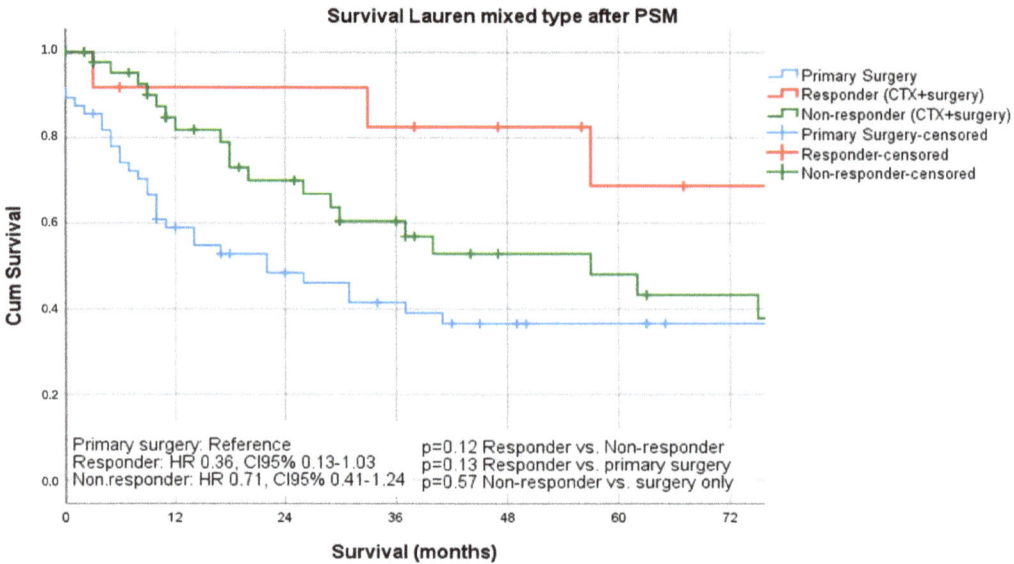

Figure 6. Survival curves for mixed subtype after PSM differentiated by responders, non-responders and surgery only.

Recurrence rates and disease free survival were analyzed for the PS-matched groups. In the intestinal type subgroup, the recurrence rates were 79/170 (46.5%) in the surgery only group as compared to 89/170 (52.4%) in the chemotherapy + surgery group ($p = 0.33$). Disease free median survival was 30 months (1–176) in the primary surgery group and 29.5 months (1–242) in the chemotherapy + surgery group (HR 1.12; CI95% 0.83–1.12; $p = 0.45$). In the diffuse type subgroup, the recurrence rates were 62/105 (59%) in the surgery only group compared to 67/105 (63.8%) in the chemotherapy + surgery group ($p = 0.57$). Disease free median survival was 24 months (1–176) in the primary surgery group and 17 months (1–204) in the chemotherapy+surgery group (HR 1.28; CI95% 0.91–1.81; $p = 0.16$). In the mixed type subgroup, the recurrence rates were 35/56 (62.5%) in the surgery only group when compared to 25/56 (44.6%) in the chemotherapy + surgery group ($p = 0.09$). The disease free median survival was 15.5 months (1–171) in the primary surgery group and 38 months (3–202) in the chemotherapy+surgery group (HR 0.52; CI95% 0.31–0.87; $p = 0.01$).

3. Discussion

This analysis of a large single center cohort, including 1209 patients, demonstrates an association between the benefit of neoadjuvant chemotherapy and the Lauren subtype. Based on the presented data, only those patients demonstrating the intestinal subtype benefit from the application of neoadjuvant chemotherapy for locally advanced gastric cancer. However, this only holds true for those patients developing histopathologic regression. In contrast, there was no benefit for those patients with diffuse subtype. In the diffuse type group, those patients undergoing neoadjuvant chemotherapy even demonstrated a deterioration of survival when compared to patients who had primary surgery. Patients with Lauren mixed type features revealed a potential benefit, especially those responding to chemotherapy; however, this was not statistically significant. Neoadjuvant/perioperative chemotherapy has become standard of care in Europe and it has become manifest in most of the guidelines for locally advanced gastric and gastroesophageal junction cancers [3,11–13]. However, in recent years, it has become increasingly clear that chemotherapy may not be effective for all patients in the same manner. The overall survival rates still range between 20–40% after five years [7,11,14,15]. This analysis surprisingly demonstrates that patients having undergone surgery only revealed survival rates around 40%, and this was improved to over 70% when intestinal subtype tumors demonstrated good histopathologic response. In many studies, the histological subtype was described as an independent factor of survival [15–18], but it also determines the effectiveness of the chemotherapy administered. However, the histological subtypes are so far not sufficiently respected in regard of therapeutic decisions, for which the clinical tumor stage is still the only tool to be applied when multimodal therapies are recommended. This is underlined by the present analysis, in which patients were subjected to neoadjuvant/multimodal chemotherapy without respect to the Lauren subtype. Taking into account that only 49 of 331 patients (15%) demonstrated real benefit from preoperative chemotherapy, it has to be stated that 85% of the patients were treated ineffectively and may even have been harmed by (ineffective) cytotoxic drugs (Figure S5). The Spanish AGAMENON research group already published a correlation between the response to chemotherapy and the Lauren subtype in 2017. They also pointed out that there were no subgroup analyses in the large therapy trials for locally advanced stomach cancer, although there were indications of a link [7]. Further, the AGAMENON study incorporated almost only patients undergoing treatment for metastatic disease, which is not comparable to the present analysis. Another important analysis was the multicentric retrospective FREGAT study, which analyzed a similar cohort [19]. However, the French analysis was related to the impact of signet ring cell differentiation on oncologic outcomes and not exactly to Lauren diffuse types. In the present analysis it was found that there was not a single Lauren diffuse type cancer without signet ring cells. None the less, Lauren diffuse types should not be equalized to signet ring cell differentiation. An international European group proposed a new definition for signet ring cell containing gastric cancer, as this is still a matter of debate between surgeons, oncologists, and pathologists [9]. However, this new consensus is neither ratified nor prospectively analyzed nor evaluated in patients undergoing neoadjuvant/multimodal chemotherapy. Biological and prognostic differences for gastric cancer are difficult to evaluate in studies due to the fact that there are different histological classifications for gastric carcinoma histological phenotypes and there is no uniform classification. This is considerably relevant when new chemotherapeutic regimens (FLOT) are propagated as effective in signet ring cell gastric cancer. The prospective FREGAT study (PRODIGE-19-FFCD1103-ADCI002) is currently the only trial that is going to elucidate whether direct surgery is a potential option for signet ring cell type gastric cancer [20]. Another factor that does not allow for direct comparisons is the issue that there is no broad consensus on which tumor regression classification to use (Becker, Mandard, Cologne, etc.). Certainly, this analysis should be replicated by different centers, applying different tumor regression systems in order to determine whether the Lauren diffuse subtype is a non-responding entity. Therefore, the aim of future studies should be to unify the different histological classifications for gastric cancer in order to further investigate the influence of histology on survival and prognosis.

The limitations of this analysis are certainly the monocentric character of the study, the long observation period during which both surgical and perioperative regimens have changed, different chemotherapy regimens having been used, and the fact that FLOT, as the current standard of care, is still underrepresented in this analysis. Although potential biases inherent to the Lauren type subgroups were possibly corrected by PSM, this method cannot compensate for unconscious and biological biases or those factors not having been determined. More than that, it is critical that the PSM resulted in a relatively small number of patients per group. Therefore, no exact statements can be made about unmatched patients. Another limitation is that the PS-matching did not balance adequately for the UICC stages in the Lauren diffuse type subgroup, so the balance is skewed towards more advanced cases in the nCTx+surgery group, which might limit further conclusions regarding survival prognosis. Further, the generalizability of the present results is certainly restricted, as the practice of neoadjuvant/multimodal chemotherapy is only evident in the Western (mostly European) world and the findings are not transferable to Asian patients, due to ethnicity and, more importantly, due to the fact that preoperative chemotherapy is not a standard of care in countries, such as Korea, Japan, and China.

Molecular markers, including microsatellite instability (MSI-H) and the Cancer Genome Atlas (TCGA) molecular subtypes [21], which could have influenced the results of our study were not assessed and is a limitation of our study. A recently published meta-analysis demonstrated that MSI-H could predict outcomes to neoadjuvant chemotherapy [22]. However, this same meta-analysis revealed that MSI-H comprised a very small proportion (2.4%) of non-intestinal type gastric cancers. In the present analysis the number of patients not responding to chemotherapy in the diffuse type group was markedly higher (>80% for non-intestinal type cancer), which does not explain the influence of MSI-status only. Beyond molecular factors, the amount of chemotherapy administered may have also been a confounding factor. Although most of the patients received neoadjuvant chemotherapy only (94.6%), relatively few patients (5.4%) received the perioperative FLOT/MAGIC regimens (i.e., pre-operative + post-operative). We are unable to determine the influence of post-operative chemotherapy on the outcomes in our study due to incomplete data available about the administration of post-operative chemotherapy. Nevertheless, despite these limitations, the results of our study raise questions regarding the benefit of neoadjuvant/perioperative chemotherapy in diffuse-type gastric cancer. Complete surgical resection remains the only curative option for gastric cancer patients, even if overall survival is markedly shorter for patients with diffuse-type histology as compared to intestinal or mixed type histologies. To the authors' knowledge, except for possibly MSI status, which represents a small proportion of patients, there is no existing biomarker in clinical practice that can adequately predict clinical and histopathologic response to neoadjuvant chemotherapy, and future research on identifying other molecular markers are needed.

The clinical implications of this analysis would be to carefully evaluate the application of neoadjuvant/perioperative chemotherapy in diffuse type patients. It remains speculative as to whether a multimodal treatment concept would be harmful for those patients, but it was demonstrated here that it is not beneficial either. Certainly, R0-surgery remains the only option of curation in these patients, even if the overall survival is markedly shorter than in intestinal or mixed type patients.

4. Materials and Methods

4.1. Patients

Data from patients who underwent curative surgery for gastroesophageal cancer at the Surgical Department of TUM School of Medicine from 1987 to 2017 were extracted from a prospectively documented database. The data were obtained from the medical records and then transferred to the institutional databases as soon as the patients were discharged from inpatient hospital care. The inclusion criteria for this analysis were: histologically proven gastroesophageal cancer (Siewert type II/III, all non-cardia cancers) staged cT2-cT4cN$_{any}$ undergoing neoadjuvant/perioperative chemotherapy after multidisciplinary team review, the Lauren histotype confirmed by expert pathologist (intestinal, diffuse or mixed type). The exclusion criteria were: Siewert type I, metastatic disease, hospital mortality within 30 days, loss of follow-up within a 60 months period, macroscopic residual cancer after surgery (R2), and indeterminate Lauren histotypes. Neoadjuvant/perioperative treatment consisted of either preoperative two cycles cisplatin or oxaliplatin/leucovorin/5-FU (PLF/OLF) only or perioperative three cycles of ECX/ECF (MAGIC) or perioperative four cycles FLOT [12,23]. All of the surgical procedures were performed according to the Japanese guidelines for GC treatment, including standardized D2-lymphnode dissection [24]. In the case of GE junction cancer (Siewert type II and III), the surgical procedure was extended to the distal esophagus. All of the patients received intraoperative frozen sections for the oral resection margin in order to confirm R0 resection. If the resection margin was positive, the surgical procedure was extended to the distal esophagus and esophagectomy was carried out whenever necessary. Circumferential and aboral resection margins were not determined intraoperatively on a routine basis. All of the resected specimens were examined by one or two specialized pathologists, being classified according to the TNM-classification and staged according to UICC-recommendations (8th edition) [25]. The histopathologic response was graded according to the Becker classification. Patients with 0–10% remnant viable tumor cells within the tumor area were graded as histopathologic responders (Becker Ia/Ib), whereas all other patients (Becker II (10–50% remnant viable tumor cells) and Becker III (>50% remnant viable tumor cells)) were graded as histopathologic non-responders [26]. Except for patients receiving FLOT or MAGIC regimens (n = 64, 5.4%, adjuvant chemotherapy was not considered on a routine basis. Following oncologic surgery, all of the patients were followed up every six to twelve months in an outpatient department (Roman Herzog Comprehensive Cancer Center) over the next five years by EGD and CT scans according to the institutional protocol.

Only deceased or surviving patients with a complete follow-up of at least 60 months were included in this analysis. Survival was computed from the day of surgery. The dataset consisted of patients' gender, age, location (upper, middle, lower third), clinical stages (cT2N0, cT1/cT2cN+, cT3/cT4cN0, cT3/cT4N+), number of dissected lymph nodes, postoperative complications (none, Clavien–Dindo Grade I/II and III/IV), pT-(pT1/pT2/pT3/pT4), pN-(pN0/pN1/pN2/pN3), and UICC-stages (UICC-I/-II/-III), grading (G1/2, G3/4), R-status (R0/R1), Lauren subtype (intestinal, diffuse, mixed), and follow-up period with survival status. Institutional Review Board (IRB)-approval for this study was obtained according to local guidelines (IRB Registration: 364/20 S).

4.2. Statistical Analysis

Descriptive statistics on demographic and clinical tumor characteristics were calculated as the mean ± standard deviation (continuous variables) and frequencies (categorical variables). The survival time was calculated from the day of surgery to death or last follow up date (at least 60 months after surgery for survivors). The Kaplan–Meier method was used in order to estimate the survival probabilities stratified by the application of neoadjuvant/perioperative chemotherapy. The log-rank test was used to compare the estimated survival. Survival prognosticators were analyzed by uni- and multivariate cox regression analyses. The variables that entered into the model were age, tumor location (all locations), all UICC-stages, Lauren intestinal and diffuse subtypes, R-status, grading, and occurrence of postoperative complications. After univariate analysis, all of the variables were entered in the multivariate model. Statistical analyses were performed while using SPSS version 25 (IBM Inc., Ehningen, Germany). PSM was performed with R and the MatchIt Plugin (Version 3.01, Vienna, Austria, URL http://www.R-project.org/). p-values of less than 0.05 were considered to be statistically significant. This retrospective analysis was approved by the local IRB (No.364/20s; Ethikkommission der Fakultät für Medizin, TUM School of Medicine).

5. Conclusions

In conclusion, the present findings demonstrate that the Lauren subtype might be a relevant prognostic factor in relation to overall survival after neoadjuvant/perioperative chemotherapy for locally advanced gastric or gastroesophageal cancer. Data from this analysis suggest that patients with a diffuse subtype may not benefit from neoadjuvant chemotherapy, but further exploration of other factors (e.g., molecular markers, MSI status, EBV-status, etc.), validation in prospective studies, and evaluation of other novel treatments (e.g., immune checkpoint inhibitors) are urgently required.

Supplementary Materials: The following are available online at https://www.mdpi.com/2072-6694/13/2/290/s1, Figure S1: Love plot for propensity-score matching of confounding variables within the respective Lauren type subgroups, Figure S2. Kaplan Meier curve for OS in UICC stage I of PSM-cohort, Figure S3. Kaplan Meier curve for OS in UICC stage II of PSM-cohort, Figure S4. Kaplan Meier curve for OS in UICC stage III of PSM-cohort, Figure S5. From 331 patients only 49 (15%) revealed histopathologic response and thus survival benefit.

Author Contributions: Conceptualization: A.N. and D.R.; Methodology: D.R.; Software: D.R.; Validation, R.S., D.R., A.N., J.S.-H., C.O. and H.F.; formal analysis: D.R. and R.S.; investigation: C.O., R.S. and D.R.; Data curation: C.O., R.S. and D.R., writing—original draft preparation: R.S. and D.R., writing—review and editing: R.S., A.N., C.O., J.S.-H., H.F., D.R.; supervision: A.N. and H.F.; project administration D.R.; All authors have read and agreed to the published version of the manuscript.

Funding: This research received no external funding

Institutional Review Board Statement: Institutional Review Board (IRB)-approval for this study was obtained according to local guidelines (IRB Registration: 364/20 S).

Informed Consent Statement: Informed consent was not required due to the retrospective nature of this study according to §27 Bayerisches Krankenhausgesetz.

Data Availability Statement: The data presented in this study are available on request from the corresponding author. The data are not publicly available due to European data protection regulation.

Conflicts of Interest: The authors declare no conflict of interest.

References

1. Guggenheim, D.E.; Shah, M.A. Gastric cancer epidemiology and risk factors. *J. Surg. Oncol.* **2013**, *107*, 230–236. [CrossRef] [PubMed]
2. Lagarde, S.M.; ten Kate, F.W.; Reitsma, J.B.; Busch, O.R.C.; van Lanschot, J.J.B. Prognostic factors in adenocarcinoma of the esophagus or gastroesophageal junction. *J. Clin. Oncol.* **2006**, *24*, 4347–4355. [CrossRef]
3. Cunningham, D.; Allum, W.H.; Stenning, S.P.; Thompson, J.N.; Van de Velde, C.J.H.; Nicolson, M.; Scarffe, J.H.; Lofts, F.J.; Falk, S.J.; Iveson, T.J.; et al. Perioperative chemotherapy versus surgery alone for resectable gastroesophageal cancer. *N. Engl. J. Med.* **2006**, *355*, 11–20. [CrossRef] [PubMed]
4. Ychou, M.; Boige, V.; Pignon, J.-P.; Conroy, T.; Bouche, O.; Lebreton, G.; Ducourtieux, M.; Bedenne, L.; Fabre, J.-M.; Saint-Aubert, B.; et al. Perioperative Chemotherapy Compared With Surgery Alone for Resectable Gastroesophageal Adenocarcinoma: An FNCLCC and FFCD Multicenter Phase III Trial. *J. Clin. Oncol.* **2011**, *29*, 1715–1721. [CrossRef] [PubMed]
5. Van Hagen, P.; Hulshof, M.C.; van Lanschot, J.J.; Steyerberg, E.W.; van Berge Henegouwen, M.I.; Wijnhoven, B.P.; Richel, D.J.; Nieuwenhuijzen, G.A.; Hospers, G.A.; Bonenkamp, J.J.; et al. Preoperative chemoradiotherapy for esophageal or junctional cancer. *N. Engl. J. Med.* **2012**, *366*, 2074–2084. [CrossRef] [PubMed]
6. Hass, H.G.; Smith, U.; Jäger, C.; Schäffer, M.; Wellhäuber, U.; Hehr, T.; Markmann, H.U.; Nehls, O.; Denzlinger, C. Signet ring cell carcinoma of the stomach is significantly associated with poor prognosis and diffuse gastric cancer (Lauren's): Single-center experience of 160 cases. *Onkologie* **2011**, *34*, 682–686. [CrossRef]
7. Jiménez Fonseca, P.; Carmona-Bayonas, A.; Hernández, R.; Custodio, A.; Cano, J.M.; Lacalle, A.; Echavarria, I.; Macias, I.; Mangas, M.; Visa, L.; et al. Lauren subtypes of advanced gastric cancer influence survival and response to chemotherapy: Real-world data from the AGAMENON National Cancer Registry. *Br. J. Cancer* **2017**, *117*, 775–782. [CrossRef]
8. Piessen, G.; Messager, M.; Robb, W.B.; Bonnetain, F.; Mariette, C. Gastric signet ring cell carcinoma: How to investigate its impact on survival. *J. Clin. Oncol.* **2013**, *31*, 2059–2060. [CrossRef]
9. Mariette, C.; Carneiro, F.; Grabsch, H.I.; van der Post, R.S.; Allum, W.; de Manzoni, G.; European Chapter of International Gastric Cancer, A. Consensus on the pathological definition and classification of poorly cohesive gastric carcinoma. *Gastric Cancer* **2019**, *22*, 1–9. [CrossRef]
10. LAURÉN, P. The two histological main types of gastric carcinoma: Diffuse and so-called intestinal-type carcinoma. *Acta Pathol. Microbiol. Scand.* **1965**, *64*, 31–49. [CrossRef]
11. Ronellenfitsch, U.; Schwarzbach, M.; Hofheinz, R.; Kienle, P.; Kieser, M.; Slanger, T.E.; Burmeister, B.; Kelsen, D.; Niedzwiecki, D.; Schuhmacher, C.; et al. Preoperative chemo(radio)therapy versus primary surgery for gastroesophageal adenocarcinoma: Systematic review with meta-analysis combining individual patient and aggregate data. *Eur. J. Cancer* **2013**, *49*, 3149–3158. [CrossRef] [PubMed]
12. Schuhmacher, C.; Gretschel, S.; Lordick, F.; Reichardt, P.; Hohenberger, W.; Eisenberger, C.F.; Haag, C.; Mauer, M.E.; Hasan, B.; Welch, J.; et al. Neoadjuvant chemotherapy compared with surgery alone for locally advanced cancer of the stomach and cardia: European Organisation for Research and Treatment of Cancer randomized trial 40954. *J. Clin. Oncol* **2010**, *28*, 5210–5218. [CrossRef]
13. Moehler, M.; Al-Batran, S.E.; Andus, T.; Anthuber, M.; Arends, J.; Arnold, D.; Aust, D.; Baier, P.; Baretton, G.; Bernhardt, J.; et al. German S3-guideline "Diagnosis and treatment of esophagogastric cancer". *Z Gastroenterol.* **2011**, *49*, 461–531. [CrossRef]
14. Petrelli, F.; Berenato, R.; Turati, L.; Mennitto, A.; Steccanella, F.; Caporale, M.; Dallera, P.; de Braud, F.; Pezzica, E.; Di Bartolomeo, M.; et al. Prognostic value of diffuse versus intestinal histotype in patients with gastric cancer: A systematic review and meta-analysis. *J. Gastrointest Oncol.* **2017**, *8*, 148–163. [CrossRef]
15. Lee, J.H.; Chang, K.K.; Yoon, C.; Tang, L.H.; Strong, V.E.; Yoon, S.S. Lauren Histologic Type Is the Most Important Factor Associated With Pattern of Recurrence Following Resection of Gastric Adenocarcinoma. *Ann. Surg.* **2018**, *267*, 105–113. [CrossRef]

16. Pattison, S.; Mitchell, C.; Lade, S.; Leong, T.; Busuttil, R.A.; Boussioutas, A. Early relapses after adjuvant chemotherapy suggests primary chemoresistance in diffuse gastric cancer. *PLoS ONE* **2017**, *12*, e0183891. [CrossRef] [PubMed]
17. Huang, S.C.; Ng, K.F.; Yeh, T.S.; Cheng, C.T.; Lin, J.S.; Liu, Y.J.; Chuang, H.C.; Chen, T.C. Subtraction of Epstein-Barr virus and microsatellite instability genotypes from the Lauren histotypes: Combined molecular and histologic subtyping with clinicopathological and prognostic significance validated in a cohort of 1248 cases. *Int. J. Cancer* **2019**, *145*, 3218–3230. [CrossRef]
18. Van der Kaaij, R.T.; Snaebjornsson, P.; Voncken, F.E.; van Dieren, J.M.; Jansen, E.P.; Sikorska, K.; Cats, A.; van Sandick, J.W. The prognostic and potentially predictive value of the Lauren classification in oesophageal adenocarcinoma. *Eur. J. Cancer* **2017**, *76*, 27–35. [CrossRef] [PubMed]
19. Messager, M.; Lefevre, J.H.; Pichot-Delahaye, V.; Souadka, A.; Piessen, G.; Mariette, C. The impact of perioperative chemotherapy on survival in patients with gastric signet ring cell adenocarcinoma: A multicenter comparative study. *Ann. Surg.* **2011**, *254*, 684–693. [CrossRef]
20. Piessen, G.; Messager, M.; Le Malicot, K.; Robb, W.B.; Di Fiore, F.; Guilbert, M.; Moreau, M.; Christophe, V.; Adenis, A.; Mariette, C. Phase II/III multicentre randomised controlled trial evaluating a strategy of primary surgery and adjuvant chemotherapy versus peri-operative chemotherapy for resectable gastric signet ring cell adenocarcinomas—PRODIGE 19—FFCD1103—ADCI002. *BMC Cancer* **2013**, *13*, 281. [CrossRef] [PubMed]
21. Cancer Genome Atlas Research Network. Comprehensive molecular characterization of gastric adenocarcinoma. *Nature* **2014**, *513*, 202–209. [CrossRef] [PubMed]
22. Pietrantonio, F.; Miceli, R.; Raimondi, A.; Kim, Y.W.; Kang, W.K.; Langley, R.E.; Choi, Y.Y.; Kim, K.M.; Nankivell, M.G.; Morano, F.; et al. Individual Patient Data Meta-Analysis of the Value of Microsatellite Instability As a Biomarker in Gastric Cancer. *J. Clin. Oncol.* **2019**, *37*, 3392–3400. [CrossRef] [PubMed]
23. Al-Batran, S.E.; Homann, N.; Pauligk, C.; Goetze, T.O.; Meiler, J.; Kasper, S.; Kopp, H.G.; Mayer, F.; Haag, G.M.; Luley, K.; et al. Perioperative chemotherapy with fluorouracil plus leucovorin, oxaliplatin, and docetaxel versus fluorouracil or capecitabine plus cisplatin and epirubicin for locally advanced, resectable gastric or gastro-oesophageal junction adenocarcinoma (FLOT4): A randomised, phase 2/3 trial. *Lancet* **2019**, *393*, 1948–1957. [CrossRef] [PubMed]
24. Japanese Gastric Cancer Association. Japanese gastric cancer treatment guidelines 2014 (ver. 4). *Gastric Cancer* **2017**, *20*, 1–19. [CrossRef]
25. Sano, T.; Coit, D.G.; Kim, H.H.; Roviello, F.; Kassab, P.; Wittekind, C.; Yamamoto, Y.; Ohashi, Y. Proposal of a new stage grouping of gastric cancer for TNM classification: International Gastric Cancer Association staging project. *Gastric Cancer* **2017**, *20*, 217–225. [CrossRef]
26. Becker, K.; Mueller, J.D.; Schulmacher, C.; Ott, K.; Fink, U.; Busch, R.; Böttcher, K.; Siewert, J.R.; Höfler, H. Histomorphology and grading of regression in gastric carcinoma treated with neoadjuvant chemotherapy. *Cancer* **2003**, *98*, 1521–1530. [CrossRef]

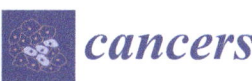

Review

Progress in Multimodal Treatment for Advanced Esophageal Squamous Cell Carcinoma: Results of Multi-Institutional Trials Conducted in Japan

Kazuo Koyanagi *, Kohei Kanamori, Yamato Ninomiya, Kentaro Yatabe, Tadashi Higuchi, Miho Yamamoto, Kohei Tajima and Soji Ozawa

Department of Gastroenterological Surgery, Tokai University School of Medicine, Isehara 259-1193, Japan; heyhey.cohey@gmail.com (K.K.); yamato.ninomiya@gmail.com (Y.N.); k-yatabe@tokai-u.jp (K.Y.); tadashi.h@tsc.u-tokai.ac.jp (T.H.); miho-n@is.icc.u-tokai.ac.jp (M.Y.); tadidas0203@gmail.com (K.T.); sozawa@tokai.ac.jp (S.O.)
* Correspondence: kkoyanagi@tsc.u-tokai.ac.jp; Tel.: +81-463-93-1121

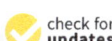

Citation: Koyanagi, K.; Kanamori, K.; Ninomiya, Y.; Yatabe, K.; Higuchi, T.; Yamamoto, M.; Tajima, K.; Ozawa, S. Progress in Multimodal Treatment for Advanced Esophageal Squamous Cell Carcinoma: Results of Multi-Institutional Trials Conducted in Japan. *Cancers* **2021**, *13*, 51. https://dx.doi.org/10.3390/cancers13010051

Received: 26 October 2020
Accepted: 24 December 2020
Published: 27 December 2020

Publisher's Note: MDPI stays neutral with regard to jurisdictional claims in published maps and institutional affiliations.

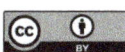

Copyright: © 2020 by the authors. Licensee MDPI, Basel, Switzerland. This article is an open access article distributed under the terms and conditions of the Creative Commons Attribution (CC BY) license (https://creativecommons.org/licenses/by/4.0/).

Simple Summary: In Japan, the therapeutic strategies for esophageal squamous cell carcinoma (ESCC) are based on the results of multi-institutional trials conducted by the Japan Esophageal Oncology Group (JEOG), a subgroup of the Japan Clinical Oncology Group (JCOG). Since there are several differences in the factors influencing the treatment approach for esophageal cancer between Eastern and Western countries, the therapeutic strategies adopted in Asian countries, especially Japan, are often different from those in Western countries. Because a transthoracic esophagectomy with three-field lymph node dissection has been performed as a standard surgical procedure for advanced thoracic ESCC in Japan, multimodal treatment for ESCC has been developed to improve the surgical outcomes after this relatively invasive surgical procedure. In this review, we describe the history and current status of therapeutic strategies for ESCC in Japan with a focus on the results of clinical trials conducted by the JEOG.

Abstract: In Japan, the therapeutic strategies adopted for esophageal carcinoma are based on the results of multi-institutional trials conducted by the Japan Esophageal Oncology Group (JEOG), a subgroup of the Japan Clinical Oncology Group (JCOG). Owing to the differences in the proportion of patients with squamous cell carcinoma among all patients with esophageal carcinoma, chemotherapeutic drugs available, and surgical procedures employed, the therapeutic strategies adopted in Asian countries, especially Japan, are often different from those in Western countries. The emphasis in respect of postoperative adjuvant therapy for patients with advanced esophageal squamous cell carcinoma (ESCC) shifted from postoperative radiotherapy in the 1980s to postoperative chemotherapy in the 1990s. In the 2000s, the optimal timing of administration of perioperative adjuvant chemotherapy returned from the postoperative adjuvant setting to the preoperative neoadjuvant setting. Recently, the JEOG commenced a three-arm randomized controlled trial of neoadjuvant therapies (cisplatin + 5-fluorouracil (CF) vs. CF + docetaxel (DCF) vs. CF + radiation therapy (41.4 Gy) (CRT)) for localized advanced ESCC, and patient recruitment has been completed. Salvage and conversion surgeries for ESCC have been developed in Japan, and the JEOG has conducted phase I/II trials to confirm the feasibility and safety of such aggressive surgeries. At present, the JEOG is conducting several trials for patients with resectable and unresectable ESCC, according to the tumor stage. Herein, we present a review of the JEOG trials conducted for advanced ESCC.

Keywords: esophageal squamous cell carcinoma; multimodal treatment; neoadjuvant chemotherapy; neoadjuvant chemoradiotherapy; definitive chemoradiotherapy

1. Introduction

Multimodal treatment approaches have led to improved oncological outcomes of patients with esophageal squamous cell carcinoma (ESCC) worldwide [1]. Since there are several differences in the factors influencing the treatment approach for esophageal cancer, such as differences in the proportion of patients with squamous cell carcinoma among all patients with esophageal carcinoma, chemotherapeutic drugs available, and surgical procedures employed, between Eastern and Western countries, the therapeutic strategies adopted in Asian countries, especially Japan, are often different from those in Western countries [2]. In Japan, a transthoracic esophagectomy with cervical, mediastinal, and abdominal (three-field) lymph node dissection has been established and still performed as a standard surgical procedure for advanced thoracic ESCC [3]. Therefore, multimodal treatment for esophageal squamous cell carcinoma has been developed to improve the surgical outcomes after this relatively invasive surgical procedure. On the other hand, in many Western countries, the Ivor Louis esophagectomy is the standard perioperative treatment. In addition to the surgical procedures, the strategy of multimodal treatment for advanced ESCC, such as tumors invading deeper than the muscle layer and/or with regional lymph node metastasis, has evolved differently in Japan and in Western countries.

Considering these characteristics of surgical procedures in Japan, the Japan Esophageal Oncology Group (JEOG), a subgroup of the Japan Clinical Oncology Group (JCOG) has developed the optimal therapeutic strategies for advanced ESCC that were determined by multi-institutional trials [4]. We describe the history and current status of therapeutic strategies for esophageal squamous cell carcinoma in Japan and also the differences to those of Western countries, with a focus on the results of clinical trials conducted by the JEOG.

2. Postoperative and Preoperative Therapies Used for ESCC in Japan

2.1. History of Postoperative Therapy

2.1.1. Preoperative and Postoperative Radiotherapy

Preoperative radiation therapy was the predominantly employed postoperative treatment for ESCC in the 1970s. It was generally believed that this approach would improve the resectability of the primary tumor and prevent local tumor recurrence [5]. On the other hand, the superiority of postoperative radiotherapy was highlighted by some research groups, who reported lower postoperative morbidity and improved survival rates, based on a retrospective comparison with a control group [6]. Therefore, the JEOG conducted a randomized controlled trial (RCT) to determine which mode of radiotherapy, preoperative or postoperative radiotherapy, would provide better survival. This study (JCOG 8201, 1981–1983) compared preoperative radiotherapy (30 Gy) plus postoperative radiotherapy (24 Gy) with postoperative radiotherapy (50 Gy) only (Table 1). The results revealed significantly better survival rates in the surgery plus postoperative radiotherapy alone group as compared to that in the surgery plus preoperative radiotherapy plus postoperative radiotherapy group [7]. The results prompted a switch of the timing of administration of postoperative therapy for ESCC from preoperative to postoperative, and there was a general movement away from preoperative radiotherapy to postoperative radiotherapy.

Table 1. Overview of clinical trials of adjuvant therapy for ESCC in Japan.

Trial	Year	Stage Enrollment [†]	Phase	Group	n	Primary Endpoint	p Value	Summary
JCOG8201	1981–1983	I–III	III	Preoperative + postoperative RT	104	OS *: 13.1	<0.01	Postoperative RT alone group was superior.
				Postoperative RT alone	103	OS *: 21.6		
JCOG8503	1984–1987	I–IV (resectable)	III	Postoperative RT	127	5-year OS: 44%	N.S.	
				Postoperative CT (CV)	126	5-year OS: 42%		
JCOG8806	1988–1991	I–IV (resectable)	III	Surgery alone	100	5-year OS: 44.9%	N.S.	
				Surgery + postoperative CT (CV)	105	5-year OS: 48.1%		
JCOG9204	1992–1997	II/III, excluding T4	III	Surgery alone	122	5-year DFS: 45%	0.04	Surgery plus postoperative CT group was superior.
				Surgery + postoperative CT (CF)	120	5-year DFS: 55%		
JCOG9907	2000–2006	II/III, excluding T4	III	Preoperative CT (CF)	164	5-year OS: 55%	0.04	Preoperative CT group was superior.
				Postoperative CT (CF)	161	5-year OS: 43%		
JCOG1109	2012–2018	II/III, excluding T4	III	Preoperative CT (CF)		OS		Follow-up is ongoing.
				Preoperative CT (DCF)				
				Preoperative CRT				

ESCC, esophageal squamous cell carcinoma; RT, radiotherapy; OS, overall survival; CT, chemotherapy; CV, cisplatin plus vindesine; N.S., not significant; DFS, disease-free survival; CF, cisplatin + 5-FU; DCF, docetaxel, cisplatin plus 5-FU; CRT, chemoradiotherapy; [†] UICC at the time; * median, month.

2.1.2. Postoperative Radiotherapy versus Postoperative Chemotherapy

In Japan, cisplatin has been considered a useful drug for the treatment of esophageal cancer since the early 1980s. The JEOG conducted a RCT to determine whether postoperative radiation therapy or postoperative chemotherapy might provide the better survival rate. This study (JCOG8503, 1984–1987) compared postoperative radiotherapy (50 Gy) with postoperative chemotherapy (cisplatin 70 mg/m^2 + vindesine 3 mg/m^2 × 2 courses). At the time of this trial, 5-FU was not yet widely available, and the combination of cisplatin plus vindesine, which was the standard treatment for non-small-cell lung cancer at that time, was used in the study. Although the study did not reveal any significant difference in the 5-year overall survival (OS) between the two treatment arms, the results at least suggested that postoperative chemotherapy was not inferior to postoperative radiotherapy, which was the standard of care in the world at the time [8]. Therefore, chemotherapy with cisplatin became generally accepted as the postoperative treatment regimen for ESCC in Japan.

2.1.3. Postoperative Chemotherapy versus Surgery Alone

There have been marked advances in the surgical techniques used for esophageal cancer surgery, especially in regard to lymphadenectomy, including specific resection of the superior mediastinal cervical lymph nodes, which has become a standard procedure in Japan since the late 1980s. Therefore, the JEOG conducted a RCT to investigate whether postoperative chemotherapy could improve the survival in patients undergoing esophagectomy with three-field lymphadenectomy. This study (JCOG 8806, 1988–1991) compared surgery alone with surgery plus postoperative chemotherapy (cisplatin 70 mg/m^2 + vindesine 3 mg/m^2 × 2 courses) and revealed no significant difference in the 5-year OS rate between the two groups, so that esophagectomy with three-field lymphadenectomy alone was adopted as the standard of care for ESCC at that time [9].

Thereafter, two phase II trials indicated that CF was superior to combined cisplatin plus vindesine as postoperative therapy for advanced esophageal cancer. Therefore, the JEOG initiated a RCT to determine whether postoperative chemotherapy with CF was additively effective in improving survival as compared to surgery with two- or three-field lymphadenectomy alone for ESCC, pathologic stage II/III, except T4. This trial (JCOG 9204, 1992–1997) compared surgery alone with surgery plus postoperative chemotherapy (80 mg/m^2 cisplatin on day 1 + 800 mg/m^2 5-FU on days 1–5 × 2 courses). The primary endpoint of the study was the 5-year disease-free survival (DFS) rate, and the DFS rate in the postoperative chemotherapy group (120 patients) was better than that in the surgery-alone group (122 patients) (55% vs. 45%, $p = 0.04$); the 5-year OS rates were 61% and 52% ($p = 0.13$), respectively. The improved outcomes with postoperative chemotherapy were more pronounced in the subgroup with lymph node metastases [10]. Based on these findings, surgery followed by postoperative CF chemotherapy was considered as the standard of care for advanced ESCC patients in the late 1990s.

2.1.4. Postoperative Chemotherapy versus Preoperative Chemotherapy

While postoperative chemotherapy had been the standard of care for esophageal cancer in Japan, in the West, preoperative chemotherapy had remained the mainstay of treatment due to the high invasiveness of and morbidity associated with surgery [11]. Therefore, it remained controversial as to whether preoperative chemotherapy might have a superior effect on the survival of esophageal cancer patients as compared to surgery alone or surgery plus postoperative chemotherapy. Therefore, the JEOG conducted a RCT to determine the optimal timing of chemotherapy (preoperative vs. postoperative) in patients with locally advanced ESCC. In this study (JCOG9907, 2000–2006), patients with clinical stage II/III ESCC, excluding T4 cases, were randomly assigned to groups that received either preoperative or postoperative chemotherapy (cisplatin 80 mg/m^2 on day 1 and 5-FU 800 mg/m^2 continuous infusion over days 1–5, up to 2 courses with a 3-week interval). The primary endpoint of progression-free survival did not reach the discontinuation boundary, but the OS was better in the preoperative chemotherapy group (164 patients) than in the postoperative chemotherapy group (166 patients) ($p = 0.01$). An updated analysis showed that the 5-year OS rate was 43% in the postoperative chemotherapy group and 55% in the preoperative chemotherapy group (hazard ratio (HR), 0.73, 95% confidence interval (CI), 0.54–0.99, $p = 0.04$) [12]. In addition, preoperative chemotherapy was not associated with an increased risk of postoperative complications or hospital mortality [13].

There were three possible reasons for the favorable results of preoperative chemotherapy in this trial. First, downstaging was achieved with preoperative chemotherapy in some patients. The proportion of patients with clinical stage II was similar in the two groups, but the proportion of patients with pathological stage II or less was higher in the preoperative than in the postoperative chemotherapy group. Second, the frequency of complete resection (R0) was slightly higher in the preoperative chemotherapy group than in the postoperative chemotherapy group. Third, the completion rate of the protocol treatment was much higher in the preoperative chemotherapy group than in the postoperative chemotherapy group; protocol-based treatment with two courses of chemotherapy and R0 resection was completed in 85.4% of patients in the preoperative chemotherapy group, but in only 75.0% of patients of the postoperative chemotherapy group [14]. These results led to preoperative chemotherapy with CF becoming established as the standard of care for patients with stage II/III ESCC in Japan (Figure 1). Thus, the optimal timing of chemotherapy again changed from postoperative chemotherapy to preoperative chemotherapy.

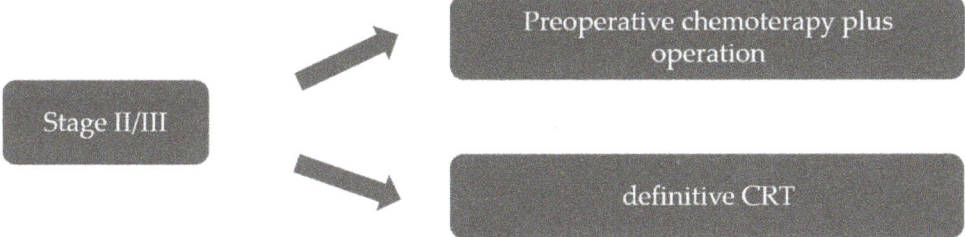

Figure 1. Treatment strategies for stage II/III ESCC, adapted and modified from guidelines of the Japan Esophageal Society. ESCC, esophageal squamous cell carcinoma; CRT, chemoradiotherapy.

2.1.5. Postoperative Chemotherapy for ESCC in Western Countries

Reports of postoperative chemotherapy for ESCC were very few. The French Association for Surgical Research performed a randomized controlled trial comparing surgery alone with postoperative chemotherapy using CF for patients with ESSC [15] (Table 2). Before randomization, they separated 120 patients into two groups, curative complete resection and palliative resection leaving residual macroscopic or microscopic tumor tissue. As a result, OS was similar in the two groups, with almost identical medians of 13 months in the postoperative group and 14 months in the surgery-alone group. The survival curves with or without chemotherapy were similar in the curative resection group and also in the palliative resection group. Based on these data, it was concluded that CF followed by surgery is not useful for patients with ESCC.

2.1.6. Preoperative Chemotherapy for ESCC in Western Countries

Ancona and colleagues compared surgery alone with preoperative chemotherapy using CF plus surgery for stage II/III ESCC [16]. The surgical procedure adopted in this study was transthoracic esophagectomy combined with two-field lymphadenectomy. The 5-year OS (primary endpoint) was 22% in the surgery-alone group and 34% in the preoperative chemotherapy group ($p = 0.55$). They concluded that improved long-term survival was obtained in patients with clinically resectable ESCC who underwent preoperative chemotherapy and obtained a pathologic complete response. They also emphasized the necessity of major efforts to identify patients who are likely to respond to preoperative chemotherapy.

Two pivotal RCTs in terms of preoperative chemotherapy are known worldwide, the Radiation Therapy Oncology Group (RTOG) and the Medical Research Council (MRC) trials, although both squamous cell carcinoma and adenocarcinoma were included. The RTOG trial compared surgery alone with preoperative chemotherapy using CF plus surgery followed by two courses of postoperative chemotherapy in operable esophageal cancer cases [17]. More than 50% of patients (53% in the surgery-alone group and 54% in the preoperative chemotherapy group) consisted of adenocarcinoma, and both transthoracic and transhiatal esophagectomy were performed as the surgical procedures without limiting the extent of lymphadenectomy. The median survival was 16.1 months in the surgery-alone group and 14.9 months in the preoperative chemotherapy group ($p = 0.53$). There were no differences in survival between patients with squamous cell carcinoma and those with adenocarcinoma. They concluded that preoperative chemotherapy with a combination of CF did not improve OS among patients with squamous cell carcinoma or adenocarcinoma. They reported, in a long-term update, that the median survival times were 1.3 years for patients receiving preoperative chemotherapy versus 1.3 years for those undergoing surgery alone [18]. They described similar outcomes to those described by other researchers, with objective response to preoperative chemotherapy being associated with better survival. Investigators in the Medical Research Council Oesophageal Cancer Working Party compared surgery alone with preoperative chemotherapy using CF plus surgery for resectable esophageal cancer [19]. Two-thirds of patients (67% in the surgery-alone group and 66% in the preoperative chemotherapy group) consisted of adenocarcinoma, and the surgical procedure was chosen by the operating surgeon. The median survival was 13.3 months in the surgery-alone group and 16.8 months in the preoperative chemotherapy group ($p = 0.004$), and the 2-year survival rates were 34% and 43%, respectively. Hazard ratios for treatment effect in patients with squamous cell carcinoma and those with adenocarcinoma were the same, showing that the effects of treatment were extremely similar for both histologic types. They concluded that preoperative chemotherapy improved survival in patients with resectable esophageal cancer. In long-term update results of this trial, they reported that the 5-year survival was 17.1% in the surgery-alone group and 23.0% in the preoperative chemotherapy group, with consistent treatment effect achieved in both histologic types [20]. They emphasized that preoperative chemotherapy is an essential standard of care for patients with resectable esophageal cancer. Because two pivotal studies demonstrated completely different conclusions, the benefit of preoperative chemotherapy, even when limited to patients with ESCC was controversial, and there seems to be no current worldwide consensus as to the optimal preoperative chemotherapy.

2.1.7. Preoperative Chemoradiotherapy for ESCC in Western Countries

A Dutch group (Chemoradiotherapy for Oesophageal Cancer Followed by Surgery Study (CROSS) Group) compared surgery alone with preoperative chemoradiotherapy followed by surgery for potentially curable squamous cell carcinoma (23%) or adenocarcinoma (75%) of the esophagus or the esophagogastric junction. A transthoracic esophagectomy with two-field lymphadenectomy was performed. A transhiatal resection was preferred for the tumors involving the esophagogastric junction. The median survival was 48.6 months in the preoperative chemoradiotherapy group and 24.0 months in the surgery-alone group ($p = 0.003$), and 81.6 months and 21.1 months, respectively, for patients with squamous cell carcinoma. The 5-year OS was 47% and 33%, respectively. They concluded that preoperative chemoradiotherapy improved survival among patients with potentially curable esophageal or esophagogastric junction cancer, regardless of histologic subtype [21]. The result of this study supported preoperative chemoradiotherapy as a standard of care for locally advanced esophageal cancer in Western countries in which adenocarcinoma is predominant histologic type.

The most recent meta-analysis by Sjoquist et al. [22] included 12 RCTs comparing preoperative chemoradiotherapy vs. surgery alone, with a total of 1854 patients. A significant survival benefit was evident for preoperative chemoradiotherapy with an HR of 0.78 (0.70–0.88; $p < 0.0001$). In a subgroup analysis, the HR for squamous cell carcinoma was 0.80 (0.68–0.93; $p = 0.004$) and for adenocarcinoma it was 0.75 (0.59–0.95; $p = 0.02$). This updated meta-analysis provided stronger evidence for a survival benefit than the former meta-analysis conducted by the same group [23]. This analysis also compared preoperative chemotherapy to preoperative chemoradiotherapy and demonstrated a non-statistically significant survival benefit for preoperative chemoradiotherapy (HR 0.88, 0.76–1.01; $p = 0.07$). Therefore, controversy still exists as to whether preoperative chemotherapy or preoperative chemoradiotherapy is more beneficial [24]. A RCT comparing preoperative chemotherapy using CF (91 patients including 25 SCC patients) with preoperative chemoradiotherapy (90 patients including 25 SCC patients) was conducted in Sweden and Norway. They revealed that the addition of radiotherapy to preoperative chemotherapy resulted in higher pathological complete response (pCR) rate and higher R0 resection rate, without significantly affecting survival [25].

2.2. Future Candidates for Preoperative Therapy for ESCC

2.2.1. Adequate Preoperative Therapy

The results of a subgroup analysis in the JCOG9907 study showed that preoperative chemotherapy was more effective in clinical stage II or T1–2 esophageal cancer patients than in stage III or T3 patients, i.e., in patients with relatively early-stage disease. Furthermore, the low single-site recurrence rates of 31% and 25% in cases of tumor recurrence in the two groups could be attributable to our elaborate surgical technique. The results of this study suggested that preoperative chemotherapy with cisplatin plus 5-FU would be a good treatment strategy when aggressive surgery provides adequate local tumor control, but when the local tumor control is inadequate, more aggressive adjuvant therapy, such as more intensive preoperative chemotherapy or preoperative chemoradiotherapy, may be the preferable treatment strategy to obtain adequate local tumor control as well as systemic disease control. Docetaxel is one of the most promising agents for esophageal cancer, and an exploratory study of preoperative chemotherapy with DCF for locally advanced ESCC showed a favorable response rate (61.5%), with no treatment-related deaths. The therapeutic promise of docetaxel was demonstrated in a randomized phase II trial [26]. However, the clinical question of whether preoperative chemotherapy or preoperative chemoradiotherapy is superior still remained unresolved.

Under this circumstance, the JEOG initiated a three-arm randomized controlled trial (JCOG1109) in 2012, to confirm the superiority of DCF and chemoradiotherapy with CF (CF-RT) over CF as preoperative therapy for locally advanced ESCC in terms of the OS [27]. Patients in group A were treated with two courses of preoperative CF (cisplatin 80 mg/m^2 on day 1, 5-FU 800 mg/m^2 on days 1–5) repeated every three weeks; group B received three courses of preoperative DCF (70 mg/m^2 docetaxel on day 1, 70 mg/m^2 cisplatin on day 1, 750 mg/m^2 5-FU on days 1–5) repeated every three weeks; group C received two courses of preoperative chemoradiation (41.4 Gy/23 fractions) with two courses of CF (75 mg/m^2 cisplatin on day 1 plus 5-FU 1000 mg/m^2 on days 1–4) repeated every four weeks. Both transthoracic open esophagectomy and minimally invasive esophagectomy were acceptable in all three groups, and surgery should be performed within 56 days after completion of the preoperative treatment. Patient enrollment was completed in 2018 and follow-up of the enrolled patients is ongoing.

Table 2. Overview of clinical trials of adjuvant therapy for ESCC in Western countries.

Authors	Year	Stage Enrollment [†]	Phase	Group	n	Primary Endpoint	p Value	Summary
Pouliquen [15]	1987–1992	II–IV	III	Surgery alone	68	OS *: 14	N.S.	CF followed by surgery is not useful.
				Preoperative CT (CF)	52	OS *: 13		
Ancona [16]	1992–1997	II/III	III	Surgery alone	47	5-year OS: 22%	N.S.	OS was improved only in the patients with pCR.
				Surgery + postoperative CT (CF)	47	5-year OS: 34%		
Kelsen [17] (RTOG trial)	1990–1995	I/II/III (AC: 53%)	III	Surgery + postoperative CT (CF)	100	OS *: 16.1	N.S.	Preoperative chemotherapy with CF did not improve OS.
				Surgery + pre and postoperative CT (CF)	105	OS *: 14.9		
Working group [‡] [19] (MRC trial)	1992–1998	I/II/III (AC: 67%)	III	Surgery alone	402	OS *: 13.3	<0.01	Preoperative CT improved survival.
				Surgery + preoperative CT (CF)	400	OS *: 16.8		
Shapiro [21]	2000–2004	I/II/III (AC: 75%)	III	Surgery alone	188	OS *: 81.6	<0.01	Preoperative CRT was effective.
				Preoperative CRT	180	OS *: 21.1		
Sjoquist [22]			meta-analysis	Surgery alone	952	OS HR: 0.78 (0.70–0.88) §		Strong evidence for a benefit of preoperative CRT.
				Preoperative CRT	980			
				Preoperative CT	1141	OS HR: 0.88 (0.76–1.01) §		Advantage of preoperative CRT was unclear.
				Preoperative CRT	1079			
Klevebro [25]	2006–2013	I/II/III (AC: 72%)	III	Preoperative CT	91	pCR rate: 9%	<0.01	Preoperative CRT had higher pCR rate.
				Preoperative CRT	90	pCR rate: 28%		

ESCC, esophageal squamous cell carcinoma; CT, chemotherapy; CF, cisplatin plus 5-FU; OS, overall survival; N.S., not significant; pCR, pathological complete response; AC, adenocarcinoma; CRT, chemoradiotherapy; [‡] UICC at the time; * median, month; [‡] Medical Research Council Oesophageal Cancer Working Party; § 95% confidence interval.

2.2.2. Preoperative Therapy with Immune Checkpoint Inhibitors

Nivolumab and pembrolizumab are immune checkpoint inhibitors, newly developed drugs with antitumor activity. Until recently, no molecular-targeted drugs were approved for the treatment of advanced esophageal cancer, but in 2019, the FDA approved pembrolizumab as a second- or subsequent-line treatment for PD-L1-positive cases [28]. Strong PD-L1 expression is generally observed in esophageal cancers, with reported expression levels in the tumor cells of 15–83% and in immune cells of 13–31% [28–31]. Furthermore, in 2019, an international phase III trial (ATTRACTION-3) showed that nivolumab significantly prolonged the OS in patients with unresectable advanced or recurrent esophageal cancer who were refractory or intolerant to fluoropyrimidine and platinum as compared to the existing taxanes in an international phase III trial [32]. Thus, in Japan, nivolumab was approved in 2020 for use as second-line chemotherapy for patients with unresectable advanced or recurrent esophageal cancer. Based on these results, the JEOG has initiated a phase I trial (JCOG1804E) to evaluate the efficacy of preoperative chemotherapy with the addition of nivolumab to CF and DCF [33].

3. Surgery for ESCC in Japan

3.1. Techniques of Esohagectomy in Japan

3.1.1. Approach to Esophagectomy

Open thoracic and abdominal surgery remained the only surgical strategies adopted for esophageal cancer, before Cuschieri first reported thoracoscopic esophagectomy in 1992 [34]. Since then, thoracoscopic/laparoscopic surgery has been developed rapidly and is now considered as a less-invasive approach than open surgery. To date, several thoracoscopic or laparoscopic approaches for resection of thoracic esophageal cancer have come to be defined as minimally invasive esophagectomy (MIE), based on the tumor location, clinical stage, and patient demographics [35,36]. Although, total thoracoscopic esophagectomy and laparoscopic esophagectomy are representative of (total) MIE in a narrow sense, video-assisted thoracoscopic surgery (VATS) [37], esophagectomy with mini thoracotomy (up to an approximately 5-cm incision) in a wider sense, and laparoscopic approaches are also considered as falling within the scope of MIE [38]. In Japan, Akaishi et al. were the first to report the use of thoracoscopic total esophagectomy with en bloc mediastinal lymphadenectomy in 1996 [39]. After these exploratory studies, the number of MIEs performed has increased and there have been advances towards the standardization of surgical techniques.

We reviewed studies that compared the surgical outcomes of open transthoracic esophagectomy (OE) and MIE and found that MIE was not inferior to OE in terms of the accuracy of lymph node dissection and surgical invasiveness, and might also be associated with a reduced risk of respiratory complications [40].

Robot-assisted MIE (RAMIE) was first described in 2004 by Kernstine et al. [41]. In 2006, they published an account of their first experience with the use of RAMIE in combination with conventional laparoscopic surgery and showed that this new surgical procedure is technically feasible and associated with lower blood loss [42].

The da Vinci Robotic Systems (Intuitive, Sunnyvale, CA, USA) provides a three-dimensional magnified view of the surgical field [43]. Because of the theoretical advantages of robot-assisted surgery, including articulation of the instruments, tremor filtering, features allowing minimization of large movements for the surgeon, and better ergonomics, it has the potential to accelerate the MIE learning curve. The increased degree of freedom provided by the articulation of the surgical instruments might overcome the movement restrictions caused by the rib cage and improve the accuracy of lymph node dissection around the recurrent laryngeal nerves [44], which could be expected to lead to better outcomes and avoidance of recurrent laryngeal paralysis. Although RAMIE is spreading rapidly in Japan based on these theoretical advantages, there are still several issues to be investigated—the expensive cost of da Vinci Robotic Systems and the clinical usefulness compared with thoracoscopic surgery.

3.1.2. Three-Field Lymph Nodes Dissection

The importance of lymphadenectomy in esophageal cancer surgery has been well established around the world. Ever since Torek reported the first case of successful esophagectomy in 1913 [45], the safety and efficacy of esophagectomy for esophageal cancer have been reported by numerous researchers, and the range of lymph node (LN) dissection has been extended. Three-field LN dissection (3FD) was initiated by two Japanese Surgeons. Kajitani was the first to perform systematic dissection of the LNs around the recurrent laryngeal nerves and developed upper mediastinal LN dissection [46]. Sannohe then reported cervical LN dissection and the incidence of metastases in patients who underwent 3FD [47]. Following these reports, the safety and survival rates of 3FD were also shown by a number of reports in Japan [48–51]. Initially, surgical procedures were performed without considering recurrent laryngeal nerves, and recurrent laryngeal nerve paralysis occurred in many patients. However, with the improvement in surgical technique around recurrent laryngeal nerves, the frequency of recurrent laryngeal nerve paralysis had gradually decreased. In the 1990's, 3FD was accepted worldwide and its safety was established [52–54]. Kato et al. reported that patients with esophageal cancer who underwent 3FD showed better OS rates than those who received 2FD [55]. Igaki et al. showed that neck dissection is also important in patients with lower thoracic ESCC. They reported that 3FD for patients with LN metastases in the upper and/or central mediastinum can improve the survival rate as compared to 2FD, even in patients with lower thoracic ESCC [3]. Moreover, Altorki et al. reported 80 patients who underwent esophagectomy with 3FD, in 30% of whom the disease was upstaged following 3FD [52]. Based on these previous reports, esophagectomy with 3FD is currently adopted as the standard procedure for thoracic esophageal cancer in Japan.

We speculate the following reasons for the prolonged postoperative survival associated with 3FD. First, extended LN dissections may increase the curative potential of esophagectomy. Esophageal cancer can cause LN metastasis extending from the cervical to the abdominal fields, and an extended range of LN dissection could be expected to lead to better elimination of tumor cells. Second, extended LN dissection improves the accuracy of staging and leads to better postoperative survival in patients with each disease stage. Even if an upper mediastinal LN dissection could be performed with both 3FD and 2FD, the number of dissected LNs in the upper mediastinum would be higher in 3FD, because of the added cervical approach in 3FD. Therefore, 3FD may be beneficial for obtaining better postoperative survival.

Recently, several systematic reviews and meta-analyses have been reported. Shang et al. analyzed the long-term survival of the patients and showed that 3FD was superior to 2FD in patients with LN metastasis in the cervical or upper mediastinal LNs [56]. Ma et al. also conducted a meta-analysis and reported that 3FD was associated with improved survival rates following esophagectomy [57].

3.2. Salvage and Conversion Surgery

3.2.1. Terminology

Salvage surgery is generally considered as a surgical procedure for radical resection of a lesion that has failed to resolve, or that has resurfaced after radiation and/or chemotherapy, with the intent of cure. Conversion surgery, on the other hand, is considered to be a procedure that involves a change in treatment, such as from chemotherapy and/or radiation to surgical resection. The concept of induction chemotherapy, especially for patients with borderline resectable esophageal cancer, which involves deciding whether to perform conversion surgery or chemoradiotherapy after chemotherapy, has also been becoming popular recently, and clinical trials are under way in Japan. As described below, chemoradiation therapy for unresectable advanced esophageal cancer is also widely used. Salvage surgery and conversion surgery are playing increasingly important roles in the multimodal treatment of advanced esophageal cancer (Figure 2).

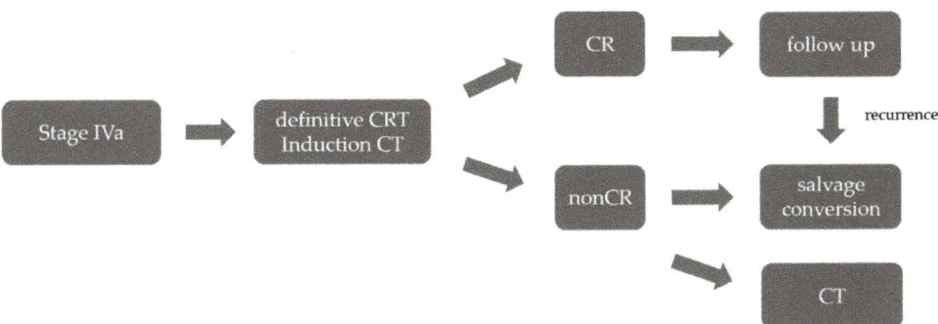

Figure 2. Treatment strategies for stage IVa ESCC, adapted and modified from guidelines of the Japan Esophageal Society. ESCC, esophageal squamous cell carcinoma; CRT, chemoradiotherapy; CT, chemotherapy; CR complete response.

3.2.2. Clinical Trials for Resectable ESCC

In 1999, a phase III trial conducted in the US in patients with T1-3N0-1M0 ESCC showed that CRT with CF concurrently with 50.4 Gy radiation yielded a significantly improved 5-year OS of 26%, as compared to 0% for radiation alone [58]. This made CRT a standard noninvasive treatment for patients who did not wish to undergo surgery. Therefore, the JEOG conducted a phase II study (JCOG9906, 2000–2002) to evaluate the efficacy and safety of CRT in patients with Stage II/III ESCC (Table 3). CRT was performed in 96 patients and the outcomes in the CRT arm were comparable to those in the preoperative chemotherapy plus surgery arm, and the toxicity was manageable. However, late toxicities, comprising Grade 3/4 esophagitis (13%), pericardial (16%) and pleural (9%) effusion, and radiation pneumonitis (4%), were observed, causing four deaths, and it was concluded that further improvement was required for reduction in the incidence of late toxicities [59].

In Japan, based on the results of trials, definitive CRT (dCRT) with 60 Gy of radiation in combination with CF therapy is adopted for patients with Stage II/III ESCC who do not wish to undergo surgery. However, the high incidence of late toxicities and of complications after salvage surgery have made dCRT for Stage II/III ESCC an option that could be considered. For this reason, the JEOG conducted a single-arm confirmatory study (JCOG 0909, 2010–2014) to evaluate the reduction in the incidence of late toxicities with a reduced radiation dose to 50.4 Gy, the improvement in the outcomes with the inclusion of salvage therapy, and the safety of salvage therapy. The 3-year OS rate was 74.2% (90% CI: 65.9–80.8), which was higher than the expected rate of 55%. Salvage surgery resulted in Grade 3/4 postoperative mobility in five patients (20%) and postoperative death in one patient (4%), but R0 surgery was possible in 76% of cases [60]. Salvage surgery was considered as an effective treatment option for limited indications, and CRT, consisting of radiotherapy at 50.4 Gy plus CF, became the standard of care for esophageal cancer patients in Japan who preferred nonsurgical treatment.

3.2.3. Clinical Trials for Unresectable ESCC

The JEOG conducted a phase II/III trial (JCOG0303, 2004–2009) of CRT for esophageal cancer patients with T4b disease or unresectable lymph nodes with standard-dose CF (Arm A) versus low-dose CF (Arm B). Because there were no differences in the toxicities between the two arms, Arm B was judged as not worthy of further evaluation in the phase III setting and the study was terminated [61]. Daily RT plus low-dose CF chemotherapy did not qualify for further evaluation as a new treatment option for patients with locally advanced unresectable esophageal cancer.

Table 3. Summary of clinical trials of CRT or induction chemotherapy for ESCC conducted in Japan.

Trial	Year	Stage Enrollment [†]	Phase	Group	n	Primary Endpoint	p Value	Summary
JCOG9906	2000–2002	II/III, excluding T4	II	CRT	76	OS *: 29		CRT was effective.
JCOG0909	2010–2014	II/III, excluding T4	II	CRT with/without salvage	94	3-year OS: 74.2%		CRT with salvage was effective and safe.
JCOG0303	2004–2009	T4b or unresectable LN	II	CRT (standard-dose CF)	71	OS *: 14.4	N.S.	Low-dose group was slightly inferior.
				CRT (low-dose CF)	71	OS *: 13.1		
COSMOS	2013–2014	T4b or unresectable LN	II	indDCF and CS/CRT	48	1-year OS: 67.9%		IndDCF and CS showed tolerability and efficacy.
JCOG1510	2016 -	T4b or unresectable LN	III	CRT indDCF and CS/CRT		OS		Patient enrollment is ongoing.

CRT, chemoradiotherapy; ESCC, esophageal squamous cell carcinoma; OS, overall survival; CF, cisplatin plus 5-fluorouracil; LN, lymph node; N.S., not significant; indDCF, induction therapy with docetaxel, cisplatin, and 5-fulorouracil; CS, conversion surgery; [†] UJCC at the time; * median, month.

In 2013, a multicenter phase II trial (COSMOS trial) was performed to assess the safety and efficacy of induction DCF chemotherapy and subsequent conversion surgery for initially unresectable locally advanced ESCC. Conversion surgery was performed in 41.7% of patients after induction chemotherapy or subsequent CRT, and R0 resection was achieved in 95% of these patients, with no serious postoperative complications. Induction DCF chemotherapy followed by conversion surgery as a multidisciplinary treatment strategy showed promise in terms of both the tolerability and efficacy in patients with locally advanced unresectable ESCC [62]. Based on these results, the JEOG designed a phase III trial (JCOG1510) to determine the outcomes of conversion surgery after induction chemotherapy [63]. The purpose of this study was to confirm the superiority, in terms of the OS, of induction chemotherapy with DCF followed by conversion surgery or dCRT over dCRT alone OS in patients with locally advanced unresectable ESCC, and patient enrollment is ongoing.

4. Discussion

In this review, we have shown the history and results of RCTs for advanced ESCC in Japan and also presented ongoing RCT conducted by JEOG. Thanks to the JEOG's continued efforts, we have been able to achieve better outcomes for advanced ESCC. Rationale for multimodal treatment for advanced ESCC in Japan is different from other Western countries—multimodal treatment for ESCC has been shown to improve the outcomes after surgical treatment. Non-surgical treatment has not been considered as standard treatment, therefore, RCT that compared the superiority or non-inferiority of non-surgical treatment over the esophagectomy has not been conducted. There are two possible reasons for this. One is that the prognosis of the patients was dramatically improved after introduction of three-field lymph node dissection. The other is that few drugs have been approved by national insurance and used for ESCC in Japan. In addition to cisplatin and 5-FU, until 2019, only docetaxel and paclitaxel could be used. In 2020, nivolumab was approved and is now available for unresectable and/or recurrent ESCC. Given these backgrounds, we believe that new perspectives should be considered for multimodal treatment of advanced ESCC. Quality of life (QOL) is considered as an important issue. Although three-field lymph node dissection could contribute the better prognosis, this kind of invasive procedure might reduce the patient's QOL. We also need to investigate new drugs that can be used for ESCC.

Identification of responders and non-responders for chemotherapy and radiotherapy is an urgent need based on the evidence that histological complete response is predictive of long overall survival. If it were possible to predict responders and non-responders, unnecessary toxicity, and time caused by unnecessary preoperative chemotherapy or chemoradiotherapy, could be avoided. Therefore, future RCT should focus on the identification of prognostic and predictive biomarkers as well as the integration of molecular targets. Clinical trials incorporating molecularly targeted therapeutics into multimodal treatment for esophageal cancer are being initiated. Although promising results have not been demonstrated yet, development of molecularly targeted drugs could contribute the progress of multimodal treatment for advanced ESCC.

Immune checkpoint inhibitors are already available in ESCC and are another promising candidate for multimodal treatment because strong PD-L1 expression is generally observed in esophageal cancers, with reported expression levels in the tumor cells of 15–83% and in immune cells of 13–31% [28–31]. Furthermore, in 2019, an international phase III trial (ATTRACTION-3) showed that nivolumab significantly prolonged the OS in patients with unresectable advanced or recurrent esophageal cancer who were refractory or intolerant to fluoropyrimidine and platinum as compared to the existing taxanes in an international phase III trial [32]. Immune checkpoint inhibitors have a different mechanism of action in cancer tissues to that of traditional anticancer drugs. Thus, nivolumab as well as well as pembrolizumab are expected to be studied as very promising candidates for multimodal treatment for advanced ESCC.

5. Conclusions

We have summarized the history and current status of multidisciplinary treatment for ESCC in Japan, mainly based on the results of clinical trials conducted by the JEOG. We are expecting the results of a three-arm randomized controlled trial of preoperative chemotherapy (JCOG1109) and a phase I trial (JCOG1804E) to evaluate the efficacy of adding nivolumab to preoperative CF and DCF.

Funding: This research received no external funding.

Institutional Review Board Statement: Not applicable.

Informed Consent Statement: Not applicable.

Data Availability Statement: The data presented in this study are openly available.

Conflicts of Interest: The authors declare no conflict of interest.

References

1. Mariette, C.; Piessen, G.; Triboulet, J.P. Therapeutic strategies in oesophageal carcinoma: Role of surgery and other modalities. *Lancet Oncol.* **2007**, *8*, 545–553. [CrossRef] [PubMed]
2. Law, S.; Wong, J. Changing disease burden and management issues for esophageal cancer in the Asia-Pacific region. *J. Gastroenterol. Hepatol.* **2002**, *17*, 374–381. [CrossRef] [PubMed]
3. Igaki, H.; Tachimori, Y.; Kato, H. Improved survival for patients with upper and/or middle mediastinal lymph node metastasis of squamous cell carcinoma of the lower thoracic esophagus treated with 3-field dissection. *Ann. Surg.* **2004**, *239*, 483–490. [CrossRef] [PubMed]
4. Fukuda, H. Development of cancer cooperative groups in Japan. *Jpn. J. Clin. Oncol.* **2010**, *40*, 881–890. [CrossRef] [PubMed]
5. Akakura, I.; Nakamura, Y.; Kakegawa, T.; Nakayama, R.; Watanabe, H.; Yamashita, H. Surgery of carcinoma of the esophagus with preoperative radiation. *Chest* **1970**, *57*, 47–57. [CrossRef] [PubMed]
6. Kasai, M. Surgical treatment for carcinoma of the esophagus. *J. Jpn. Surg. Soc.* **1980**, *81*, 845–853.
7. Iizuka, T.; Ide, H.; Kakegawa, T.; Sasaki, K.; Takagi, I.; Ando, N.; Mori, S.; Arimori, M.; Tsugane, S. Preoperative radioactive therapy for esophageal carcinoma. Randomized evaluation trial in eight institutions. *Chest* **1988**, *93*, 1054–1058. [CrossRef]
8. Japanese Esophageal Oncology Group. A comparison of chemotherapy and radiotherapy as adjuvant treatment to surgery for esophageal carcinoma. *Chest* **1993**, *104*, 203–207. [CrossRef]
9. Ando, N.; Iizuka, T.; Kakegawa, T.; Isono, K.; Watanabe, H.; Ide, H.; Tanaka, O.; Shinoda, M.; Takiyama, W.; Arimori, M.; et al. A randomized trial of surgery with and without chemotherapy for localized squamous carcinoma of the thoracic esophagus: The Japan Clinical Oncology Group Study. *J. Thorac. Cardiovasc. Surg.* **1997**, *114*, 205–209. [CrossRef]
10. Ando, N.; Iizuka, T.; Ide, H.; Ishida, K.; Shinoda, M.; Nishimaki, T.; Takiyama, W.; Watanabe, H.; Isono, K.; Aoyama, N.; et al. Surgery plus chemotherapy compared with surgery alone for localized squamous cell carcinoma of the thoracic esophagus: A Japan Clinical Oncology Group Study—JCOG9204. *J. Clin. Oncol.* **2003**, *21*, 4592–4596. [CrossRef]
11. Kleinberg, L.; Forastiere, A.A. Chemoradiation in the management of esophageal cancer. *J. Clin. Oncol.* **2007**, *25*, 4110–4117. [CrossRef] [PubMed]
12. Ando, N.; Kato, H.; Igaki, H.; Shinoda, M.; Ozawa, S.; Shimizu, H.; Nakamura, T.; Yabusaki, H.; Aoyama, N.; Kurita, A.; et al. A randomized trial comparing postoperative adjuvant chemotherapy with cisplatin and 5-fluorouracil versus preoperative chemotherapy for localized advanced squamous cell carcinoma of the thoracic esophagus (JCOG9907). *Ann. Surg. Oncol.* **2012**, *19*, 68–74. [CrossRef] [PubMed]
13. Hirao, M.; Ando, N.; Tsujinaka, T.; Udagawa, H.; Yano, M.; Yamana, H.; Nagai, K.; Mizusawa, J.; Nakamura, K. Influence of preoperative chemotherapy for advanced thoracic oesophageal squamous cell carcinoma on perioperative complications. *Br. J. Surg.* **2011**, *98*, 1735–1741. [CrossRef] [PubMed]
14. Tsukada, Y.; Higashi, T.; Shimada, H.; Kikuchi, Y.; Terahara, A. The use of neoadjuvant therapy for resectable locally advanced thoracic esophageal squamous cell carcinoma in an analysis of 5016 patients from 305 designated cancer care hospitals in Japan. *Int. J. Clin. Oncol.* **2018**, *23*, 81–91. [CrossRef]
15. Pouliquen, X.; Levard, H.; Hay, J.M.; McGee, K.; Fingerhut, A.; Langlois-Zantain, O. 5-fluorouracil and cisplatin therapy after palliative surgical resection of squamous cell carcinoma of the esophagus. A multicenter randomized trial. French associations for surgical research. *Ann. Surg.* **1996**, *223*, 127–133. [CrossRef]
16. Ancona, E.; Ruol, A.; Santi, S.; Merigliano, S.; Sileni, V.C.; Koussis, H.; Zaninotto, G.; Bonavina, L.; Peracchia, A. Only pathologic complete response to neoadjuvant chemotherapy improves significantly the long term survival of patients with resectable esophageal squamous cell carcinoma. Final report of randomized, controlled trial of preoperative chemotherapy versus surgery alone. *Cancer* **2001**, *91*, 2165–2174.
17. Kelsen, D.P.; Ginsberg, R.; Pajak, T.F.; Sheahan, D.G.; Gunderson, L.; Mortimer, J.; Estes, N.; Haller, D.G.; Ajani, J.; Kocha, W.; et al. Chemotherapy followed by surgery compared with surgery alone for localized esophageal cancer. *N. Engl. J. Med.* **1998**, *339*, 1979–1984. [CrossRef]

18. Kelsen, D.P.; Winter, K.A.; Gunderson, L.L.; Mortimer, J.; Estes, N.C.; Haller, D.G.; Ajani, J.A.; Kocha, W.; Minsky, B.D.; Roth, J.A.; et al. Radiation Therapy Oncology Group; USA Intergroup. Long-term results of RTOG trial 8911 (USA intergroup 113): A random assignment trial comparison of chemotherapy followed by surgery compared with surgery alone for esophageal cancer. *J. Clin. Oncol.* **2007**, *25*, 3719–3725. [CrossRef]
19. Medical Research Council Oesophageal Cancer Working Party. Surgical resection with or without preoperative chemotherapy in oesophageal cancer: A randomised controlled trial. *Lancet* **2002**, *359*, 1727–1733. [CrossRef]
20. Allum, W.H.; Stenning, S.P.; Bancewicz, J.; Clark, P.I.; Langley, R.E. Long-term results of a randomized trial of surgery with or without preoperative chemotherapy in esophageal cancer. *J. Clin. Oncol.* **2009**, *27*, 5062–5067. [CrossRef]
21. Shapiro, J.; van Lanschot, J.J.B.; Hulshof, M.C.C.M.; van Hagen, P.; van Berge Henegouwen, M.I.; Wijnhoven, B.P.L.; van Laarhoven, H.W.M.; Nieuwenhuijzen, G.A.P.; Hospers, G.A.P.; Bonenkamp, J.J.; et al. CROSS study group. Neoadjuvant chemoradiotherapy plus surgery versus surgery alone for esophageal or junctional cancer (CROSS): Long-term results of a randomized controlled trial. *Lancet Oncol.* **2015**, *16*, 1090–1098. [CrossRef]
22. Sjoquist, K.M.; Burmeister, B.H.; Smithers, B.M.; Zalcberg, J.R.; Simes, R.J.; Barbour, A.; Gebski, V.; Australasian Gastro-Intestinal Trials Group. Survival after neoadjuvant chemotherapy or chemoradiotherapy for resectable oesophageal carcinoma: An updated meta-analysis. *Lancet Oncol.* **2011**, *12*, 681–692. [CrossRef]
23. Gebski, V.; Burmeister, B.; Smithers, B.M.; Foo, K.; Zalcberg, J.; Simes, J.; Australasian Gastro-Intestinal Trials Group. Survival benefits from neoadjuvant chemoradiotherapy or chemotherapy in oesophageal carcinoma: A meta-analysis. *Lancet Oncol.* **2007**, *8*, 226–234. [CrossRef]
24. Hamilton, E.; Vohra, R.S.; Griffiths, E.A. What is the best neoadjuvant regimen prior to oesophagectomy: Chemotherapy or chemoradiotherapy? *Int. J. Surg.* **2014**, *12*, 196–199. [CrossRef]
25. Klevebro, F.; Alexandersson von Dobeln, G.; Wang, N.; Johnsen, G.; Jacobsen, A.B.; Friesland, S.; Hatlevoll, I.; Glenjen, N.I.; Lind, P.; Tsai, J.A.; et al. A randomized clinical trial of neoadjuvant chemotherapy versus neoadjuvant chemoradiotherapy for cancer of the oesophagus or gastro-oesophageal junction. *Ann. Oncol.* **2016**, *27*, 660–667. [CrossRef]
26. Hara, H.; Tahara, M.; Daiko, H.; Kato, K.; Igaki, H.; Kadowaki, S.; Tanaka, Y.; Hamamoto, Y.; Matsushita, H.; Nagase, M.; et al. Phase II feasibility study of preoperative chemotherapy with docetaxel, cisplatin, and fluorouracil for esophageal squamous cell carcinoma. *Cancer Sci.* **2013**, *104*, 1455–1460. [CrossRef]
27. Nakamura, K.; Kato, K.; Igaki, H.; Ito, Y.; Mizusawa, J.; Ando, N.; Udagawa, H.; Tsubosa, Y.; Daiko, H.; Hironaka, S.; et al. Three-arm phase III trial comparing cisplatin plus 5-FU (CF) versus docetaxel, cisplatin plus 5-FU (DCF) versus radiotherapy with CF (CF-RT) as preoperative therapy for locally advanced esophageal cancer (JCOG1109, NExT study). *Jpn. J. Clin. Oncol.* **2013**, *43*, 752–755. [CrossRef]
28. Shah, M.A.; Kojima, T.; Hochhauser, D.; Enzinger, P.; Raimbourg, J.; Hollebecque, A.; Lordick, F.; Kim, S.B.; Tajika, M.; Kim, H.T.; et al. Efficacy and Safety of Pembrolizumab for Heavily Pretreated Patients with Advanced, Metastatic Adenocarcinoma or Squamous Cell Carcinoma of the Esophagus: The Phase 2 KEYNOTE-180 Study. *JAMA Oncol.* **2019**, *5*, 546–550. [CrossRef]
29. Jiang, Y.; Lo, A.W.I.; Wong, A.; Chen, W.; Wang, Y.; Lin, L.; Xu, J. Prognostic significance of tumor-infiltrating immune cells and PD-L1 expression in esophageal squamous cell carcinoma. *Oncotarget* **2017**, *8*, 30175–30189. [CrossRef]
30. Guo, W.; Wang, P.; Li, N.; Shao, F.; Zhang, H.; Yang, Z.; Li, R.; Gao, Y.; He, J. Prognostic value of PD-L1 in esophageal squamous cell carcinoma: A meta-analysis. *Oncotarget* **2018**, *9*, 13920–13933. [CrossRef]
31. Qu, H.X.; Zhao, L.P.; Zhan, S.H.; Geng, C.X.; Xu, L.; Xin, Y.N.; Jiang, X.J. Clinicopathological and prognostic significance of programmed cell death ligand 1 (PD-L1) expression in patients with esophageal squamous cell carcinoma: A meta-analysis. *J. Thorac. Dis.* **2016**, *8*, 3197–3204. [CrossRef] [PubMed]
32. Kato, K.; Cho, B.C.; Takahashi, M.; Okada, M.; Lin, C.Y.; Chin, K.; Kadowaki, S.; Ahn, M.J.; Hamamoto, Y.; Doki, Y.; et al. Nivolumab versus chemotherapy in patients with advanced oesophageal squamous cell carcinoma refractory or intolerant to previous chemotherapy (ATTRACTION-3): A multicentre, randomised, open-label, phase 3 trial. *Lancet Oncol.* **2019**, *20*, 1506–1517. [CrossRef]
33. Yamamoto, S.; Kato, K.; Daiko, H.; Kojima, T.; Hara, H.; Abe, T.; Tsubosa, Y.; Nagashima, K.; Aoki, K.; Mizoguchi, Y.; et al. Feasibility study of nivolumab as neoadjuvant chemotherapy for locally esophageal carcinoma: FRONTiER (JCOG1804E). *Future Oncol.* **2020**, *16*, 1351–1357. [CrossRef] [PubMed]
34. Cuschieri, A.; Shimi, S.; Banting, S. Endoscopic oesophagectomy through a right thoracoscopic approach. *J. R. Coll. Surg. Edinb.* **1992**, *37*, 7–11. [PubMed]
35. Shichinohe, T.; Hirano, S.; Kondo, S. Video-assisted esophagectomy for esophageal cancer. *Surg. Today* **2008**, *38*, 206–213. [CrossRef]
36. Ozawa, S.; Ito, E.; Kazuno, A.; Chino, O.; Nakui, M.; Yamamoto, S.; Shimada, H.; Makuuchi, H. Thoracoscopic esophagectomy while in a prone position for esophageal cancer: A preceding anterior approach method. *Surg. Endosc.* **2013**, *27*, 40–47. [CrossRef]
37. Nagpal, K.; Ahmed, K.; Vats, A.; Yakoub, D.; James, D.; Ashrafian, H.; Darzi, A.; Moorthy, K.; Athanasiou, T. Is minimally invasive surgery beneficial in the management of esophageal cancer? A meta-analysis. *Surg. Endosc.* **2010**, *24*, 1621–1629. [CrossRef]
38. Osugi, H.; Takemura, M.; Higashino, M.; Takada, N.; Lee, S.; Kinoshita, H. A comparison of video-assisted thoracoscopic oesophagectomy and radical lymph node dissection for squamous cell cancer of the oesophagus with open operation. *Br. J. Surg.* **2003**, *90*, 108–113. [CrossRef]

39. Akaishi, T.; Kaneda, I.; Higuchi, N.; Kuriya, Y.; Kuramoto, J.; Toyoda, T.; Wakabayashi, A. Thoracoscopic en bloc total esophagectomy with radical mediastinal lymphadenectomy. *J. Thorac. Cardiovasc. Surg.* **1996**, *112*, 1533–1540, discussion 1531–1540. [CrossRef]
40. Koyanagi, K.; Ozawa, S.; Tachimori, Y. Minimally invasive esophagectomy performed with the patient in a prone position: A systematic review. *Surg. Today* **2016**, *46*, 275–284. [CrossRef]
41. Kernstine, K.H.; DeArmond, D.T.; Karimi, M.; Van Natta, T.L.; Campos, J.H.; Yoder, M.R.; Everett, J.E. The robotic, 2-stage, 3-field esophagolymphadenectomy. *J. Thorac. Cardiovasc. Surg.* **2004**, *127*, 1847–1849. [CrossRef] [PubMed]
42. van Hillegersberg, R.; Boone, J.; Draaisma, W.A.; Broeders, I.A.; Giezeman, M.J.; Borel Rinkes, I.H. First experience with robot-assisted thoracoscopic esophagolymphadenectomy for esophageal cancer. *Surg. Endosc.* **2006**, *20*, 1435–1439. [CrossRef] [PubMed]
43. Camarillo, D.B.; Krummel, T.M.; Salisbury, J.K., Jr. Robotic technology in surgery: Past, present, and future. *Am. J. Surg.* **2004**, *188*, 2–15. [CrossRef] [PubMed]
44. Suda, K.; Ishida, Y.; Kawamura, Y.; Inaba, K.; Kanaya, S.; Teramukai, S.; Satoh, S.; Uyama, I. Robot-assisted thoracoscopic lymphadenectomy along the left recurrent laryngeal nerve for esophageal squamous cell carcinoma in the prone position: Technical report and short-term outcomes. *World J. Surg.* **2012**, *36*, 1608–1616. [CrossRef] [PubMed]
45. Torek, F. The first successful case of resection of the thoracic portion of the oesophagus for carcinoma. *Surg. Gynecol. Obstet.* **1913**, *16*, 614–617.
46. Fujita, H. History of lymphadenectomy for esophageal cancer and the future prospects for esophageal cancer surgery. *Surg. Today* **2015**, *45*, 140–149. [CrossRef] [PubMed]
47. Sannohe, Y.; Hiratsuka, R.; Doki, K. Lymph node metastases in cancer of the thoracic esophagus. *Am. J. Surg.* **1981**, *141*, 216–218. [CrossRef]
48. Kato, H.; Tachimori, Y.; Mizobuchi, S.; Igaki, H.; Ochiai, A. Cervical, mediastinal, and abdominal lymph node dissection (three-field dissection) for superficial carcinoma of the thoracic esophagus. *Cancer* **1993**, *72*, 2879–2882. [CrossRef]
49. Baba, M.; Aikou, T.; Yoshinaka, H.; Natsugoe, S.; Fukumoto, T.; Shimazu, H.; Akazawa, K. Long-term results of subtotal esophagectomy with three-field lymphadenectomy for carcinoma of the thoracic esophagus. *Ann. Surg.* **1994**, *219*, 310–316. [CrossRef]
50. Fujita, H.; Kakegawa, T.; Yamana, H.; Shima, I.; Toh, Y.; Tomita, Y.; Fujii, T.; Yamasaki, K.; Higaki, K.; Noake, T.; et al. Mortality and morbidity rates, postoperative course, quality of life, and prognosis after extended radical lymphadenectomy for esophageal cancer. Comparison of three-field lymphadenectomy with two-field lymphadenectomy. *Ann. Surg.* **1995**, *222*, 654–662. [CrossRef]
51. Ando, N.; Ozawa, S.; Kitagawa, Y.; Shinozawa, Y.; Kitajima, M. Improvement in the results of surgical treatment of advanced squamous esophageal carcinoma during 15 consecutive years. *Ann. Surg.* **2000**, *232*, 225–232. [CrossRef] [PubMed]
52. Altorki, N.; Kent, M.; Ferrara, C.; Port, J. Three-field lymph node dissection for squamous cell and adenocarcinoma of the esophagus. *Ann. Surg.* **2002**, *236*, 177–183. [CrossRef] [PubMed]
53. Lerut, T.; Nafteux, P.; Moons, J.; Coosemans, W.; Decker, G.; De Leyn, P.; Van Raemdonck, D.; Ectors, N. Three-field lymphadenectomy for carcinoma of the esophagus and gastroesophageal junction in 174 R0 resections: Impact on staging, disease-free survival, and outcome: A plea for adaptation of TNM classification in upper-half esophageal carcinoma. *Ann. Surg.* **2004**, *240*, 962–972. [CrossRef] [PubMed]
54. Fang, W.T.; Chen, W.H.; Chen, Y.; Jiang, Y. Selective three-field lymphadenectomy for thoracic esophageal squamous carcinoma. *Dis. Esophagus* **2007**, *20*, 206–211. [CrossRef] [PubMed]
55. Kato, H.; Watanabe, H.; Tachimori, Y.; Iizuka, T. Evaluation of neck lymph node dissection for thoracic esophageal carcinoma. *Ann. Thorac. Surg.* **1991**, *51*, 931–935. [CrossRef]
56. Shang, Q.X.; Chen, L.Q.; Hu, W.P.; Deng, H.Y.; Yuan, Y.; Cai, J. Three-field lymph node dissection in treating the esophageal cancer. *J. Thorac. Dis.* **2016**, *8*, E1136–E1149. [CrossRef]
57. Ma, G.W.; Situ, D.R.; Ma, Q.L.; Long, H.; Zhang, L.J.; Lin, P.; Rong, T.H. Three-field vs two-field lymph node dissection for esophageal cancer: A meta-analysis. *World J. Gastroenterol.* **2014**, *20*, 18022–18030. [CrossRef]
58. Cooper, J.S.; Guo, M.D.; Herskovic, A.; Macdonald, J.S.; Martenson, J.A., Jr.; Al-Sarraf, M.; Byhardt, R.; Russell, A.H.; Beitler, J.J.; Spencer, S.; et al. Chemoradiotherapy of locally advanced esophageal cancer: Long-term follow-up of a prospective randomized trial (RTOG 85-01). Radiation Therapy Oncology Group. *JAMA* **1999**, *281*, 1623–1627. [CrossRef]
59. Kato, K.; Muro, K.; Minashi, K.; Ohtsu, A.; Ishikura, S.; Boku, N.; Takiuchi, H.; Komatsu, Y.; Miyata, Y.; Fukuda, H. Phase II study of chemoradiotherapy with 5-fluorouracil and cisplatin for Stage II-III esophageal squamous cell carcinoma: JCOG trial (JCOG 9906). *Int J. Radiat Oncol. Biol. Phys.* **2011**, *81*, 684–690. [CrossRef]
60. Ito, Y.; Takeuchi, H.; Ogawa, G.; Kato, K.; Onozawa, M.; Minashi, K.; Yano, T.; Nakamura, K.; Tsushima, T.; Hara, H.; et al. A single-arm confirmatory study of definitive chemoradiotherapy (dCRT) including salvage treatment in patients (pts) with clinical (c) stage II/III esophageal carcinoma (EC) (JCOG0909). *J. Clin. Oncol.* **2018**, *36*, 4051. [CrossRef]
61. Shinoda, M.; Ando, N.; Kato, K.; Ishikura, S.; Kato, H.; Tsubosa, Y.; Minashi, K.; Okabe, H.; Kimura, Y.; Kawano, T.; et al. Randomized study of low-dose versus standard-dose chemoradiotherapy for unresectable esophageal squamous cell carcinoma (JCOG0303). *Cancer Sci.* **2015**, *106*, 407–412. [CrossRef] [PubMed]

62. Yokota, T.; Kato, K.; Hamamoto, Y.; Tsubosa, Y.; Ogawa, H.; Ito, Y.; Hara, H.; Ura, T.; Kojima, T.; Chin, K.; et al. Phase II study of chemoselection with docetaxel plus cisplatin and 5-fluorouracil induction chemotherapy and subsequent conversion surgery for locally advanced unresectable oesophageal cancer. *Br. J. Cancer* **2016**, *115*, 1328–1334. [CrossRef] [PubMed]
63. Terada, M.; Hara, H.; Daiko, H.; Mizusawa, J.; Kadota, T.; Hori, K.; Ogawa, H.; Ogata, T.; Sakanaka, K.; Sakamoto, T.; et al. Phase III study of tri-modality combination therapy with induction docetaxel plus cisplatin and 5-fluorouracil versus definitive chemoradiotherapy for locally advanced unresectable squamous-cell carcinoma of the thoracic esophagus (JCOG1510: TRIANgLE). *Jpn. J. Clin. Oncol.* **2019**, *49*, 1055–1060. [CrossRef] [PubMed]

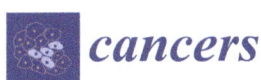

Article

Role of Postoperative Complications in Overall Survival after Radical Resection for Gastric Cancer: A Retrospective Single-Center Analysis of 1107 Patients

Christian Galata [1], Susanne Blank [1], Christel Weiss [2], Ulrich Ronellenfitsch [3], Christoph Reissfelder [1] and Julia Hardt [1,*]

1. Department of Surgery, Universitätsmedizin Mannheim, Medical Faculty Mannheim, Heidelberg University, 68167 Mannheim, Germany; christian.galata@umm.de (C.G.); susanne.blank@umm.de (S.B.); christoph.reissfelder@umm.de (C.R.)
2. Department of Medical Statistics and Biomathematics, Medical Faculty Mannheim, Heidelberg University, 68167 Mannheim, Germany; christel.weiss@medma.uni-heidelberg.de
3. Department of Visceral, Vascular and Endocrine Surgery, University Hospital Halle (Saale), Martin-Luther-University Halle-Wittenberg, 06120 Halle (Saale), Germany; ulrich.ronellenfitsch@uk-halle.de
* Correspondence: julia.hardt@umm.de

Received: 3 November 2019; Accepted: 25 November 2019; Published: 27 November 2019

Abstract: *Background:* The aim of this study was to investigate the impact of postoperative complications on overall survival (OS) after radical resection for gastric cancer. *Methods:* A retrospective analysis of our institutional database for surgical patients with gastroesophageal malignancies was performed. All consecutive patients who underwent R0 resection for M0 gastric cancer between October 1972 and February 2014 were included. The impact of postoperative complications on OS was evaluated in the entire cohort and in a subgroup after exclusion of 30 day and in-hospital mortality. *Results:* A total of 1107 patients were included. In the entire cohort, both overall complications ($p < 0.001$) and major surgical complications ($p = 0.003$) were significant risk factors for decreased OS in univariable analysis. In multivariable analysis, overall complications were an independent risk factor for decreased OS ($p < 0.001$). After exclusion of patients with complication-related 30 day and in-hospital mortality, neither major surgical ($p = 0.832$) nor overall complications ($p = 0.198$) were significantly associated with decreased OS. *Conclusion:* In this study, postoperative complications influenced OS due to complication-related early postoperative deaths. In patients successfully rescued from early postoperative complications, neither overall complications nor major surgical complications were risk factors for decreased survival.

Keywords: gastric cancer; gastrectomy; complications; outcome; survival

1. Introduction

Even today, surgery for gastric cancer remains challenging, and patients undergoing radical resection are reported to have high complication and failure-to-rescue rates [1,2]. Failure-to-rescue rates are reported to be even higher after surgery for gastric cancer than after esophageal resections [3]. Recently, several studies have reported adverse effects of postoperative complications on overall survival (OS) in these patients. Such studies have attracted particular interest as they suggest that postoperative complications have a negative impact on oncologic outcomes. However, to understand the importance of postoperative morbidity for oncologic outcomes, patients with complication-related early postoperative mortality must be critically considered. A recent systematic review and meta-analysis including 16 retrospective studies found that postoperative complications are correlated with poor prognosis after radical gastrectomy [4]. Thirteen of these studies reported effects of postoperative complications on OS, but only eight excluded influences from in-hospital death in the survival analysis. This is of particular interest because the pooled hazard ratio in this meta-analysis was notably lower after the exclusion of in-hospital mortality (1.40 vs. 1.79). Moreover, of the six studies reporting correlations between postoperative infectious complications and OS, only four excluded in-hospital mortality. Furthermore, the authors found a lower pooled hazard ratio (1.47 vs. 1.86) depending on whether in-hospital mortality was excluded from their analysis. They also reported different 95% confidence intervals (CI) for these two scenarios (1.22–2.83 for included in-hospital mortality vs. 0.90–2.40 for excluded in-hospital mortality).

In general, studies investigating the effect of postoperative morbidity on OS after surgery for gastric cancer either exclude or include patients with complication-related early postoperative deaths. Data on how the inclusion or exclusion of in-hospital mortality affects the role of postoperative complications in decreased OS within the same study population are scarce. The aim of this study was to investigate risk factors for decreased OS in patients undergoing radical resection for gastric cancer with special regard to the effect of postoperative complications. Therefore, we investigated two different cohorts, one including and one excluding patients with complication-related postoperative deaths.

2. Results

2.1. Patient Characteristics

Data of 1107 consecutive patients who underwent R0 resection for M0 gastric cancer at our institution between October 1972 and February 2014 were included in the analysis. Patient characteristics are shown in Table 1. There were more males than females (54.9% vs. 45.1%) and the median age was 65 years old. Most tumors were proximally located (60.9%) and predominantly classified as non-diffuse type (59.1%) according to the Laurén classification. The proportion of signet-ring cell carcinomas was 27.6%. As a rigorous standard at our institution, all oncologic resections with curative intent were performed by senior surgeons specialized in upper gastrointestinal surgery. During the study period, the standard approach for radical resection of gastric cancer at our department was open total or subtotal (4/5) gastrectomy with D2 lymphadenectomy (LAD). Total gastrectomy was performed in 47.1% of the cases and subtotal gastrectomy in 52.9% of the cases. Types of reconstruction after total gastrectomy were Roux-en-Y (n = 313, 28.3%), Longmire's reconstruction (n = 143, 12.9%), Schloffer's reconstruction (n = 69, 5.7%) and esophago-duodenostomy (n = 2, 0.2%). For subtotal gastrectomies, the type of reconstruction was documented in 489 cases (83.5%). Most patients received Billroth II procedures (total: n = 447, 40.3%; retrocolic: n = 234, 21.1%; antecolic: n = 213, 19.2%), whereas Billroth I procedures were performed in 42 patients (3.8%). The remaining 97 patients (16.5%) underwent subtotal gastrectomy without documentation of the reconstruction method. Multivisceral resections were performed in 45.9% of the patients, with splenectomies (34.2%) and cholecystectomies (10.9%) being the most common procedures.

Locally advanced tumor stages (pT2–4) were observed in 75.9% of the patients, and positive lymph nodes at the final pathology workup (pN1–3) were present in 52.1%. While pN stages were documented from the inception of the database, for over more than four decades, the extent of LAD and the number of harvested lymph nodes were not documented until 1998. However, when the 214 cases where the number of harvested lymph nodes was available were analyzed, the median number of harvested lymph nodes was 21 (17–27), indicating an adequate extent of LAD. Of the 136 patients where D1–3 LAD was documented, the vast majority underwent D2 LAD (n = 120, 86.9%) while D1 LAD and D3 LAD was performed in 10 (7.3%) and 8 (5.8%) patients, respectively. Data on the American Society of Anesthesiologists (ASA) physical status classification system was not documented before 2008. When patients with data on ASA grading (n = 46) were evaluated, 13.0% were categorized as ASA I, 37.0% as ASA II, 45.7% as ASA III and 4.3% as ASA IV.

Table 1. Patient characteristics.

Variable	n or Median	% or IQR
Gender		
Female	499	45.1
Male	608	54.9
Age (years)	65	56–72
Gastrectomy		
Total	521	47.1
Subtotal	586	52.9
Multivisceral resection	503	45.9
Splenectomy	375	34.2
Cholecystectomy	120	10.9
Intestinal resection	29	2.6
Pancreatic procedure	29	2.6
Hepatic procedure	20	1.8
Tumor location		
Non-antropyloric	674	60.9
Antropyloric	433	39.1
Laurén classification		
Diffuse	442	40.9
Non-diffuse	638	59.1
Signet-ring cell carcinoma	306	27.6
pT stage		
T1	267	24.1
T2	579	52.3
T3	211	19.1
T4	50	4.5
pN stage		
N0	530	47.9
N1	366	33.1
N2	181	16.4
N3	29	2.6
AJCC/UICC stage		
IA	229	20.7
IB	286	25.9
II	263	23.8
IIIA	187	16.9
IIIB	76	6.9
IV	65	5.9

IQR: interquartile range; AJCC: American Joint Committee on Cancer; UICC: Union Internationale Contre le Cancer.

2.2. Postoperative Outcomes

Postoperative outcomes are reported in Table 2. The median length of hospital stay was 14 (13–19) days. An overall complication rate of 25.3% was observed. Major surgical complications (defined as anastomotic leak, postoperative abdominal abscess, fascial dehiscence, peritonitis, sepsis, secondary hemorrhage, and relaparotomy for any reason during the postoperative course) were observed in 10.6% of the patients. The number of overall ($p = 0.126$) and major ($p = 0.238$) postoperative complications between total and subtotal gastrectomies was not significantly different. Postoperative 30 day mortality rate and in-hospital mortality rate were 4.7% and 5.7%, respectively. The median follow-up time was 27 (10–70) months with an estimated 5 year survival rate of 53.7%. OS was significantly different across American Joint Committee on Cancer/Union for International Cancer Control (AJCC/UICC) stages ($p < 0.001$). Median OS of all patients was 61 (95% CI: 50.05–71.95) months. Figure 1 shows the corresponding Kaplan–Meier survival curves. Operating times and intraoperative blood loss were not documented before 2004 and 2005, respectively. However, when patients with data on operating time (n = 132) were analyzed, the median operating time was 248 (213–298) min. For patients with data on intraoperative blood loss (n = 82), a median blood loss of 300 (200–600) mL was observed.

Table 2. Patient outcomes.

Variable	n or Median	% or IQR
Length of stay (days)	14	13–19
Overall complications	277	25.3
Major surgical complications	116	10.6
Anastomotic leak	50	43.1
Abdominal abscess/fascial dehiscence	36	31.0
Secondary hemorrhage	18	15.5
Relaparotomy (other than above)	6	5.2
Relaparotomy (not specified)	5	4.3
General sepsis (not specified)	1	0.9
Postoperative mortality		
30 day mortality	52	4.7
In-hospital mortality	63	5.7
Median follow-up (months) [a]	27	10–70
5 year survival rate [a]		53.7
5 year survival rate [b]		50.1

[a] Patients with in-hospital mortality excluded [b] All patients.

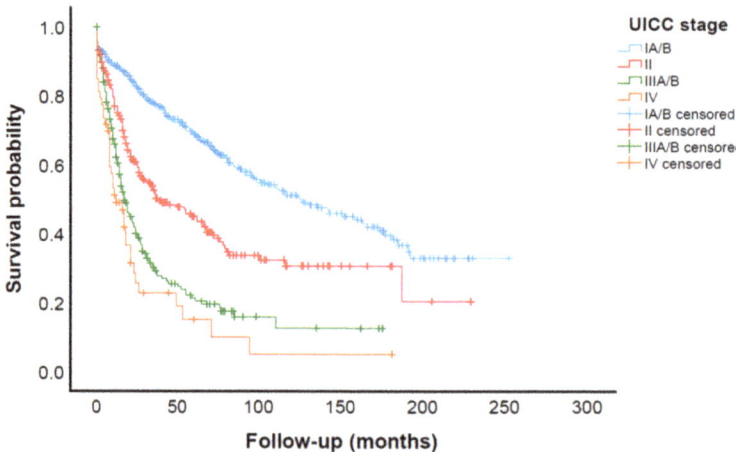

Figure 1. Kaplan–Meier survival curves. OS was significantly different across UICC stages ($p < 0.001$). Median OS of all patients was 61 (95% CI: 50.05–71.95) months. OS: overall survival; UICC: Union Internationale Contre le Cancer.

To investigate the impact of postoperative complications on OS, patients were stratified into two cohorts: one cohort consisting of all patients in the study and one cohort comprising only patients without complication-related postoperative deaths (30 day mortality and in-hospital mortality). Univariable and multivariable Cox regression analyses were performed to determine the parameters that might influence OS.

2.3. Risk Factors for Decreased Overall Survival in the Entire Cohort

The impact of clinically relevant variables on OS of all patients in the study is shown in Table 3. Overall complications ($p < 0.001$), major surgical complications ($p = 0.003$) and anastomotic leak ($p < 0.001$) were significant risk factors for decreased OS in univariable analysis. Other significant risk factors in univariable analysis were higher pT ($p < 0.001$), higher pN ($p < 0.001$), and higher AJCC/UICC stages ($p < 0.001$), older patient age ($p < 0.001$), earlier year of surgery ($p = 0.003$), non-antropyloric compared to antropyloric tumor location ($p = 0.025$), multivisceral resection ($p = 0.041$), splenectomy ($p = 0.012$), additional intestinal resections ($p < 0.001$), and additional pancreatic procedures ($p = 0.010$). When multivariable analysis was performed, the occurrence of overall postoperative complications was an independent risk factor for decreased OS ($p < 0.001$) together with advanced pT ($p < 0.001$) and pN ($p < 0.001$) stages, older patient age ($p < 0.001$), and earlier year of surgery ($p < 0.001$). For patients with data on operating time and intraoperative blood loss were available, neither parameter had a significant impact on OS in univariable analysis (operating time: $p = 0.327$, HR 0.997; blood loss: $p = 0.147$; HR 0.999).

Table 3. Factors associated with OS (all patients).

Variable	Univariable		Multivariable ($n = 935$)	
	p Value	Hazard Ratio	p Value	Hazard Ratio (95% CI)
Overall complications	<0.001	1.904	**<0.001**	1.968 (1.617–2.396)
Major surgical complications	0.003	1.506	0.327	
Anastomotic leak	<0.001	2.252	0.360	
pT stage	<0.001	1.892	**<0.001**	1.604 (1.414–1.819)
pN stage	<0.001	1.726	**<0.001**	1.518 (1.356–1.698)
AJCC/UICC stage	<0.001	1.485	0.124	
Age	<0.001	1.021	**<0.001**	1.020 (1.011–1.029)
Year of surgery	0.003	0.984	**<0.001**	0.973 (0.963–0.984)
Tumor location (distal vs. proximal)	0.025	1.236	0.289	
Multivisceral resection	0.041	1.204	0.135	
Splenectomy	0.012	1.263	0.149	
Intestinal resection	<0.001	2.487	0.096	
Pancreatic procedure	0.010	1.896	0.335	
Gender (male vs. female)	0.297	1.099		
Laurén type (diffuse vs. non-diffuse)	0.114	0.864		
Signet-ring cell carcinoma	0.367	0.911		
Gastrectomy (total vs. subtotal)	0.149	0.877		
Hepatic procedure	0.806	1.098		
Cholecystectomy	0.984	1.003		

AJCC: American Joint Committee on Cancer; OS: Overall survival; UICC: Union Internationale Contre le Cancer. p values in bold type indicate statistical significance in multivariable analysis.

2.4. Risk Factors for Decreased Survival after Exclusion of Early Postoperative Mortality

For this subgroup analysis (n = 1042), patients with complication-related early postoperative mortality (30 day mortality and in-hospital mortality) were excluded (Table 4). Overall complications ($p = 0.198$), major surgical complications ($p = 0.832$) and anastomotic leak ($p = 0.396$) did not reach statistical significance as risk factors for decreased OS in univariable analysis. Significant risk factors in univariable analysis were advanced pT ($p < 0.001$), pN ($p < 0.001$), and AJCC/UICC ($p < 0.001$) stages, older patient age ($p < 0.001$), proximal tumor location ($p = 0.008$), multivisceral resection ($p = 0.007$), splenectomy ($p = 0.004$), additional intestinal resections ($p < 0.001$), additional pancreatic procedures ($p = 0.006$), diffuse histologic type according to the Laurén classification ($p = 0.046$), and performance of a total vs. subtotal gastrectomy ($p = 0.027$). Earlier year of surgery did not reach statistical significance on the $\alpha = 0.050$ level in univariable analysis but showed a trend towards shorter OS ($p = 0.064$) and was therefore included in the multivariable analysis. In a multivariable Cox regression analysis, independent risk factors associated with decreased OS were advanced pT ($p < 0.001$) and pN ($p < 0.001$) stage, older patient age ($p < 0.001$), earlier year of surgery ($p = 0.010$), proximal tumor location ($p = 0.040$), and diffuse histologic type according to the Laurén classification (p = 0.013). For patients with data on operating time and intraoperative blood loss available, neither parameter had a significant impact on OS in univariable analysis (operating time: $p = 0.821$, HR 0.999; blood loss: $p = 0.290$; HR 0.999).

Table 4. Factors associated with OS (in-hospital mortality excluded).

Variable	Univariable		Multivariable (n = 862)	
	p Value	Hazard Ratio	*p* Value	Hazard Ratio (95% CI)
pT stage	<0.001	2.022	**<0.001**	1.638 (1.428–1.879)
pN stage	<0.001	1.830	**<0.001**	1.578 (1.399–1.779)
AJCC/UICC stage	<0.001	1.546	0.052	
Age	<0.001	1.019	**<0.001**	1.022 (1.012–1.032)
Year of surgery	0.064	0.990	**0.010**	0.985 (0.973–0.996)
Tumor location (distal vs. proximal)	0.008	1.308	**0.040**	1.236 (1.009–1.515)
Multivisceral resection	0.007	1.297	0.893	
Splenectomy	0.004	1.333	0.679	
Intestinal resection	<0.001	2.645	0.117	
Pancreatic procedure	0.006	2.061	0.557	
Laurén type (diffuse vs. non-diffuse)	0.046	0.821	**0.013**	0.771 (0.629–0.946)
Gastrectomy (total vs. subtotal)	0.027	0.807	0.170	
Overall complications	0.198	1.168		
Major surgical complications	0.832	1.038		
Anastomotic leak	0.396	1.250		
Signet-ring cell carcinoma	0.403	0.911		
Gender (male vs. female)	0.401	1.085		
Hepatic procedure	0.511	1.285		
Cholecystectomy	0.762	1.054		

AJCC: American Joint Committee on Cancer; OS: Overall survival; UICC: Union Internationale Contre le Cancer.
p values in bold type indicate statistical significance in multivariable analysis.

2.5. Neoadjuvant and Adjuvant Treatment

Administration of neoadjuvant and adjuvant chemotherapy was not documented in the database before the year 2005 and 2007, respectively. When patients treated with neoadjuvant (n = 106) and adjuvant (n = 75) therapy were investigated, neither treatment had a significant impact on OS in univariable analysis, neither before (neoadjuvant: $p = 0.104$, HR 0.466; adjuvant: $p = 0.698$, HR 1.229) nor after exclusion of in-hospital mortality (neoadjuvant: $p = 0.214$, HR 0.550; adjuvant: $p = 0.501$, HR 1.461).

2.6. Subgroup Analysis of AJCC/UICC Stages after Exclusion of Early Postoperative Mortality

As the impact of postoperative complications on OS might vary between patients with different tumor stages, subgroup analyses for AJCC/UICC stages I–IV were performed after exclusion of early postoperative mortality. For patients with AJCC/UICC stage I (n = 489) and IV (n = 57), neither overall complications ($p = 0.452$, HR 0.843; $p = 0.669$, HR 1.219), nor major postoperative complications ($p = 0.274$, HR 0.698; $p = 0.521$, HR 0.519) or anastomotic leak ($p = 0.420$, HR 0.624; $p = 0.743$, HR 0.713) reached statistical significance in univariable analysis. For patients with AJCC/UICC stage II (n = 249) no influence of overall complications ($p = 0.100$), anastomotic leak ($p = 0.234$) nor major surgical complications ($p = 0.061$) on OS was observed in univariable analysis. When multivariable analysis was performed (Appendix A Table A1), only the type of gastrectomy ($p = 0.037$) and the year of surgery ($p = 0.001$) remained in the model as factors with significant impact on OS. For patients with AJCC/UICC stage III (n = 246), no significant influence of overall complications ($p = 0.288$), major surgical complications ($p = 0.705$), or anastomotic leak ($p = 0.097$) on OS was observed in univariable analysis. When multivariable analysis was performed (Appendix A Table A2), older patient age ($p = 0.012$) was the only significant factor associated with OS.

3. Discussion

This study examined factors associated with OS after radical resection for gastric cancer over a time period of more than four decades in a cohort of 1107 consecutive patients at a European university surgical center. In our previous work, we investigated trends in postoperative morbidity, mortality, and failure to rescue in this study population (Christian Galata, Ulrich Ronellenfitsch, Susanne Blank, Christoph Reissfelder, Julia Hardt: Postoperative morbidity and failure to rescue in surgery for gastric cancer: A single center analysis of 1107 patients from 1972 to 2014; submitted and under review, November 2019). Here, we aimed to investigate risk factors for decreased OS with particular consideration for the role of postoperative overall complications and major surgical complications.

The main finding of this study was that postoperative complications had a significant impact on OS in the entire cohort in both univariable and multivariable analysis. However, when complication-related early postoperative deaths (30 day mortality and in-hospital mortality) were excluded, a statistically significant effect of postoperative complications on patient survival was no longer observed. This also holds true for all AJCC/UICC stages subgroups.

The clinicopathological features of the patients in our study are comparable to those of other long-term evaluations [5]. Multivariable analysis identified overall complications, advanced pT stage, advanced pN stage, older patient age, and earlier year of surgery as risk factors for decreased OS in the entire cohort. After exclusion of patients with early postoperative mortality, multivariable analysis rendered advanced pT stage, advanced pN stage, older patient age, earlier year of surgery, proximal tumor location, and diffuse histologic type according to the classification of Laurén as risk factors for decreased OS. The risk factors identified in our cohort are in line with those reported by other authors [6,7]. Possible reasons for the association of an earlier year of surgery with worse OS are improvements in surgical strategy, perioperative management, and oncologic therapy. Notably, when complication-related postoperative deaths were excluded neither major surgical complications nor anastomotic leak or overall complications were significant risk factors for decreased OS in univariable and multivariable analysis.

Recently, a number of studies have investigated the impact of postoperative complications on OS after surgery for gastric cancer, but the way in which the results have been reported is inconsistent. Some studies excluded patients with in-hospital mortality [6,8–11], while others did not exclude in-hospital mortality, thus potentially increasing the chance of detecting significant correlations between postoperative morbidity and patient survival [7,12–16]. A meta-analysis by Wang et al. found postoperative complications to correlate with poor prognosis after radical gastrectomy [4]. However, this effect was markedly weaker when the authors analyzed the subgroup of studies in which patients with in-hospital mortality were excluded.

In general, studies on this topic usually either include or exclude early postoperative mortality. Data on the effects of including or excluding surgery-related mortality are rarely reported for the same study population. In our analysis, we show that postoperative complications have a significant impact on OS if complication-related early postoperative deaths are not excluded. After exclusion of 30 day and in-hospital mortality, neither overall complications nor major surgical complications or anastomotic leak showed a significant effect on OS in the entire cohort. Likewise, no significant effect of these parameters on OS was observed in multivariable analysis when subgroup analyses of AJCC/UICC stages were performed. Thus, our data suggest that the identification of postoperative complications as a risk factor for inferior oncologic outcomes after radical resection for gastric cancer may have been overestimated depending on whether and how early postoperative mortality is excluded. These results are not in line with the study results by Jin et al. who report that postoperative complications remained an independent risk factor for decreased OS after curative resection for gastric cancer, even after exclusion of patients who died within 30 days postoperatively. Moreover, patients who experienced postoperative complications were 50% less likely to receive adjuvant therapy. The combination of postoperative complications and failure to receive adjuvant therapy increased the risk of death more than twice compared to patients without postoperative morbidity who successfully underwent adjuvant therapy [17]. To summarize, the currently available evidence on the impact of postoperative morbidity on long-term oncologic outcome is still heterogeneous.

Some limitations of this study must be mentioned. The study was retrospective and, thus, the inherent potential for misclassification may limit the validity of our data. In addition, the median OS exceeded the median follow-up which may limit the conclusions. There may be confounding variables that were not available for analysis, in particular preoperative ECOG (Eastern Cooperative Oncology Group) performance status, which might impact patient outcomes. However, since we investigated a cohort that underwent radical resection with curative intent, it may seem justified to assume that the vast majority of our patients were in a general condition that allows for extensive upper abdominal surgery. This is supported by the data of patients for whom ASA grading was available, which were categorized as ASA II and III in 82.7% of the cases. No continuous documentation of the extent of LAD, the number of harvested lymph nodes or the administration of perioperative chemotherapy was available over the long period covered in this study, but data of patients for whom the extent of LAD or the number of harvested lymph nodes were available indicate that D2 LAD with adequate extent was performed for the vast majority of patients in our cohort. When patients with data on neoadjuvant and adjuvant therapy were analyzed, neither of the treatments had a significant impact on OS in univariable analysis, neither before nor after exclusion of in-hospital mortality. These data must be interpreted cautiously, as the small sample size and lack of data on the completeness of chemotherapy and chemotherapy regimens used may have led to a bias. Neoadjuvant treatment, which was introduced at our institution in 2005, was not found to increase postoperative morbidity or mortality in several other studies [18,19], but in itself improves the prognosis of patients with locally advanced gastric cancer [20]. Concerning the extent of LAD, a more aggressive (D 1–3 or D 1–2 instead of D1 alone) surgical procedure might be associated with an increase in postoperative morbidity [21,22]. On the other hand, a more radical lymph node dissection (D 1–2 vs. D1 alone) has been shown to prolong OS [23,24].

4. Materials and Methods

4.1. Ethics Approval

Ethics board approval was obtained from the Medical Ethics Commission II of the Medical Faculty Mannheim, Heidelberg University, Mannheim, Germany (2019–849R). All patient data used in this analysis were completely anonymized. The study was performed according to the Declaration of Helsinki.

4.2. Patients

A retrospective analysis of our institutional database for surgical patients with gastroesophageal malignancies was performed. Medical records of 2252 consecutive patients operated on between October 1972 and February 2014 were examined, and 1107 patients with M0 gastric cancer who underwent R0 resection were included in the analysis. Patients with Barrett carcinoma, gastric remnant cancer, atypical gastric resections, esophageal resections or pT0 stage on final histology workup were excluded. Tumors of the subcardial stomach (Siewert type III) were included, whereas esophagogastric junctional adenocarcinomas (Siewert type I and II) were excluded, as these are classified and staged according to the esophageal scheme in the current AJCC/UICC system [25]. A flow chart of the study population is shown in Figure 2.

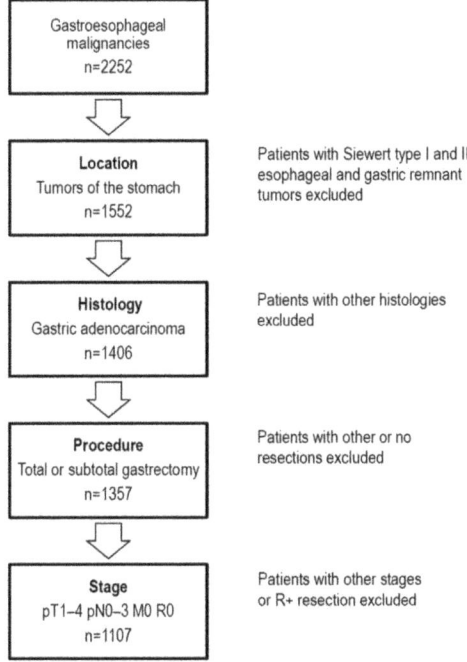

Figure 2. Flow chart of the study population.

4.3. AJCC/UICC Stages

For gastric cancer patients operated on between 1972 and 2001, AJCC/UICC stages according to the 5th edition of the AJCC/UICC staging system were available. The 6th and 7th edition of the AJCC/UICC classification were used from 2002 until 2009 and from 2010 until 2014, respectively. Before analysis, all patients in this study were restaged according to the 6th edition of the AJCC/UICC staging system for gastric cancer.

4.4. Postoperative Complications

Data on postoperative complications were extracted from the database, where they had been documented based on medical records. Major surgical complications were defined as one of the following events during the postoperative course: anastomotic leak (including duodenal stump insufficiency), postoperative abdominal abscess, fascial dehiscence, peritonitis, sepsis, secondary hemorrhage, and relaparotomy for any reason. When multiple complications occurred, the most severe complication was used for classifying if a patient had major surgical complications. Complication-related postoperative mortality is presented as early postoperative (30 day) and in-hospital mortality.

4.5. Follow-Up and Overall Survival

Follow-up in the database was based on medical records and direct contact with the patient or with the treating physicians. OS time was defined as the interval from surgery to death or latest time point the patient was known to be alive.

4.6. Statistical Analysis

Mean and standard deviations were calculated for quantitative variables. Qualitative variables were quoted as absolute numbers and relative frequencies. Median and interquartile range (IQR) are presented for skewed or ordinal scaled parameters. All statistical tests for the comparison of two groups were two-tailed. In general, a test result was considered statistically significant if $p < 0.050$. For qualitative variables, a Fisher's exact test was used. Univariable and multivariable Cox regression analyses were performed to identify factors that might influence OS. Variables reaching a significance level of $\alpha = 0.100$ in univariable Cox regression analyses were used as covariates in multivariable Cox regression analyses. In the multiple analyses, the backward stepwise selection based on the probability of the Wald statistic was used, and a significance level of $\alpha = 0.050$ was chosen to detect several parameters that might influence the outcome. Hazard ratios in the multiple analyses are presented together with their 95% CI. The Kaplan–Meier method was used to present survival data and the log-rank test was used to compare survival distributions. Statistical analyses were performed using the SAS statistical analysis software (release 9.4, Cary, NC, USA).

5. Conclusions

In summary, our data support the evidence that postoperative complications are a significant risk factor for poor OS in patients undergoing radical resection for gastric cancer. However, our study shows that this was an effect caused by complication-related early postoperative mortality. Indeed, postoperative complications did not have an impact on OS in patients who were successfully rescued from postoperative overall or major surgical complications.

Author Contributions: Conceptualization, C.G., S.B., U.R., C.R. and J.H.; Formal analysis, C.G. and C.W.; Methodology, C.G., S.B., C.W., U.R., C.R. and J.H.; Software, C.G. and C.W.; Supervision, U.R. and C.R.; Writing—original draft, C.G., S.B., U.R., C.R. and J.H.; Writing—review and editing, C.G., S.B., U.R., C.R. and J.H.

Funding: This research received no external funding.

Conflicts of Interest: The authors declare no conflict of interest.

Appendix A

Table A1. Factors associated with OS in patients with AJCC/UICC stage II (in-hospital mortality excluded).

Variable	Univariable		Multivariable (n = 218)	
	p Value	Hazard Ratio	p Value	Hazard Ratio (95% CI)
Year of surgery	0.005	0.970	**0.001**	0.963 (0.941–0.986)
Gastrectomy (total vs. subtotal)	0.096	0.726	**0.037**	0.665 (0.453–0.976)
Intestinal resection	0.041	3.358	0.057	
Major surgical complications	0.061	1.739	0.079	
Splenectomy	0.089	1.375	0.356	
Overall complications	0.100	1.447		
Anastomotic leak	0.234	1.724		
pT stage	0.691	0.901		
pN stage	0.691	1.110		
Tumor location (distal vs. proximal)	0.890	0.974		
Laurén type (diffuse vs. non-diffuse)	0.196	0.784		
Signet-ring cell carcinoma	0.644	1.113		
Gender (male vs. female)	0.471	1.145		
Age	0.350	1.008		
Multivisceral resection	0.243	1.248		
Pancreatic procedure	0.739	0.788		
Hepatic procedure	0.974	0.981		
Cholecystectomy	0.962	0.984		

AJCC: American Joint Committee on Cancer; OS: Overall survival; UICC: Union Internationale Contre le Cancer. p values in bold type indicate statistical significance in multivariable analysis.

Table A2. Factors associated with OS in AJCC/UICC stage III (in-hospital mortality excluded).

Variable	Univariable		Multivariable (n = 196)	
	p Value	Hazard Ratio	*p* Value	Hazard Ratio (95% CI)
Age	0.012	1.023	**0.012**	1.023 (1.005–1.041)
Splenectomy	0.086	1.351	0.061	
Anastomotic leak	0.097	2.018	0.069	
Overall complications	0.288	1.246		
Major surgical complications	0.705	1.122		
pT stage	0.102	1.315		
pN stage	0.670	0.938		
Tumor location (distal vs. proximal)	0.220	1.266		
Laurén type (diffuse vs. non-diffuse)	0.275	0.825		
Signet-ring cell carcinoma	0.733	1.067		
Gender (male vs. female)	0.445	0.874		
Year of surgery	0.340	0.990		
Gastrectomy (total vs. subtotal)	0.358	0.850		
Multivisceral resection	0.161	1.282		
Intestinal resection	0.495	1.366		
Pancreatic procedure	0.819	0.908		
Hepatic procedure	0.551	0.549		
Cholecystectomy	0.811	1.082		

AJCC: American Joint Committee on Cancer; OS: Overall survival; UICC: Union Internationale Contre le Cancer. *p* values in bold type indicate statistical significance in multivariable analysis.

References

1. Tu, R.H.; Lin, J.X.; Zheng, C.H.; Li, P.; Xie, J.W.; Wang, J.B.; Lu, J.; Chen, Q.Y.; Cao, L.L.; Lin, M.; et al. Complications and failure to rescue following laparoscopic or open gastrectomy for gastric cancer: A propensity-matched analysis. *Surg. Endosc.* **2017**, *31*, 2325–2337. [CrossRef]
2. Weledji, E.P.; Verla, V. Failure to rescue patients from early critical complications of oesophagogastric cancer surgery. *Ann. Med. Surg.* **2016**, *7*, 34–41. [CrossRef] [PubMed]
3. Busweiler, L.A.; Henneman, D.; Dikken, J.L.; Fiocco, M.; van Berge Henegouwen, M.I.; Wijnhoven, B.P.; van Hillegersberg, R.; Rosman, C.; Wouters, M.W.; van Sandick, J.W.; et al. Failure-to-rescue in patients undergoing surgery for esophageal or gastric cancer. *Eur. J. Surg. Oncol.* **2017**, *43*, 1962–1969. [CrossRef]
4. Wang, S.; Xu, L.; Wang, Q.; Li, J.; Bai, B.; Li, Z.; Wu, X.; Yu, P.; Li, X.; Yin, J. Postoperative complications and prognosis after radical gastrectomy for gastric cancer: A systematic review and meta-analysis of observational studies. *World J. Surg. Oncol.* **2019**, *17*, 18–20. [CrossRef]
5. Rosa, F.; Alfieri, S.; Tortorelli, A.P.; Fiorillo, C.; Costamagna, G.; Doglietto, G.B. Trends in clinical features, postoperative outcomes, and long-term survival for gastric cancer: A Western experience with 1,278 patients over 30 years. *World J. Surg. Oncol.* **2014**, *12*, 1–11. [CrossRef]
6. Climent, M.; Hidalgo, N.; Vidal Puig, S.; Iglesias, M.; Cuatrecasas, M.; Ramón, J.M.; García-Albéniz, X.; Grande, L.; Pera, M. Postoperative complications do not impact on recurrence and survival after curative resection of gastric cancer. *Eur. J. Surg. Oncol.* **2016**, *42*, 132–139. [CrossRef]
7. Ohashi, M.; Morita, S.; Fukagawa, T.; Kushima, R.; Katai, H. Surgical treatment of non-early gastric remnant carcinoma developing after distal gastrectomy for gastric cancer. *J. Surg. Oncol.* **2015**, *111*, 208–212. [CrossRef]
8. Kim, S.-H.; Son, S.-Y.; Park, Y.-S.; Ahn, S.-H.; Park, D.J.; Kim, H.-H. Risk Factors for Anastomotic Leakage: A Retrospective Cohort Study in a Single Gastric Surgical Unit. *J. Gastric Cancer* **2015**, *15*, 167–175. [CrossRef]
9. Watanabe, M.; Kinoshita, T.; Tokunaga, M.; Kaito, A.; Sugita, S. Complications and their correlation with prognosis in patients undergoing total gastrectomy with splenectomy for treatment of proximal advanced gastric cancer. *Eur. J. Surg. Oncol.* **2018**, *44*, 1181–1185. [CrossRef]
10. Tsujimoto, H.; Ichikura, T.; Ono, S.; Sugasawa, H.; Hiraki, S.; Sakamoto, N.; Yaguchi, Y.; Yoshida, K.; Matsumoto, Y.; Hase, K. Impact of postoperative infection on long-term survival after potentially curative resection for gastric cancer. *Ann. Surg. Oncol.* **2009**, *16*, 311–318. [CrossRef]

11. Li, Z.; Bai, B.; Zhao, Y.; Yu, D.; Lian, B.; Liu, Y.; Zhao, Q. Severity of complications and long-term survival after laparoscopic total gastrectomy with D2 lymph node dissection for advanced gastric cancer: A propensity score-matched, case-control study. *Int. J. Surg.* **2018**, *54*, 62–69. [CrossRef] [PubMed]
12. Yoo, H.M.; Lee, H.H.; Shim, J.H.; Jeon, H.M.; Park, C.H.; Song, K.Y. Negative impact of leakage on survival of patients undergoing curative resection for advanced gastric cancer. *J. Surg. Oncol.* **2011**, *104*, 734–740. [CrossRef]
13. Nagasako, Y.; Satoh, S.; Isogaki, J.; Inaba, K.; Taniguchi, K.; Uyama, I. Impact of anastomotic complications on outcome after laparoscopic gastrectomy for early gastric cancer. *Br. J. Surg.* **2012**, *99*, 849–854. [CrossRef] [PubMed]
14. Li, Q.-G.; Li, P.; Tang, D.; Chen, J.; Wang, D.-R. Impact of postoperative complications on long-term survival after radical resection for gastric cancer. *World J. Gastroenterol.* **2013**, *19*, 4060–4065. [CrossRef] [PubMed]
15. Tokunaga, M.; Tanizawa, Y.; Bando, E.; Kawamura, T.; Terashima, M. Poor survival rate in patients with postoperative intra-abdominal infectious complications following curative gastrectomy for gastric cancer. *Ann. Surg. Oncol.* **2013**, *20*, 1575–1583. [CrossRef]
16. Kubota, T.; Hiki, N.; Sano, T.; Nomura, S.; Nunobe, S.; Kumagai, K.; Aikou, S.; Watanabe, R.; Kosuga, T.; Yamaguchi, T. Prognostic significance of complications after curative surgery for gastric cancer. *Ann. Surg. Oncol.* **2014**, *21*, 891–898. [CrossRef] [PubMed]
17. Jin, L.X.; Sanford, D.E.; Squires, M.H.; Moses, L.E.; Yan, Y.; Poultsides, G.A.; Votanopoulos, K.I.; Weber, S.M.; Bloomston, M.; Pawlik, T.M.; et al. Interaction of Postoperative Morbidity and Receipt of Adjuvant Therapy on Long-Term Survival After Resection for Gastric Adenocarcinoma: Results From the U.S. Gastric Cancer Collaborative. *Ann. Surg. Oncol.* **2016**, *23*, 2398–2408. [CrossRef]
18. Marcus, S.G.; Cohen, D.; Lin, K.; Wong, K.; Thompson, S.; Rothberger, A.; Potmesil, M.; Hiotis, S.; Newman, E. Complications of gastrectomy following CPT-11 based neoadjuvant chemotherapy for gastric cancer. *Gastroenterology* **2003**, *124*, A789. [CrossRef]
19. Luo, H.; Wu, L.; Huang, M.; Jin, Q.; Qin, Y.; Chen, J. Postoperative morbidity and mortality in patients receiving neoadjuvant chemotherapy for locally advanced gastric cancers. *Medicine (Baltimore)*. **2018**, *97*, e12932. [CrossRef]
20. Ronellenfitsch, U.; Schwarzbach, M.; Hofheinz, R.; Kienle, P.; Kieser, M.; Slanger, T.E.; Burmeister, B.; Kelsen, D.; Niedzwiecki, D.; Schuhmacher, C.; et al. Preoperative chemo(radio)therapy versus primary surgery for gastroesophageal adenocarcinoma: systematic review with meta-analysis combining individual patient and aggregate data. *Eur. J. Cancer* **2013**, *49*, 3149–3158. [CrossRef]
21. Bonenkamp, J.J.; Hermans, J.; Sasako, M.; Welvaart, K.; Songun, I.; Meyer, S.; Plukker, J.T.M.; Van Elk, P.; Obertop, H.; Gouma, D.J.; et al. Extended Lymph-Node Dissection for Gastric Cancer. *N. Engl. J. Med.* **1999**, *340*, 908–914. [CrossRef]
22. Cuschieri, A.; Joypaul, V.; Fayers, P.; Cook, P.; Fielding, J.; Craven, J.; Bancewicz, J. Postoperative morbidity and mortality after D1 and D2 resections for gastric cancer: preliminary results of the MRC randomised controlled surgical trial. *Lancet* **1996**, *347*, 995–999. [CrossRef]
23. Coimbra, F.J.F.; de Jesus, V.H.F.; Ribeiro, H.S.C.; Diniz, A.L.; de Godoy, A.L.; de Farias, I.C.; Felismino, T.; Mello, C.A.L.; Almeida, M.F.; Begnami, M.D.F.S.; et al. Impact of ypT, ypN, and Adjuvant Therapy on Survival in Gastric Cancer Patients Treated with Perioperative Chemotherapy and Radical Surgery. *Ann. Surg. Oncol.* **2019**, 1–9. [CrossRef] [PubMed]
24. Songun, I.; Putter, H.; Kranenbarg, E.M.-K.; Sasako, M.; van de Velde, C.J.H. Surgical treatment of gastric cancer: 15-year follow-up results of the randomised nationwide Dutch D1D2 trial. *Lancet. Oncol.* **2010**, *11*, 439–449. [CrossRef]
25. Brierley, J.D.; Gospodarowicz, M.K.; Wittekind, C. *TNM Classification of Malignant Tumours*; Wiley Blackwell: Oxford, UK, 2017; ISBN 978-1-119-26357-9.

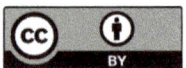

© 2019 by the authors. Licensee MDPI, Basel, Switzerland. This article is an open access article distributed under the terms and conditions of the Creative Commons Attribution (CC BY) license (http://creativecommons.org/licenses/by/4.0/).

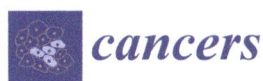

Article

Clinical Pathways for Oncological Gastrectomy: Are They a Suitable Instrument for Process Standardization to Improve Process and Outcome Quality for Patients Undergoing Gastrectomy? A Retrospective Cohort Study

Patrick Téoule [1], Emrullah Birgin [1], Christina Mertens [2], Matthias Schwarzbach [3], Stefan Post [1], Nuh N. Rahbari [1], Christoph Reißfelder [1] and Ulrich Ronellenfitsch [4,*]

1. Department of Surgery, Universitätsmedizin Mannheim, Medical Faculty Mannheim, Heidelberg University, Theodor-Kutzer-Ufer 1-3, 68167 Mannheim, Germany; patrick.teoule@umm.de (P.T.); emrullah.birgin@umm.de (E.B.); st.post@icloud.com (S.P.); nuh.rahbari@umm.de (N.N.R.); christoph.reissfelder@umm.de (C.R.)
2. Department of General and Visceral Surgery, Städtisches Klinikum Karlsruhe, Moltkestr.90, 76133 Karlsruhe, Germany; christina.mertens@klinikum-karlsruhe.de
3. Department of General, Visceral, Vascular, and Thoracic Surgery, Klinikum Frankfurt Höchst, Gotenstraße 6-8, 65929 Frankfurt, Germany; matthias.schwarzbach@klinikumfrankfurt.de
4. Department of Visceral, Vascular and Endocrine Surgery, University Hospital Halle (Saale), Ernst-Grube-Str.40, 06120 Halle (Saale), Germany
* Correspondence: ulrich.ronellenfitsch@uk-halle.de; Tel.: +49-345-557-2314; Fax: +49-345-557-2551

Received: 7 January 2020; Accepted: 12 February 2020; Published: 13 February 2020

Abstract: (1) *Background*: Oncological gastrectomy requires complex multidisciplinary management. Clinical pathways (CPs) can potentially facilitate this task, but evidence related to their use in managing oncological gastrectomy is limited. This study evaluated the effect of a CP for oncological gastrectomy on process and outcome quality. (2) *Methods*: Consecutive patients undergoing oncological gastrectomy before ($n = 64$) or after ($n = 62$) the introduction of a CP were evaluated. Assessed parameters included catheter and drain management, postoperative mobilization, resumption of diet and length of stay. Morbidity, mortality, reoperation and readmission rates were used as indicators of outcome quality. (3) *Results*: Enteral nutrition was initiated significantly earlier after CP implementation (5.0 vs. 7.0 days, $p < 0.0001$). Readmission was more frequent before CP implementation (7.8% vs. 0.0%, $p = 0.05$). Incentive spirometer usage increased following CP implementation (100% vs. 90.6%, $p = 0.11$). Mortality, morbidity and reoperation rates remained unchanged. (4) *Conclusions*: After implementation of an oncological gastrectomy CP, process quality improved, while indicators of outcome quality such as mortality and reoperation rates remained unchanged. CPs are a promising tool to standardize perioperative care for oncological gastrectomy.

Keywords: clinical pathways; gastric surgery; oncological gastrectomy; quality of care; outcomes; standardization

1. Introduction

Gastric cancer is the fifth most common neoplasm and still ranks third among the world's leading causes of cancer deaths, affecting approximately 783,000 people annually [1]. Regardless of improvements in surgical technique and perioperative management, surgery for gastric cancer remains challenging and patients who undergo radical resection are reported to have high complication rates [2,3]. One reason is that more and more elderly and multimorbid patients are resected [4,5].

On the other hand, due to preoperative malnutrition of patients with gastric neoplasms and chronic comorbidities, perioperative mortality can reach up to 8.8% [6]. Therefore, multidisciplinary perioperative management is required to reduce the risk of possibly severe perioperative complications during and after oncological gastrectomy. The implementation of clinical pathways (CPs) can potentially improve the quality of perioperative management [7]. CPs are specific instruments developed to improve the quality of outcomes of care by standardizing treatment processes. They can be defined as a protocol stipulating all tasks that should be carried out during a defined treatment [8–10]. The designated goal of CPs is to transfer evidence to the bedside. They comprise all disciplines involved in patient care [11,12]. For several gastrointestinal operations, CPs have proven advantageous with regard to perioperative outcomes [13]. Several studies have reported the results of patients undergoing oncological gastrectomy and treated with CPs. These studies showed a reduction in the length of stay (LOS) and reported a non-significant decrease in total complications, mortality and reoperation [14]. However, all of these studies were conducted in Asian countries. In Europe only a few studies have assessed the influence of multimodal management after gastrectomy. They were focused on laparoscopic gastrectomy or a comparative pre-CP group was missing [15–18].

Given that the expected effects of CPs must be considered specific to health systems, we performed a study in a German tertiary care hospital to evaluate an oncological gastrectomy CP with respect to its effects on process and outcome quality.

2. Results

2.1. Patient Characteristics

A total of 126 patients underwent oncological gastrectomy during the study period. The pre-CP group comprised 64 patients and the CP group involved 62 patients. Patient characteristics are displayed in Table 1. The clinical and demographic characteristics of both groups were comparable. The proportion of total gastrectomies was non-significantly higher in the pre-CP group, and correspondingly, there were proportionally more tumors extending to the entire stomach in this group. The type of surgical reconstruction differed significantly between the two groups. While all patients received a Roux-en-Y reconstruction, the proportion of handsewn esophagojejunostomies was higher in the pre-CP group (23.4%) than in the CP group (8.1%; $p = 0.01$).

Table 1. Characteristics of the study groups.

Patient Characteristic	Pre-CP Group (n = 64) %	CP Group (n = 62) %	p-Value
Age in years; median (range; IQR)	65.5 (30-85; 20)	65.0 (25-89; 21)	0.79
Sex			0.88
Male	40 (62.5)	38 (61.3)	
ASA score			0.16
I	6 (10.0)	1 (1.8)	
II	26 (43.3)	23 (40.3)	
III	28 (46.7)	32 (56.1)	
IV	0 (0)	1 (1.8)	
X	4	5	
Type of tumor			0.12
Adenocarcinoma	61 (95.3)	58 (93.5)	
Other	3 (4.7)	4 (6.5)	
Tumor location			0.05
Proximal part	21 (32.8)	26 (41.9)	
Middle part	1 (1.6)	3 (4.8)	
Distal part	13 (20.3)	9 (14.5)	
Entire stomach	28 (43.7)	19 (30.7)	

Table 1. Cont.

Patient Characteristic	Pre-CP Group (n = 64) %	CP Group (n = 62) %	p-Value
Remnant cancer	1 (1.6)	5 (8.1)	
Neoadjuvant chemotherapy	38 (59.4)	35 (56.5)	0.85
TNM classification for Adenocarcinoma	61 (95.3)	58 (93.5)	
Tumor stage			0.57
T0	3 (4.9)	5 (8.6)	
T1	11 (18.0)	14 (24.1)	
T2	9 (14.8)	10 (17.2)	
T3	27 (44.3)	21 (36.2)	
T4	11 (18.0)	8 (13.8)	
Nodal status			0.46
N0	25 (41.0)	32 (55.2)	
N1	11 (18.0)	8 (13.8)	
N2	13 (21.3)	8 (13.8)	
N3	12 (19.7)	10 (17.2)	
Metastasis			0.66
M0	53 (85.5)	52 (88.1)	
M1	9 (14.5)	7 (11.9)	
X	2	3	
Resectional status			0.74
R0	57 (93.4)	55 (91.7)	
R1	4 (6.6)	5 (8.3)	
X	3	2	
Type of resection			0.07
Total	40 (62.5)	26 (41.9)	
Subtotal	9 (14.0)	10 (15.1)	
Completion gastrectomy	1 (1.6)	5 (8.1)	
Trans-hiatally extended	14 (21.9)	21 (33.9)	
Type of lymphadenectomy			0.19
D2	40 (67.8)	28 (60.8)	
Partial D3	14 (23.7)	15 (32.6)	
Local	1 (1.7)	2 (4.3)	
None	4 (6.8)	0 (0)	0.07
X	5	17	
Associated procedure #	6 (9.4)	11 (17.4)	0.16
Liver resection	2 (3.1)	2 (3.1)	1
Colon resection	2 (3.2)	5 (8.1)	0.36
Distal pancreatectomy and splenectomy	4 (6.3)	5 (8.1)	0.36
Reconstruction			
Roux-en-Y	64 (100)	62 (100)	1
Stapler	49 (76.6)	57 (92.9)	0.01 *
Handsewn	15 (23.4)	5 (8.1)	
Preoperative albumin mean (g/L)	35.1	35.9	0.4
(standard deviation)	(4.75)	(4.40)	
Mean number of resected lymph nodes	26.6	25.1	0.43
(standard deviation)	(10.11)	(10.70)	
Mean lymph node ratio (positive LN/ total LN)	18	12	0.43
(range)	(0–92)	(0–89)	

ASA = American Society of Anesthesiology; X = missing data; Pre-CP group = Pre-Clinical pathway group; CP group = Clinical pathway group; dignity others Pre-CP-Group = in declining order: two neuroendocrine tumors, one leiomyosarcoma; dignity others CP-Group = in declining order: two leiomyosarcomas, one leiomyoma, one gastric metastasis of kidney cell carcinoma; IQR = interquartile range; # = multiple answers are possible; g/l = gram/liter; * = p-value ≤ 0.05.

2.2. Process Quality

Table 2 gives an overview of the comparison of the outcomes that reflect process quality. In the CP group, patients received liquid nutritional supplements significantly earlier (median 5.0 vs. 7.0 days in the pre-CP group; $p < 0.0001$). The usage of incentive spirometers increased following CP implementation, although the difference did not reach statistical significance (100% vs. 90.6% in the pre-CP group; $p = 0.11$). Foley and arterial catheters were removed significantly earlier in the pre-CP group (median of 1.0 vs. 4.0 and 2.0 vs. 5.0 days, respectively; $p = 0.01$).

Table 2. Parameters of process quality.

Patient Characteristic	Pre-CP Group (n = 64) %	CP Group (n = 62) %	p-Value
Usage of incentive spirometer	58 (90.6)	62 (100)	0.11
Median day of oral toluidine test	5	5	0.72
(range; IQR]	(5–6; 0.0)	(4.0–7.0; 0.0)	
Number of patients with positive oral toluidine test	1 (1.6)	0 (0)	1
X	10	8	
Median day of peripheral venous catheter removal	6.5	4	0.35
(range; IQR)	(1–44; 10)	(0–24; 4.5)	
Median day of PDA catheter removal	6	6	0.71
(range; IQR)	(1–10; 2)	(0–9; 3)	
Number of patients with PDA catheter	59 (92.2)	53 (85.5)	0.47
Median day of central venous catheter removal	7	7	0.57
(range; IQR)	(1–19; 3.0)	(1–33; 4.0)	
Number of patients with central venous catheter	61 (95.3)	58 (93.5)	0.71
Median day of arterial catheter removal	1	2	0.01 *
(range; IQR)	(0–7; 1.0)	(1–8; 2.0)	
Number of patients with arterial catheter	55 (88.7)	59 (95.1)	0.11
Median day of foley catheter removal	4	5	0.01 *
(range; IQR)	(1–11; 3.0)	(1–3; 3.0)	
Number of patients with foley catheter	61 (95.3)	57 (91.9)	0.7
Median day of nasogastric tube removal	1	1	0.42
(range; IQR)	(0–3; 0.0)	(0–3; 0.0)	
Number of patients with nasogastric tube	54 (84.4)	57 (91.9)	0.67
Median day of EF drain removal	7	7	0.81
(range; IQR)	(4–32; 2.0)	(5–55; 2.0)	
Number of patients with EF drain	49 (76.5)	55 (88.7)	0.07
Median day of first intake of liquid nutritional supplement	7	5	<0.0001 *
(range, IQR)	(2–14; 4.0)	(4–10; 2.0)	
Median day of first intake of soft diet	6	6	0.62
(range, IQR)	(2–15; 1.0)	(3–7; 1.0)	
Median day of first intake of full diet	9	8	0.34
(range, IQR)	(6–16; 3.0)	(6–46; 4.0)	
Median day of full mobilization	1	1	0.75
(range; IQR)	(0–2; 0.0)	(0–5; 0.0)	
X	1	1	

Pre-CP Group = Pre-Clinical pathway group; CP group = Clinical pathway group; PDA = peridural anesthesia; IQR = interquartile range; EF = easy flow; X = missing data; * = p-value ≤ 0.05.

2.3. Outcome Quality

Table 3 summarizes the results for outcome quality. There were two postoperative fatalities in the pre-CP group. Cause of death was respiratory failure following aspiration pneumonia in one case and multiorgan failure caused by sepsis following anastomotic leakage in the other. In the CP group, four patients died due to multiorgan failure caused by sepsis: one caused by duodenal stump leakage with severe peritonitis, one caused by aspiration pneumonia and myocardial infarction, one due to anastomotic leakage, and one due to bowel leakage with severe peritonitis.

Regarding outcome quality, groups differed significantly in three parameters. Median length of hospital stay (LOS) in the intermediate care and intensive care units was significantly shorter in the pre-CP group than the CP group (median stay 2.0 vs. 3.0, $p = 0.0005$; and 0.0 vs. 0.0, $p = 0.01$, respectively). The median of the highest measured visual-analogue-scale (VAS) pain score was significantly lower in the pre-CP group (5 compared to 6 in the CP group; $p = 0.03$). The readmission rate was higher in the pre-CP group (7.8% vs. 0; $p = 0.05$). No differences could be observed between groups with regard to postoperative morbidity and mortality. Additionally, groups did not differ regarding the summary measures for specific complications. The discharge goal of the CP could not be obtained and LOS did not differ between groups.

Table 3. Parameters of outcome quality.

Patient Characteristic	Pre-CP-Group ($n = 64$) %	CP-Group ($n = 62$) %	p-Value
Readmission	5 (7.8)	0 (0.0)	0.05
Mortality	2 (3.1)	4 (6.5)	0.43
Postoperative morbidity according to the Clavien-Dindo classification			0.68
Grade 0	20 (31.3)	14 (22.6)	
Grade I	7 (10.9)	5 (8.1)	
Grade II	21 (32.8)	24 (38.7)	
Grade IIIA	10 (15.6)	10 (16.1)	
Grade IIIB	2 (3.1)	4 (6.5)	
Grade IVA	1 (1.6)	1 (1.6)	
Grade IVB	1 (1.6)	0	
Grade V	2 (3.1)	4 (6.5)	
Revisional surgery	2 (3.1)	6 (9.7)	0.16
Postoperative pneumonia	6 (9.4)	7 (11.3)	0.77
Postoperative pleural effusion	18 (28.1)	10 (16.1)	0.13
Postoperative wound infection	2 (3.1)	7 (11.3)	0.09
Anastomotic dehiscence (esophagojejunostomy)	2 (3.1)	3 (4.8)	0.67
Duodenal stump leakage	0 (0.0)	2 (3.2)	0.24
Postoperative pancreatic fistula	4 (6.3)	7 (11.3)	0.35
Patients received postoperative RBCC transfusion	15 (23.4)	13 (21.0)	0.83
Median number of postoperative transfused RBCC (range, IQR)	0 (0–4; 0.0)	0 (0–6; 0.0)	0.7
Median number of highest VAS-score of pain (range)	5 (0–10; 3.0)	6 (0–10; 3.0)	0.03 *
X	2	0	
Analgesics requested (mean number of supplemental requested doses during hospital stay)	0.24	0.31	0.31
(range)	(0–1.54)	(0–2.25)	
Median day of first defecation	4	3	0.92
(range, IQR)	(2–8; 1.0)	(1–7; 2.0)	
Median length of stay in IMC	2	3	0.0005 *
(range, IQR)	(1–26; 2.0)	(1–47; 4.0)	
Median length of stay in ICU	0	0	0.01 *
(range, IQR)	(0–29; 0.0)	(0–31; 0.0)	
Median length of stay	16	16	0.66
(range, IQR)	(8–55; 10.0)	(9–63; 11.0)	

Pre-CP-Group = pre-clinical pathway group; CP-Group = clinical pathway group; VAS = visual analogue scale; IMC = intermediate care unit; ICU = intensive care unit; RBCC = red blood cell concentrate; IQR = interquartile range; * = p-value ≤ 0.05.

3. Discussion

This study assessed the effects of an oncological gastrectomy CP with regard to parameters of perioperative process and outcome quality. Because gastric surgery and the associated perioperative care are complex, it should only be done in a specialized setting by dedicated and experienced surgeons. A reduction in perioperative mortality has been observed in recent years. However, procedure-associated morbidity remains high and this is a relevant issue for patients and treatment teams [19,20]. The fact that much older and severely co-morbid patients, as well as patients in advanced tumor stages and with compromised performance status are resected might partly explain this fact [3–5]. Nevertheless, high morbidity and mortality might also be associated with insufficient standardization of perioperative treatment, and in particular with so called "failure to rescue", a situation in which emerging complications are not detected and managed appropriately, resulting in the death of the patient [2,21–24]. Therefore, this study was designed to assess if implementing an oncological gastrectomy CP resulted in increased standardization of perioperative treatment and improved the process and outcome quality. Given that the relevant evidence is almost exclusively related to Asian countries [14,18,25], we conducted a study in a Germany tertiary care center.

In order to measure protocol adherence, process quality parameters were used as key performance indicators. Following CP implementation, we detected an improvement in some of these parameters, while others remained unaltered or even worsened.

A meta-analysis has shown that early enteral nutrition is associated with lower mortality and a shorter hospital stay after gastrectomy [26]. We observed a significantly earlier intake of liquid nutritional supplement, and a non-significantly earlier intake of soft and full diet after CP implementation. The incidence of postoperative pneumonia can be decreased by the use of incentive spirometers [27]. All patients used incentive spirometers after CP implementation, compared to only 90% in the pre-CP group. The fact that postoperative pneumonia did not decrease after CP implementation is therefore rather surprising. One potential explanation could be that more ASA III patients, who have a higher baseline risk for acquiring pneumonia, were operated on after CP implementation (56.1% vs. 46.7%). Given that ascending infections are related to indwelling catheters, early removal should be aimed for [28–30]. In our study, however, the median day when abdominal drains as well as peripheral and central venous catheters, epidural catheters and nasogastric tubes were removed remained unchanged after CP implementation. Drain fluid was checked for its amylase concentration on postoperative day 5 in all patients. Drains remained in situ in case of an elevated concentration. Therefore, a potential explanation for the delayed easy flow (EF) drain removal might be the higher proportion of pancreatic fistula in the CP group, with 11.3% vs. 6.3% for the pre-CP group, as well as duodenal stump leakage rate (3.2 vs. 0). In contrast to what was expected from CP implementation, two parameters showed an apparent decrease regarding their process quality. Foley and arterial catheters were removed on average one day later in the CP group. One hypothetical explanation for the delayed removal in patients treated with the CP could be that they stayed on average one day longer in intermediate care and intensive care units. A higher proportion of associated procedures and co-morbid patients could explain this fact.

Perioperative morbidity and mortality were not significantly different before and after CP implementation. While the 30-day mortality rate is frequently used, we employed the in-hospital mortality rate to account for prolonged treatment courses, which are common nowadays given advanced intensive care and interventional techniques. In-hospital mortality was 6.5% in the CP and 3.1% in the pre-CP group. This two-fold increase in mortality after CP implementation is worrisome. However, this observation is based on only two additional postoperative fatalities in the CP group, and the difference is not statistically significant. The result might therefore be spurious and must be interpreted with much caution. In comparison, the overall postoperative morbidity rate according to the Clavien-Dindo classification in our patients seems high. This can possibly be explained by the fact that this scheme counts every deviation from what is considered a normal postoperative course as a complication. Consequently, only 14 patients in the CP and 20 in the pre-CP group were classified as being without complications in our study.

The Enhanced Recovery After Surgery (ERAS®) society published perioperative care guidelines for gastrectomy [31]. These guidelines contain 25 care items compared to 23 items in our CP. Comparing the two documents, 17 recommendations are very similar, while six recommendations given by the ERAS guidelines are not included in our CP. Examples are as follows: surgical access type, transversus abdominis plane (TAP) block or the use of wound catheters, skin preparation, preanesthetic medication, prophylaxis for postoperative nausea and vomiting (PONV), and oral bowel preparation. In contrast to the ERAS guidelines, our CP comprises recommendations regarding vitamin B12 substitution, catheters, transfusion and nursing and rehabilitation. Possible future revisions of the CP should incorporate the evidence-based ERAS guidelines.

While the results regarding process quality were encouraging, three parameters related to outcome quality deteriorated after CP implementation. The LOS in the intermediate and intensive care units was significantly longer in the CP group. Moreover, the median of the highest visual-analogue-scale (VAS) pain score was significantly lower in the pre-CP group. This result is rather unexpected, given that the CP included a dedicated analgesia scheme according to recent recommendations. It also included epidural catheter placement, which was carried out in the overwhelming majority of patients. Additional oral analgesics were administered in a stepwise, pain-adjusted manner, so that there is no obvious explanation for higher pain levels in patients treated according to the CP. Therefore, a clear explanation for higher pain levels in the CP group is lacking. Hypothetically, nursing staff might have been more aware of possible postoperative pain after CP implementation, and consequently tended to carry out more accurate pain assessment, leading to a higher reported pain level. This would also explain why the stipulated goal of epidural catheter removal on day 3 was not met. This scenario could be regarded as ascertainment bias. On the other hand, extra requests for analgesics from patients did not differ between the groups treated with or without CP. This indicates that the stipulated analgesia scheme was quite sufficient. Inadequate pain management can lead to impaired mobilization, an increase in LOS, and ultimately, to elevated perioperative morbidity, particularly with regard to pulmonary complications.

CPs should also avoid excessively long LOS without medical reasons. In this study, we did not observe a decrease in LOS after CP implementation. However, a relevant variation in LOS was seen between individual patients. The stipulated goal for LOS in our CP might have been too ambitious, because it was clearly below the LOS reported in larger studies [14]. Moreover, the study comprised all consecutive patients, including those with severe postoperative complications. This may explain the large variation and exceedingly long LOS of some patients. The readmission rate was higher in the pre-CP group, which shows that patients treated with the CP were not discharged inappropriately early.

In summary, the implementation of a CP for oncological gastrectomy at our institution did not lead entirely to the results that were expected based on studies on gastrectomy CPs in Asian settings [32,33], and on studies on CPs for other procedures in abdominal surgery at our institution and in other settings [13,34–40]. The reasons for this apparent difference in the efficacy of gastrectomy and other abdominal surgery CPs can only be speculated on. It is known that the biology of the disease and care for patients undergoing gastrectomy for gastric cancer in Asia shows important differences compared to European settings [41], but it remains unclear which specific factors might have determined the lack of efficacy of our CP. Moreover, oncological gastrectomy potentially demands more complex perioperative care than other abdominal procedures, for which CPs have led to pronounced improvements in process and outcome quality [13,34–40,42,43]. From the results of this study, it is difficult to conclude if the lack of efficacy was mainly due to limited adherence to the CP, or due to its suboptimal content and design for the given setting.

One of the strengths of our study is that it included all consecutive patients undergoing oncological gastrectomy before and after CP implementation. This is comparable to the "intention to treat principle" in randomized trials. In the case where the individual goals of the CP were not met, the patient was not taken "off the pathway". All patients who entered the study were analyzed regardless of deviations from the CP or possible complications. Therefore, selection bias is highly unlikely.

There are several methodological limitations inherent to the study. Its design is retrospective and included a single center. Moreover, we used chart review to collect data. This could compromise the validity of the data. Furthermore, the small sample size could bias the results. Documentation was not fully complete for all patients with regard to some variables and consequently, these could not be used for the analyses. Although selectively missing documentation is unlikely, bias could result. A crossover or, in other words, contamination bias could have occurred during the development and implementation phase of the CP. Health professionals who were part of the development team could have used their knowledge of the CP content prior to its implementation in October 2012. To counteract such issues, the CP was actually designed and implemented over only three months. Due to the study design with two groups of patients operated on before and after a defined time point, i.e., implementation of the CP, patients were operated on during different periods. The treatment during these periods might have been different (beyond the usage of the CP) because of other factors that influenced the process and outcome quality. For example, it is indisputable that surgical technique, and the skills as well as the experience of the individual surgeon have an effect on perioperative outcomes [44]. During the four-year study period, the surgeons who were in charge of and operated on patients changed. Therefore, surgical performance bias cannot be excluded.

Another weakness of our study is that not all stipulated goals were achieved after CP implementation. This suggests that not all team members adhered to the CP protocol. The main reasons for non-adherence to the main subitems have been explained above. Possibly, the addition of a dedicated study nurse to the CP team, and the introduction of an electronic CP could overcome non-adherence to the CP recommendations. The study nurse could promote protocol adherence and discuss the reasons for non-adherence with the appropriate caregivers. The use of an electronic CP checklist, with reminders in case of protocol deviation, could increase adherence, and thus potentially improve process and outcome quality.

Most of these limitations would have been avoidable if the study had been conducted as a randomized controlled trial. However, this is hardly feasible for studies evaluating CP usage in a single center because it usually requires cluster randomization [36,45].

4. Materials and Methods

4.1. CP Design, Implementation, and Content

Since 2006, the Department of Surgery, University Medical Center Mannheim, Medical Faculty Mannheim, Heidelberg University has implemented CPs for different surgical procedures in a stepwise manner [34–40,42,43,46,47]. In October 2012, a CP for oncological gastrectomy was introduced.

This CP is based on CPs for colorectal and bariatric surgery that incorporate ERAS elements. Both have been previously evaluated [36,43]. Specific elements were adapted to modify the CP for use in oncological gastrectomy. Both the original colorectal and the gastrectomy CP are based on published treatment and nursing recommendations. Furthermore, the best available evidence at the time of CP design was incorporated. The CP was designed and then implemented by a multi-hierarchical and interdisciplinary (anesthesiology, surgery, nutritional services, physiotherapy) team.

A literature review was done to identify current evidence on perioperative treatment elements. Subsequently, institutional standards that existed before, were integrated. Finally, all project participants agreed to the final CP version in a consensus meeting. Prior to the definitive implementation, all involved disciplines were trained to use the CP. After implementation of the CP, continuous efforts were made to enable further development and improvements of the CP based on suggestions made by staff.

A full version of the CP is provided in the online Supplementary Materials (Table S1). Its main contents are as follows: (1) hospital admission scheduled for the day before surgery; (2) epidural catheter placement; and (3) a stepwise oral pain medication scheme, based on non-opioids for all patients and on demand medication of potent opioids. Postoperatively, patients were transferred to a surgical intermediate care unit for at least one night. ICU admission took place only if deemed necessary by the surgeon and/or anesthesiologist. All patients were encouraged to drink sweetened tea until two hours prior to scheduled full anesthesia. An oral toluidine blue swallowing test was stipulated for postoperative day five. Drains were removed in case of a negative blue test and if respective enzyme levels in the drain fluid were not elevated (target drain: amylase <250 U/l in drain fluid). Detailed instructions on how to use an incentive spirometer were provided to patients. The stipulated day of discharge was postoperative day seven. Outpatient follow-up appointments were scheduled within 14 days after discharge. Patients were told to consult our emergency room in case of clinical irregularities. The rationale for incorporating the individual elements into the CP was that they were thought to either enhance recovery and thus shorten hospital stay, or to improve perioperative outcomes such as decreasing the risk of complications. Some of the elements (preoperative nutrition and smoking cessation, preoperative fasting and treatment with carbohydrates, epidural catheter placement, antithrombotic prophylaxis, antimicrobial prophylaxis, avoidance of hypothermia, glycemic control, urine catheter management, fluid balance, early and scheduled mobilization, and stimulation of bowel movement) are recommended in the consensus guidelines for enhanced recovery after gastrectomy of the Enhanced Recovery After Surgery (ERAS®) Group [31]. The perioperative analgesia scheme was endorsed by national guidelines. Other CP elements such as the oral toluidine blue swallowing test and abdominal drain management were based on pre-existing institutional standards, which were not backed by higher-level evidence. The targeted length of hospital stay was based on the minimum stay for oncological gastrectomy defined in the German DRG system [48].

The CP was designed as a four-page paper-based document containing all designated treatment steps for each pre- and postoperative day. CPs were kept with patients' treatment charts, and therefore they were constantly available for all involved staff members.

4.2. Study Design

The study used a single-center retrospective cohort design. All consecutive patients undergoing elective oncological gastrectomy were included. The intervention group (CP group) comprised all patients operated on after CP implementation in October 2012 until September 2014. The control group (pre-CP group) included patients operated on before CP implementation (May 2010 to September 2012). No formal sample size calculation was done. Data were obtained by means of retrospective chart review.

Patients in the pre-CP group were treated according to the individual judgment and decisions taken by the treating surgeons. Several semiformal standards for selected elements of care (e.g., early removal of catheters, epidural analgesia and early mobilization) had been in place and were used prior to CP implementation, but there was no comprehensive tool covering the entire treatment continuum. In the CP group, all patients were treated according to the CP.

The study was approved by the ethical committee of the Medical Faculty of Mannheim of the University of Heidelberg (2015-823R-MA). Because of its retrospective nature, the requirement for informed consent to review medical records was waived by the ethical committee. Confidentiality of patient data was ensured. The study was conducted in compliance with the Declaration of Helsinki. Neither the individual de-identified participant data, nor the specific data are intended to be shared by the authors. The CP documents will be accessible indefinitely as online supplementary data. The study has been registered with the German Clinical Trials Register (DRKS00020323).

4.3. Patient Characteristics

Demographic and clinical characteristics included age, sex, and preoperative status of patients according to the American Society of Anesthesiologists (ASA) physical status classification [49], underlying disease, administration of neoadjuvant chemotherapy, tumor location, and serum albumin levels upon preoperative admission. Histopathological data were analyzed by the Department of Pathology, Universitätsmedizin Mannheim, Mannheim, Germany according to the 7th version of the TNM-classification [50].

4.4. Surgery

Both before and after CP implementation, surgery was carried out by dedicated upper GI surgeons with more than four years' experience. To achieve R0-resection, patients received either total, distal or completion gastrectomy, depending on the anatomic location of the tumor and possible previous gastric operations. There were no laparoscopic resections. Associated procedures were performed when necessary. The gastrointestinal passage was preferably reconstructed using a long Roux-en-Y loop. Esophagojejunostomy was performed with a 25 mm circular stapler whereas gastrojejunostomy was hand sewn. A D2 lymphadenectomy according to the guidelines of the Japanese Gastric Cancer Association should be performed in all patients.

4.5. Study Outcomes

Process and outcome quality were defined according to the Donabedian model [51,52]. Process quality was considered as the adherence to treatment specifications as detailed in the CP and was assessed using the following parameters: day of removal of the foley catheter and epidural catheter, placement of central venous line and epidural catheter, postoperative mobilization, day of removal of intra-abdominal drainage and nasogastric tube, day of oral toluidine blue test, and day of resumption of liquid and solid diet.

Outcome quality was measured with the following parameters: morbidity, mortality, reoperation rate, LOS stratified by the presence or absence of complications, day of first postoperative defecation, pain level on a numeric rating scale and readmission rate. Morbidity was assessed according to the Clavien-Dindo classification of postoperative complications [53]. Deaths were counted as postoperative if they occurred during the hospital stay or during readmission. Surgical site infections were ascertained according to the Centers for Disease Control and prevention (CDC) definition [54]. Readmission was counted as such if it occurred no later than 30 days after initial discharge and if it was considered to be related to a postoperative problem.

4.6. Statistical Analysis

All outcomes were compared between the CP and pre-CP group. Missing values were not counted in the analyses with no imputation of missing values having been performed. Dichotomous variables were compared between groups using the chi-square test. Ordinal variables were compared using the Student's *t*-test if they were normally distributed and the Mann-Whitney U-test if they were not normally distributed. For not normally distributed variables, the median was used for descriptive analyses. For normally distributed variables, the mean was used. p-values <0.05 were considered statistically significant. There was no adjustment for multiple testing. SAS 13.2 (Cary, NC, USA) was used for all statistical analyses.

5. Conclusions

This study showed that using a CP for oncological gastrectomy affects several aspects of perioperative treatment. A high degree of process standardization was achieved and the uptake of respiratory training and the timely initiation of enteral nutrition was ensured. Other expected changes such as better pain control, earlier mobilization and shorter LOS were not realized after CP implementation. Outcome quality measured with perioperative morbidity and mortality did not change after CP implementation. In conclusion, an oncological gastrectomy CP can be used to standardize perioperative care, but its utility must be carefully weighed against the anticipated cost and effort required for implementation and continuous development.

Supplementary Materials: The following are available online at http://www.mdpi.com/2072-6694/12/2/434/s1, Table S1: Clinical Pathway for oncological gastrectomy used in the CP group of the study.

Author Contributions: P.T. and U.R. participated in the conception and design of the study. P.T. performed data collection, analyzed the data and drafted the manuscript. P.T., U.R., C.M., M.S., E.B., S.P., N.N.R. and C.R. participated in the analysis and interpretation of data, and revision of the manuscript for important intellectual content. All authors have read and agreed to the published version of the manuscript and are in agreement to be accountable for all aspects of the work in ensuring that questions related to the accuracy or integrity of any part of the work are appropriately investigated and resolved.

Funding: This research received no external funding.

Acknowledgments: Sylvia Büttner from the Department of Medical Statistics, Biomathematics and Informatics Universitätsmedizin Mannheim, Medical Faculty Mannheim, Heidelberg University, Mannheim, Germany participated in the analysis of data.

Conflicts of Interest: The authors declare no conflict of interest.

References

1. Bray, F.; Ferlay, J.; Soerjomataram, I.; Siegel, R.L.; Torre, L.A.; Jemal, A. Global cancer statistics 2018: GLOBOCAN estimates of incidence and mortality worldwide for 36 cancers in 185 countries. *CA Cancer J. Clin.* **2018**, *68*, 394–424. [CrossRef]
2. Tu, R.-H.; Lin, J.-X.; Zheng, C.-H.; Li, P.; Xie, J.-W.; Wang, J.-B.; Lu, J.; Chen, Q.-Y.; Cao, L.-L.; Lin, M.; et al. Complications and failure to rescue following laparoscopic or open gastrectomy for gastric cancer: a propensity-matched analysis. *Surg. Endosc.* **2017**, *31*, 2325–2337. [CrossRef]
3. Téoule, P.; Trojan, J.; Bechstein, W.; Woeste, G. Impact of Neoadjuvant Chemotherapy on Postoperative Morbidity after Gastrectomy for Gastric Cancer. *Dig. Surg.* **2015**, *32*, 229–237. [CrossRef]
4. Hager, E.S.; Abdollahi, H.; Crawford, A.G.; Moudgill, N.; Rosato, E.L.; Chojnacki, K.A.; Yeo, C.J.; Kennedy, E.P.; Berger, A. Is gastrectomy safe in the elderly? A single institution review. *Am. Surg.* **2011**, *77*, 488–492. [PubMed]
5. Endo, S.; Yoshikawa, Y.; Hatanaka, N.; Dousei, T.; Yamada, T.; Nishijima, J.; Kamiike, W. Prognostic Factors for Gastrectomy in Elderly Patients. *Int. Surg.* **2014**, *99*, 166–173. [CrossRef] [PubMed]
6. Damhuis, R.A.M.; Wijnhoven, B.P.L.; Plaisier, P.W.; Kirkels, W.J.; Kranse, R.; van Lanschot, J.J. Comparison of 30-day, 90-day and in-hospital postoperative mortality for eight different cancer types. *Br. J. Surg.* **2012**, *99*, 1149–1154. [CrossRef] [PubMed]
7. Ronellenfitsch, U.; Rössner, E.; Jakob, J.; Post, S.; Hohenberger, P.; Schwarzbach, M. Clinical Pathways in surgery: Should we introduce them into clinical routine? A review article. *Langenbeck's Arch. Surg.* **2008**, *393*, 449–457. [CrossRef] [PubMed]
8. Weiland, D.E. Why use clinical pathways rather than practice guidelines? *Am. J. Surg.* **1997**, *174*, 592–595. [CrossRef]
9. Glenn, D.M.; Macario, A. Do clinical pathways improve efficiency? *Semin. Anesth. Perioper. Med. Pain* **1999**, *18*, 281–288. [CrossRef]
10. Pearson, S.D.; Goulart-Fisher, D.; Lee, T.H. Critical pathways as a strategy for improving care: Problems and potential. *Ann. Intern. Med.* **1995**, *123*, 941–948. [CrossRef]
11. Rotter, T.; Kinsman, L.; Machotta, A.; Zhao, F.-L.; van der Weijden, T.; Ronellenfitsch, U.; Scott, S.D. Clinical pathways for primary care: Effects on professional practice, patient outcomes, and costs. *Cochrane Database Syst. Rev.* 2013. [CrossRef]
12. Kinsman, L.; Rotter, T.; James, E.; Snow, P.; Willis, J. What is a clinical pathway? Development of a definition to inform the debate. *BMC Med.* **2010**, *8*, e31. [CrossRef] [PubMed]
13. Lemmens, L.; van Zelm, R.; Borel Rinkes, I.; van Hillegersberg, R.; Kerkkamp, H. Clinical and organizational content of clinical pathways for digestive surgery: a systematic review. *Dig. Surg.* **2009**, *26*, 91–99. [CrossRef] [PubMed]
14. Wang, L.-H.; Zhu, R.-F.; Gao, C.; Wang, S.-L.; Shen, L.-Z. Application of enhanced recovery after gastric cancer surgery: An updated meta-analysis. *World J. Gastroenterol.* **2018**, *24*, 1562–1578. [CrossRef] [PubMed]
15. Grantcharov, T.P.; Kehlet, H. Laparoscopic gastric surgery in an enhanced recovery programme. *Br. J. Surg.* **2010**, *97*, 1547–1551. [CrossRef] [PubMed]
16. Tang, J.; Humes, D.; Gemmil, E.; Welch, N.; Parsons, S.; Catton, J. Reduction in length of stay for patients undergoing oesophageal and gastric resections with implementation of enhanced recovery packages. *Ann. R. Coll. Surg. Engl.* **2013**, *95*, 323–328. [CrossRef] [PubMed]
17. Pędziwiatr, M.; Matłok, M.; Kisialeuski, M.; Major, P.; Migaczewski, M.; Budzyński, P.; Ochenduszko, S.; Rembiasz, K.; Budzyński, A. Enhanced recovery (ERAS) protocol in patients undergoing laparoscopic total gastrectomy. *Videosurgery Other Miniinvasive Tech.* **2014**, *9*, e252. [CrossRef]
18. Gianotti, L.; Fumagalli Romario, U.; De Pascale, S.; Weindelmayer, J.; Mengardo, V.; Sandini, M.; Cossu, A.; Parise, P.; Rosati, R.; Bencini, L.; et al. Association Between Compliance to an Enhanced Recovery Protocol and Outcome After Elective Surgery for Gastric Cancer. Results from a Western Population-Based Prospective Multicenter Study. *World J. Surg.* **2019**, *43*, 2490–2498. [CrossRef]
19. Siewert, J.R.; Böttcher, K.; Stein, H.J.; Roder, J.D. Relevant prognostic factors in gastric cancer: Ten-year results of the German Gastric Cancer Study. *Ann. Surg.* **1998**, *228*, 449–461. [CrossRef]

20. Galata, C.; Blank, S.; Weiss, C.; Ronellenfitsch, U.; Reissfelder, C.; Hardt, J. Role of Postoperative Complications in Overall Survival after Radical Resection for Gastric Cancer: A Retrospective Single-Center Analysis of 1107 Patients. *Cancers* **2019**, *11*, e1890. [CrossRef]
21. Messager, M.; de Steur, W.O.; van Sandick, J.W.; Reynolds, J.; Pera, M.; Mariette, C.; Hardwick, R.H.; Bastiaannet, E.; Boelens, P.G.; van deVelde, C.J.H.; et al. Variations among 5 European countries for curative treatment of resectable oesophageal and gastric cancer: A survey from the EURECCA Upper GI Group (EUropean REgistration of Cancer CAre). *Eur. J. Surg. Oncol.* **2016**, *42*, 116–122. [CrossRef] [PubMed]
22. Gruen, R.L.; Pitt, V.; Green, S.; Parkhill, A.; Campbell, D.; Jolley, D. The effect of provider case volume on cancer mortality: systematic review and meta-analysis. *CA Cancer J. Clin.* **2009**, *59*, 192–211. [CrossRef] [PubMed]
23. Busweiler, L.A.; Henneman, D.; Dikken, J.L.; Fiocco, M.; van Berge Henegouwen, M.I.; Wijnhoven, B.P.; van Hillegersberg, R.; Rosman, C.; Wouters, M.W.; van Sandick, J.W.; et al. Failure-to-rescue in patients undergoing surgery for esophageal or gastric cancer. *Eur. J. Surg. Oncol.* **2017**, *43*, 1962–1969. [CrossRef] [PubMed]
24. Dikken, J.L.; van Sandick, J.W.; Allum, W.H.; Johansson, J.; Jensen, L.S.; Putter, H.; Coupland, V.H.; Wouters, M.W.J.M.; Lemmens, V.E.P.; van de Velde, C.J.H.; et al. Differences in outcomes of oesophageal and gastric cancer surgery across Europe. *Br. J. Surg.* **2013**, *100*, 83–94. [CrossRef]
25. Mingjie, X.; Luyao, Z.; Ze, T.; YinQuan, Z.; Quan, W. Laparoscopic Radical Gastrectomy for Resectable Advanced Gastric Cancer Within Enhanced Recovery Programs: A Prospective Randomized Controlled Trial. *J. Laparoendosc. Adv. Surg. Tech. A* **2017**, *27*, 959–964. [CrossRef]
26. Yamagata, Y.; Yoshikawa, T.; Yura, M.; Otsuki, S.; Morita, S.; Katai, H.; Nishida, T. Current status of the "enhanced recovery after surgery" program in gastric cancer surgery. *Ann. Gastroenterol. Surg.* **2019**, *3*, 231–238. [CrossRef]
27. Lawrence, V.A.; Cornell, J.E.; Smetana, G.W. American College of Physicians Strategies to reduce postoperative pulmonary complications after noncardiothoracic surgery: Systematic review for the American College of Physicians. *Ann. Intern. Med.* **2006**, *144*, 596–608. [CrossRef]
28. Burnham, J.P.; Rojek, R.P.; Kollef, M.H. Catheter removal and outcomes of multidrug-resistant central-line-associated bloodstream infection. *Medicine (Baltimore)* **2018**, *97*, e12782. [CrossRef]
29. Duchalais, E.; Larson, D.W.; Machairas, N.; Mathis, K.L.; Dozois, E.J.; Kelley, S.R. Outcomes of Early Removal of Urinary Catheter Following Rectal Resection for Cancer. *Ann. Surg. Oncol.* **2018**, *26*, 79–85. [CrossRef]
30. Mermel, L.A.; Allon, M.; Bouza, E.; Craven, D.E.; Flynn, P.; O'Grady, N.P.; Raad, I.I.; Rijnders, B.J.A.; Sherertz, R.J.; Warren, D.K. Clinical Practice Guidelines for the Diagnosis and Management of Intravascular Catheter-Related Infection: 2009 Update by the Infectious Diseases Society of America. *Clin. Infect. Dis.* **2009**, *49*, 1–45. [CrossRef] [PubMed]
31. Mortensen, K.; Nilsson, M.; Slim, K.; Schäfer, M.; Mariette, C.; Braga, M.; Carli, F.; Demartines, N.; Griffin, S.M.; Lassen, K.; et al. Consensus guidelines for enhanced recovery after gastrectomy: Enhanced Recovery After Surgery (ERAS®) Society recommendations. *Br. J. Surg.* **2014**, *101*, 1209–1229. [CrossRef] [PubMed]
32. Roh, C.K.; Son, S.-Y.; Lee, S.Y.; Hur, H.; Han, S.-U. Clinical pathway for enhanced recovery after surgery for gastric cancer: A prospective single-center phase II clinical trial for safety and efficacy. *J. Surg. Oncol.* **2020**. [CrossRef] [PubMed]
33. So, J.B.Y.; Lim, Z.L.; Lin, H.-A.; Ti, T.-K. Reduction of hospital stay and cost after the implementation of a clinical pathway for radical gastrectomy for gastric cancer. *Gastric Cancer* **2008**, *11*, 81–85. [CrossRef] [PubMed]
34. Téoule, P.; Römling, L.; Schwarzbach, M.; Birgin, E.; Rückert, F.; Wilhelm, T.J.; Niedergethmann, M.; Post, S.; Rahbari, N.N.; Reißfelder, C.; et al. Clinical Pathways for Pancreatic Surgery: Are They a Suitable Instrument for Process Standardization to Improve Process and Outcome Quality of Patients Undergoing Distal and Total Pancreatectomy? - a Retrospective Cohort Study. *Ther. Clin. Risk Manag.* **2019**, *15*, 1141–1152. [CrossRef] [PubMed]
35. Téoule, P.; Kunz, B.; Schwarzbach, M.; Birgin, E.; Rückert, F.; Wilhelm, T.J.; Niedergethmann, M.; Post, S.; Rahbari, N.N.; Reißfelder, C.; et al. Influence of Clinical pathways on treatment and outcome quality for patients undergoing pancreatoduodenectomy? - a retrospective outcome cohort study. *Asian J. Surg.* **2019**. [CrossRef]

36. Ronellenfitsch, U.; Schwarzbach, M.; Kring, A.; Kienle, P.; Post, S.; Hasenberg, T. The effect of clinical pathways for bariatric surgery on perioperative quality of care. *Obes. Surg.* **2012**, *22*, 732–739. [CrossRef] [PubMed]
37. Hardt, J.; Schwarzbach, M.; Hasenberg, T.; Post, S.; Kienle, P.; Ronellenfitsch, U. The effect of a clinical pathway for enhanced recovery of rectal resections on perioperative quality of care. *Int. J. Colorectal. Dis.* **2013**, *28*, 1019–1026. [CrossRef]
38. Schwarzbach, M.; Bönninghoff, R.; Harrer, K.; Weiss, J.; Denz, C.; Schnülle, P.; Birck, R.; Post, S.; Ronellenfitsch, U. Effects of a clinical pathway on quality of care in kidney transplantation: a non-randomized clinical trial. *Langenbeck's Arch. Surg.* **2010**, *395*, 11–17. [CrossRef]
39. Schwarzbach, M.; Rössner, E.; Schattenberg, T.; Post, S.; Hohenberger, P.; Ronellenfitsch, U. Effects of a clinical pathway of pulmonary lobectomy and bilobectomy on quality and cost of care. *Langenbeck's Arch. Surg.* **2010**, *395*, 1139–1146. [CrossRef]
40. Schwarzbach, M.H.M.; Ronellenfitsch, U.; Wang, Q.; Rössner, E.D.; Denz, C.; Post, S.; Hohenberger, P. Effects of a clinical pathway for video-assisted thoracoscopic surgery (VATS) on quality and cost of care. *Langenbeck's Arch. Surg.* **2010**, *395*, 333–340. [CrossRef]
41. Russo, A.E.; Strong, V.E. Gastric Cancer Etiology and Management in Asia and the West. *Annu. Rev. Med.* **2019**, *70*, 353–367. [CrossRef]
42. De Allegri, M.; Schwarzbach, M.; Loerbroks, A.; Ronellenfitsch, U. Which factors are important for the successful development and implementation of clinical pathways? A qualitative study. *BMJ Qual. Saf.* **2011**, *20*, 203–208. [CrossRef]
43. Schwarzbach, M.; Hasenberg, T.; Linke, M.; Kienle, P.; Post, S.; Ronellenfitsch, U. Perioperative quality of care is modulated by process management with clinical pathways for fast-track surgery of the colon. *Int. J. Colorectal. Dis.* **2011**, *26*, 1567–1575. [CrossRef]
44. Fong, Y.; Gonen, M.; Rubin, D.; Radzyner, M.; Brennan, M.F. Long-term survival is superior after resection for cancer in high-volume centers. *Ann. Surg.* **2005**, *242*, 540–544. [CrossRef]
45. Brown, C.; Hofer, T.; Johal, A.; Thomson, R.; Nicholl, J.; Franklin, B.D.; Lilford, R.J. An epistemology of patient safety research: a framework for study design and interpretation. Part 2. Study design. *Qual. Saf. Health Care* **2008**, *17*, 163–169. [CrossRef]
46. Ronellenfitsch, U.; Vargas Hein, O.; Uerlich, M.; Dahmen, A.; Tuschy, S.; Schwarzbach, M. Klinische Pfade als Instrument zur Qualitätsverbesserung in der perioperativen Medizin. *Perioper. Med.* **2009**, *1*, 164–172. [CrossRef]
47. Ronellenfitsch, U.; Schwarzbach, M. [Clinical pathways in surgery]. *Zentralbl. Chir.* **2010**, *135*, 99–101.
48. DRG Systemjahr 2012 Datenjahr 2010. Available online: https://www.g-drg.de/Archiv/DRG_Systemjahr_2012_Datenjahr_2010#sm2 (accessed on 3 February 2020).
49. Saklad, M. Grading of Patients for Surgical Procedures. *Anesthesiology* **1941**, *2*, 281–284. [CrossRef]
50. Washington, K. 7th Edition of the AJCC Cancer Staging Manual: Stomach. *Ann. Surg. Oncol.* **2010**, *17*, 3077–3079. [CrossRef]
51. Donabedian, A. The quality of care. How can it be assessed? *JAMA* **1988**, *260*, 1743–1748. [CrossRef]
52. Donabedian, A.; Bashshur, R. *An Introduction to Quality Assurance in Health Care*; Oxford University Press: New York, NY, USA, 2003; ISBN 978-0-19-515809-0.
53. Dindo, D.; Demartines, N.; Clavien, P.-A. Classification of surgical complications: A new proposal with evaluation in a cohort of 6336 patients and results of a survey. *Ann. Surg.* **2004**, *240*, 205–213. [CrossRef]
54. Surgical Site Infection: Prevention and Treatment of Surgical Site Infection. Available online: https://www.ncbi.nlm.nih.gov/books/NBK53724/ (accessed on 3 February 2020).

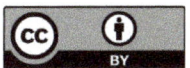

© 2020 by the authors. Licensee MDPI, Basel, Switzerland. This article is an open access article distributed under the terms and conditions of the Creative Commons Attribution (CC BY) license (http://creativecommons.org/licenses/by/4.0/).

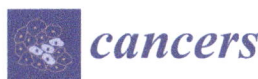

Article

The Influence of Pretherapeutic and Preoperative Sarcopenia on Short-Term Outcome after Esophagectomy

Johanna Grün [1], Lea Elfinger [1], Han Le [1], Christel Weiß [2], Mirko Otto [1], Christoph Reißfelder [1] and Susanne Blank [1,*]

[1] Department of Surgery, Universitäts Medizin Mannheim, Medical Faculty Mannheim, Heidelberg University, 68167 Mannheim, Germany; johanna.gruen@umm.de (J.G.); lea.elfinger@stud.uni-heidelberg.de (L.E.); Ngoc.Le@stud.uni-heidelberg.de (H.L.); mirko.otto@umm.de (M.O.); Christoph.reissfelder@umm.de (C.R.)
[2] Department of Medical Statistics and Biomathematics, Medical Faculty Mannheim, Heidelberg University, 68167 Mannheim, Germany; christel.weiss@medma.uni-heidelberg.de
* Correspondence: susanne.blank@umm.de

Received: 20 October 2020; Accepted: 14 November 2020; Published: 17 November 2020

Simple Summary: Although introducing minimally invasive surgery reduced postoperative morbidity after esophagectomy esophageal cancer still is a malignancy with poor prognosis. This study aimed to investigate whether preoperative sarcopenia has an influence on short-term postoperative outcome after esophagectomy in esophageal cancer patients. Our findings suggest that preoperative sarcopenia is no independent prognostic factor for postoperative outcome after esophagectomy but that patients' nutritional status consists of more factors than only body mass index (BMI) and muscle mass. Prehabilitation and preoperative optimization of the patients' nutritional status seems to be an important factor for short-term postoperative outcome after esophagectomy.

Abstract: By introducing minimally invasive surgery the rate of postoperative morbidity in esophageal cancer patients could be reduced. But esophagectomy is still associated with a relevant risk of postoperative morbidity and mortality. Patients often present with nutritional deficiency and sarcopenia even at time of diagnosis. This study focuses on the influence of skeletal muscle index (SMI) on postoperative morbidity and mortality. Fifty-two patients were included in this study. SMI was measured using computer tomographic images at the time of diagnosis and before surgery. Then, SMI and different clinicopathological and demographic features were correlated with postoperative morbidity. There was no correlation between SMI before neoadjuvant therapy ($p = 0.5365$) nor before surgery ($p = 0.3530$) with the short-term postoperative outcome. Regarding cholesterol level before surgery there was a trend for a higher risk of complications with lower cholesterol levels ($p = 0.0846$). Our findings suggest that a low preoperative SMI does not necessarily predict a poor postoperative outcome in esophageal cancer patients after esophagectomy but that there are many factors that influence the nutritional status of cancer patients. To improve nutritional status, cancer patients at our clinic receive specialized nutritional counselling during neoadjuvant treatment as well as after surgery.

Keywords: skeletal muscle index; esophagectomy; nutritional status; sarcopenia

1. Introduction

Esophageal cancer is the eighth most common type of malignancy worldwide. As diseases like reflux and obesity are increasing worldwide, the incidence of Barrett's esophagus as well as the incidence of esophageal adenocarcinomas have been increasing during the last decades. Although the outcome after curative multimodal therapy for esophageal cancer improved in the last decades, esophageal cancer still has a poor prognosis with a 10-year survival rate of approximately 16–17% and 5-year survival rate of approximately 20% [1,2].

By introducing minimally invasive procedures including the robot-assisted esophagectomy the rate of postoperative morbidity after esophagectomy could be reduced [3,4]. But esophagectomy is still associated with a relevant risk of postoperative morbidity, especially respiratory complications and anastomotic leakage including the risk of mediastinitis [5,6]. Thirty-day mortality after esophagectomy ranges between 1% and 3% and is mostly a result of postoperative complications. Postoperative complications affect short-term but also long-term survival as well as quality of life [6–8].

The Esophageal Complication Consensus Group presented an evaluation of 2704 patients with an overall complication rate of 59%. In an evaluation of 1057 total minimally invasive transthoracic esophagectomies, 56% of the patients developed at least one complication after surgery of which 26.9% were classified as Clavien Dindo grade III or more [6,9].

There are a number of studies identifying risk factors for a poor short-term outcome after surgical resection of esophageal carcinomas, such as high age, congestive heart failure, coronary artery disease, peripheral vascular disease, hypertension, body mass index <25 kg/m^2, and insulin dependent diabetes [10,11].

It has also been shown that the patient's nutritional status (including serum albumin, body mass index, muscle mass) plays an important role in determining patient outcome after surgery [12–14]. Patients with esophageal cancer often present with advanced disease and an impaired nutritional status due to dysphagia and cancer cachexia [15–17]. A good nutritional status before surgery has been proven to reduce the hypermetabolic response to surgery and to optimize wound and anastomotic healing and recovery [18–20].

Sarcopenia is defined by the European Working Group on Sarcopenia in Older People as low skeletal muscle mass and strength and is a risk factor for surgical patients in general [21,22]. It is also known as a possible risk factor for morbidity and poor prognosis after esophagectomy and could already be shown with a widespread prevalence, ranging from 16% to 79% before surgery [23–26].

A tool to measure skeletal muscle depletion is the skeletal muscle index (SMI). The skeletal muscle mass can be measured as cross-sectional area of the total skeletal muscle volume (cm^2) at L3 in computertomographic images. The SMI is calculated as total skeletal muscle volume (cm^2)/height^2 (m^2) [27,28]. It has been shown to be a prognostic factor independent from the body mass index (BMI) in oncologic patients [29].

Due to these findings the oncological patients at the Surgical Department of the University Hospital Mannheim are encouraged to take part in nutritional consulting at our clinic or at other specialized practices before and after surgery. Our clinic uses standardized protocols, guided by "Enhanced recovery after surgery"(ERAS) protocols, to improve postoperative outcome and length of hospital stay [30–33].

As a patient's nutritional status before surgery seems to play a major role for short term outcome, the aim of our study was to investigate whether sarcopenia, at the time of diagnosis or before surgery as well as BMI and serum albumin levels are risk factors for postoperative mortality and morbidity after minimally-invasive or robot-assisted esophagectomy.

2. Results

52 patients were included in the study. The demographic and clinicopathological data of these patients are presented in Table 1. Of the 52 patients in one patient the tumor could not be resected.

Twenty-eight patients (54%) were seen by the nutritional expert at our department preoperatively. All patients were seen by the nutritional expert postoperatively. Shakes with high concentration of proteins were advised to all patients preoperatively. Ten patients (19.2%) needed intravenous nutrition preoperatively.

Table 1. Demographic and clinicopathological characteristics of patient cohort.

Clinicopathological/Demographic Features	Characteristics	Total ($n = 52$)
Sex	Female	7 (13.5%)
	Male	45 (86.5%)
Age (years)	Mean	67.4 ± 12.0
	<65 years	19 (36.5%)
	≥65 years	33 (63.5%)
Histopathology	SCC	17 (32.7%)
	AEG I	17 (32.7%)
	AEG II	17 (32.7%)
	AEG III	1 (1.9%)
(y)pT	0	7 (13.73)
	1	11 (21.6%)
	2	6 (11.8%)
	3	25 (49.0%)
	4	2 (3.9%)
(y)pN	0	28 (55.0%)
	1	12 (23.5%)
	2	5 (9.8%)
	3	6 (11.8%)
(y)pM	x	50 (96.1%)
	1	2 (3.9%)
R-status	R0	50 (96.2%)
	R1	2 (3.8%)
Lymph node resection (number)	Median	21
	Range	12–56
Lymph node ratio	Median	0.07
	Range	0–0.61
Previous diseases	Cardiac	28 (53.9%)
	Pulmonary	6 (11.5%)
	Diabetes	3 (5.8%)
	Other types of cancer	10 (19.23%)
Preoperative chemotherapy		48 (92.3%)
Type of Surgery	DaVinci-assisted	26 (50%)
	Laparoscopic	20 (38.5%)
	Open	6 (11.5%)
Clavien Dindo	0–3a	36 (69.2%)
	>3a	16 (30.8%)
CCI (Comprehensive Complication Index)	Median	26.2
	Range	0–100

Mean albumin level was 35 ± 4.7 g/dL, mean cholesterol level (199.83 ± 48.18) mg/dL.

In 6 patients (11.5%) a totally minimal invasive approach was not possible, two patients had to be converted to open surgery (conversion rate 3.8%).

Mean duration of surgery was 445 min (range 303–770).

2.1. Skeletal Muscle Index

The skeletal muscle index (SMI) ranged from 29.7 to 62.6 cm^2/m^2 at time of diagnosis and from 31.9 to 62.5 cm^2/m^2 before surgery (mean values (47.7 ± 8.6 cm^2/m^2 and 42.1 ± 7.0 cm^2/m^2 respectively)).

Applying the cut-offs for sarcopenia used by Prado et al [34]. Of the patients, 54.3% were sarcopenic at time of diagnosis and 87.5% before surgery.

A moderate correlation was detected between BMI and SMI (r = 0.69855, $p < 0.001$, Pearson's correlation coefficient).

Results regarding SMI, weight and BMI are summarized in Table 2. BMI at diagnosis is missing in 10 patients.

Table 2. Skeletal muscle index (SMI), weight, and body mass index (BMI) at different time points.

SMI, BMI and Weight Reduction	Classification	Total (%)
SMI at Diagnosis	Mean (cm^2/m^2)	47.7 ± 8.6
	Range (cm^2/m^2)	29.7–62.6
SMI before surgery	Mean (cm^2/m^2)	42.1 ± 7.0
	Range (cm^2/m^2)	31.9–62.5
Reduction of SMI	Mean (cm^2/m^2)	3.3 ± 4.2
Reduction of SMI	0–5%	16 (51.6%)
	>5%	9 (29.0%)
	<0%	6 (19.4%)
Reduction of weight	0–5%	12 (29.3%)
	>5%	11 (26.8%)
	<0%	18 (44%)
BMI at diagnosis	Mean (kg/m^2)	25.87 (±3.75)
	Range (kg/m^2)	19.6–34.6
BMI before surgery	Mean (kg/m^2)	25.34 (±3.9)
	Range(kg/m^2)	18.37–34.94
BMI at diagnosis	<20 kg/m^2	2 (5%)
	20–25 kg/m^2	18 (45%)
	25–30 kg/m^2	16 (40%)
	>30 kg/m^2	4 (10%)
BMI before surgery	<20 kg/m^2	2 (3.9%)
	20–25 kg/m^2	25 (48.1%)
	25–30 kg/m^2	17 (32.7%)
	>30 kg/m^2	8 (15.4%)

2.2. Short Term Postoperative Outcome

Short term postoperative outcome was defined as complications during hospital stay and complication associated mortality.

The median length of hospital stay was 17.5 days (range 6–114 days), the length of stay at the Intensive Care Unit ranged from one to 77 days (median 17.5 days).

One patient died during the first 30 days after surgery (30-day mortality 1.9%). The 90-day mortality in our cohort did not differ from this value because there were no other patients who died within 90 days after surgery.

Four patients died because of complications of surgery, three of those after 90 days after surgery (complication associated mortality 7.69%).

The general complication rate was 59.6% (31 patients in total). Twenty-six patients had surgical complications (50%), of those 16 patients suffered from anastomosis insufficiency (30.8% anastomosis insufficiency rate). Twenty-three patients suffered from medical complications (44.2%), including cardiac complications (21.2%) and pulmonary complications (32.7%).

There was no correlation between SMI before neoadjuvant therapy nor before surgery with short-term postoperative outcome ($p = 0.5365$, $p = 0.3530$ respectively, t-test).

The BMI also had no influence on postoperative morbidity: $p = 0.4228$ (BMI before diagnosis), $p = 0.1673$ (BMI before neoadjuvant treatment), $p = 0.2810$ (BMI before surgery), t-test.

Regarding cholesterol level before surgery there was a trend for a higher risk of complications with lower cholesterol levels ((207 ± 55) mg/dL vs. (191 ± 38) mg/dL, $p = 0.0846$, t-test).

Other factors such as patient age ($p = 0.4361$, t-test), sex ($p = 0.6872$, Fisher's exact test), history of cardiac disease ($p = 0.8615$, Chi-square-test), history of pulmonary disease ($p = 1.0$, Fisher's exact test), tumor stage ((y)pT: $p = 0.7241$, (y)pN: $p = 1.0$, Cochran–Armitag-test), and preoperative albumin levels ($p = 0.3747$, t-test) had no statistically significant influence on short-term postoperative outcome. The duration of surgery however correlated with the incidence of complications ($p = 0.0034$, t-test) as patients who had longer times of surgery showed a higher risk for complications (466 vs. 392 min). Patients who had another type of cancer before developing esophageal cancer also suffered more often from complications ($p = 0.0049$, Chi-square-test).

3. Discussion

Our findings suggest that a low preoperative SMI does not necessarily predict a poor postoperative outcome in esophageal cancer patients after esophagectomy. Neither BMI before neoadjuvant therapy nor before surgery shows a correlation with postoperative outcome in our patients' collective. Only one patient presented with a BMI <20 kg/m^2. This might be due to patient selection. We included in our analysis only patients who were eligible for a thoracoabdominal surgical approach, which means that they were in a sufficient general status of health to tolerate one-lung-ventilation. We also checked all patients for nutritional deficiencies and sent them to a nutritional expert, which explains why the body weight difference between the time of diagnosis and the time of surgery is quite low and which could also explain the missing impact of BMI and SMI in our patients' collective. Often it is during neoadjuvant treatment that patients lose weight and muscle mass [35]. In our patients' collective the mean BMI before and after neoadjuvant treatment did not differ (25.87 and 25.34 kg/m^2) and most of the patients (70.95%) did not have a significant reduction of SMI (70.95% had less than 5% reduction). Of the patients, formula increase of SMI during neoadjuvant treatment. This shows that an improvement in patients' general status during neoadjuvant treatment is feasible.

As the number of patients in this cohort was relatively low it is also possible that in a greater cohort an effect of preoperative SMI on postoperative outcome might also be greater. Nevertheless, we could not see even a trend to significant correlations between SMI and complications and also there are other studies that showed similar results concerning this topic [36,37].

The level of cholesterol seems to be associated with the short-term postoperative outcome in our patients' collective, which underlines the importance of the nutritional status. The results are not statistically significant but this could be due to the relatively low number of patients included.

Malnutrition in esophageal cancer patients is caused by dysphagia and a reduced food intake but also by cancer cachexia, which is induced by systemic inflammation. Cachexia leads to loss of body weight, body fat, and skeletal muscle mass. The molecular mechanisms of cachexia are still not fully understood, additionally there exists no consistent definition [38].

It should be mentioned that only one third of our patients had a squamous cell carcinoma (SCC). Patients with SCC normally present with a more advanced malnutrition than patients with an adenocarcinoma of the esophagus as malnutrition is often already present before diagnosis of the tumor.

Different studies showed significant relations between sarcopenia and poor outcome after surgery such as the study by Elliot et al. that showed that sarcopenia is significantly associated with major complications after surgery or the study by Järvinen et al. that showed a correlation with worse overall survival [14,25,35,39–41].

Grotenhuis et al. and Siegal et al. on the other hand could not find any correlations between sarcopenia and postoperative complications or survival rates [36,37]. Nakashima et al. could find a significant correlation between sarcopenia and higher anastomotic leakage rates and also between sarcopenia and worse overall survival but these significant results were only present in a subgroup of patients older than 65 years [42].

The definition for sarcopenia is not consistent. Some studies define their own cut-offs. We used the most common cut-offs suggested by Prado et al [34], resulting in a rate of sarcopenia of 87.5% after neoadjuvant therapy. There is a huge variation in the prevalence of sarcopenia in esophageal cancer patients in the literature, varying from 16% to 75% [43].

Nevertheless, the latest meta-analysis by Papaconstantinou et al. showed a significant increase in overall morbidity, respiratory complications and anastomotic leaks in esophageal cancer patients with sarcopenia after esophagectomy. There were no statistically significant differences in overall mortality or Clavien–Dindo grade III or greater complications between patients with low and patients with normal SMI [44].

Although our findings contradict many studies that showed significant correlations between sarcopenia and higher complications or lower over-all survival there are other studies that support our findings.

There are some other important aspects of our patient cohort that should be illuminated. It has already been proven that prehabiliation and preoperative optimization of nutrition in cancer patients leads to better outcome and better quality of life after cancer surgery [45,46]. Nutrition goals include an adequate nutritional intake to prevent loss of muscle mass, modulate inflammation and the immune response, optimize glucose control, reduce the hypermetabolic response to surgery, and provide nutrients to optimize wound and anastomotic healing and recovery [18–20,47–50].

As mentioned above our cancer patients are provided with professional advice by specialized nutritional counsellors before and after surgery to improve their fitness and nutritional. This includes provision of protein shakes, dietary plans and even parenteral feeding if necessary.

It also has been shown that standardized protocols like ERAS protocols for surgical cancer patients lead to shorter in-hospital stays, decreased complications and longer overall survival [31–33,51]. Therefore, our clinic uses standardized pathways for esophageal cancer patients to improve postoperative outcomes of esophageal cancer patients.

This aspect of our preoperative treatment might be the reason for the absence of significant increase of postoperative morbidity or mortality in sarcopenic patients. One aspect that should be evaluated in further trials is, whether the outcome of esophageal cancer patients can be improved by introducing prehabilitation programs.

The presented study has some limitations. It is retrospective in nature. This increases the risk for systemic errors and selection bias. The number of patients included in this study ($n = 52$) is relatively low which may affect its statistical power, especially in regard to complication rates and specific complications.

4. Materials and Methods

4.1. Patient Selection and Study Design

The Surgical Department of the University Hospital Mannheim of Heidelberg University is a certified centre for esophageal surgery. A detailed clinico-pathologic database is prospectively maintained for all patients with esophageal cancer since January 2018 including data on short-term postoperative outcome. In this analysis we included patients having been operated between January 2018 and July 2019 in the Surgical Department of the University Hospital Mannheim of Heidelberg University. The local ethical committee "Ethikkomission II, University of Heidelberg" gave approval for the analysis (ethic code 2020-803R) and all patients gave written informed consent.

There were 52 patients who underwent surgery for treatment of esophageal cancer in whom CT scans were sufficient to determine the skeletal muscle index. Of the 52 patients, 48 underwent neoadjuvant chemotherapy before surgery (FLOT regimen).

The skeletal muscle index was measured using computer tomographic images at the time of diagnosis as well as before surgery.

Out of the 52 patients 13 did not have two usable computer tomographies either because they did not undergo neoadjuvant treatment or because imaging was not done in-hospital and was not sufficient for measurement of the SMI.

The skeletal muscle index (SMI) was calculated as the cross-sectional area of the total skeletal muscle volume (cm^2) at L3.

At the level of the third lumbar vertebra (L3) we measured the area (cm^2) of the left and right psoas major muscles, the side abdominal muscles, rectus abdominis muscles, erector spinae muscles, and quadratus lumborum muscles using "syngo.share view diagnostic" (Siemens Healthineers, Erlangen, Germany). Two adjacent axial images within the same series were selected, and total muscle cross-sectional area (cm^2) at L3 was determined and averaged for each patient (1).

$$SMI\ (cm^2/m^2) = Lean\ tissue\ area_{L3}\ (cm^2)/height^2\ (m^2) \quad (1)$$

Low SMI was defined as <52.4 cm^2/m^2 for male patients and as <38.5 cm^2/m^2 for female patients according to current literature [44].

4.2. Preoperative Treatment

All patients are seen by a surgeon specialized in upper GI surgery before admission to hospital. Education in nutrition as well as recommendation for daily physical activity and cessation of smoking is given during the consultation. Patients with nutritional deficiency are additionally sent to a nutritional consulting at the University Hospital Mannheim to compensate nutritional deficiencies before surgery.

Body weight, BMI, serum albumin levels, dysphagia, and subjective well-being are measured regularly by specialized nutritional consults. If the patients are suffering from dysphagia, weight loss or low BMI their nutritional status is treated by prescribing protein shakes, dietary plans and, if necessary parenteral feeding.

4.3. Neoadjvuant and Perioperative Therapy

Patients with locally advanced tumors (>cT2N0) receive neoadjuvant or perioperative treatment according to the FLOT protocol for adenocarcinomas and according to the CROSS protocol for squamous cell carcinomas [52].

After completion of preoperative treatment patients are reevaluated including a risk assessment and preoperative blood management.

4.4. Surgery

Surgery is performed by minimally invasive procedure, either laparoscopic and thoracoscopic approach or laparoscopic abdominal approach and robot-assisted thoracal approach. The decision for a robotic approach is taken due to availability of the DaVinci robot. Resection is done according to Ivor–Lewis procedure (right-thoracic approach). Lymphadenectomy is performed according to current guidelines including mediastinal lymphadenectomy and abdominal lymphadenectomy (D2 Lymphadenectomy). Reconstruction is done by gastric conduit and side-to-side esophagogastrostomy.

4.5. Postoperative Management

To ensure a standardized treatment of patients after surgery, the postoperative hospital management follows an in-house pathway which defines postoperative nutrition, mobilization, drainage management, laboratory tests, and dismissal after esophagectomy.

Directly after surgery patients stay in an Intermediate Care Unit (IMCU) for at least two days to ensure a balanced fluid management and to detect early postoperative complications as soon as possible.

Patients are encouraged to engage in light physical activity beginning on the day of surgery. Breathing exercises are started on the first postoperative day and should be done at least every hour for five to ten minutes.

Increased patient self-sufficiency in the general ward helps to improve mobilization and nutrition. Nutritional counselling is performed during hospital treatment to determine nutritional deficiencies and to arrange nutritional support after the dismissal.

4.6. Postoperative Complications

Postoperative complications were investigated separately as surgical and medical complications as well as complications in total. To measure complication rates the Comprehensive Complication Index (CCI) was used as well as Clavien–Dindo classification.

The Clavien–Dindo classification is a commonly used tool with which usually the single most severe complication occurring in a patient during a given episode of care is reported [53].

The CCI is a relatively new tool to measure complications based on the Clavien–Dindo classification. In contrast to the Clavien–Dindo classification the CCI integrates all postoperative complications with their respective severities, on a scale ranging from 0 (no burden from complications) to 100 (death). The CCI is calculated by adding the weights of different complications (wC) and using a defined formula (2) [54].

$$CCI = [\sqrt{(wC_1 + wC_2 \ldots + wC_x)}]/24.7 \qquad (2)$$

4.7. Statistical Analysis

For quantitative, approximately normally distributed variables, the mean and standard deviation have been calculated. Qualitative variables are given as absolute and relative frequencies. The median, together with range, are presented for skewed or ordinally scaled parameters. A Student's *t*-test was used for comparing approximately normally distributed quantitative variables. The Cochran–Armitage test for trend was used to determine the influence of (y)pT and (y)pN categories on major postoperative complications. For qualitative variables, a χ^2-test or Fisher exact test was performed, as appropriate. To determine a correlation between BMI and SMI the Pearson correlation coefficient was determined. All statistical tests for the comparison of 2 groups were two-tailed. In general, a test result was considered statistically significant if $p < 0.05$. All statistical analyses were performed using the SAS statistical analysis software, release 9.4 (SAS Institute Inc., Cary, NC, USA).

5. Conclusions

Our findings suggest that the nutritional status and physical fitness of esophageal cancer patients consist of more than BMI and skeletal muscle mass but that albumin levels, cardiac health and subjective well-being, as a consequence of adequate nutrition preoperatively, are important factors for a good postoperative outcome.

In the era of multimodal approach to esophageal cancer, treatment should consist not only of oncological treatment and surgery but also of a more systemic approach including patient education, physical exercise, and nutritional support. The period between diagnosis and surgery should be used to reduce cachexia and to better the general status of health.

Therefor prehabilitation programs as well as nutritional plans should be evaluated in clinical studies with the aim to give a consistent recommendation for patients with esophageal cancer [55].

Author Contributions: Conceptualization, M.O., C.R., and S.B.; methodology, S.B.; software, C.W.; validation, S.B.; formal analysis, C.W., S.B.; investigation, H.L., L.E.; data curation, L.E., J.G.; writing—original draft preparation, J.G.; writing—review and editing, S.B.; supervision, M.O., C.R.; project administration, S.B.; All authors have read and agreed to the published version of the manuscript.

Funding: This research received no external funding.

Conflicts of Interest: The authors declare no conflict of interest.

References

1. Robert-Koch-Institut. Gesellschaft der Epidemiologischen Krebsregister in Deutschland e.V.: Berlin. Krebs in Deutschland 2009/2010. Available online: https://www.rki.de/DE/Content/Gesundheitsmonitoring/Gesundheitsberichterstattung/GBEDownloadsB/KID2013.pdf%3F__blob%3DpublicationFile (accessed on 9 August 2013).
2. Onkologie, L. S3-Leitlinie Diagnostik und Therapie der Plattenepithelkarzinome und Adenokarzinome des Ösophagus. Available online: https://www.awmf.org/leitlinien/detail/ll/021-023OL.html (accessed on 31 December 2018).
3. Mariette, C.; Markar, S.; Dabakuyo-Yonli, T.; Meunier, B.; Pezet, D.; Collet, D.; D'Journo, X.B.; Brigand, C.; Perniceni, T.; Carrère, N.; et al. Hybrid Minimally Invasive Esophagectomy for Esophageal Cancer. *N. Engl. J. Med.* **2019**, *380*, 152–162. [CrossRef]
4. Straatman, J.; Van Der Wielen, N.; Cuesta, M.; Daams, F.; Garcia, J.R.; Bonavina, L.; Rosman, C.; van Berge Henegouwen, M.I.; Gisbertz, S.S.; van der Peet, D.L. Minimally Invasive Versus Open Esophageal Resection. *Ann. Surg.* **2017**, *266*, 232–236. [CrossRef]
5. Vetter, D.; Gutschow, C.A. Strategies to prevent anastomotic leakage after esophagectomy and gastric conduit reconstruction. *Langenbecks Arch. Surg.* **2020**. [CrossRef] [PubMed]
6. Low, D.E.; Kuppusamy, M.K.; Alderson, D.; Cecconello, I.; Chang, A.C.; Darling, G.; Davies, A.; D'Journo, X.B.; Gisbertz, S.S.; Griffin, S.M.; et al. Benchmarking Complications Associated with Esophagectomy. *Ann Surg.* **2019**, *269*, 291–298. [CrossRef] [PubMed]
7. Van der Sluis, P.C.; Tagkalos, E.; Hadzijusufovic, E.; Babic, B.; Uzun, E.; van Hillegersberg, R.; Lang, H.; Grimminger, P.P. Robot-Assisted Minimally Invasive Esophagectomy with Intrathoracic Anastomosis (Ivor Lewis): Promising Results in 100 Consecutive Patients (the European Experience). *J. Gastrointest. Surg.* **2020**. [CrossRef] [PubMed]
8. Horne, Z.D.; Wegner, R.E.; Colonias, A.; Weksler, B.; Glaser, S.M.; Kalash, R.; Beriwal, S. Drivers of 30- and 90-day Postoperative Death After Neoadjuvant Chemoradiation for Esophageal Cancer. *Ann. Thorac. Surg.* **2020**, *109*, 921–926. [CrossRef]
9. Schmidt, H.M.; Gisbertz, S.S.; Moons, J.; Rouvelas, I.; Kauppi, J.; Brown, A.; Asti, E.; Luyer, M.; Lagarde, S.M.; Berlth, F.; et al. Defining Benchmarks for Transthoracic Esophagectomy. *Ann. Surg.* **2017**, *266*, 814–821. [CrossRef]
10. Yang, Y.H.; Park, S.Y.; Kim, D.J. Chyle leakage after esophageal cancer surgery. *Korean J. Thorac. Cardiovasc. Surg.* **2020**, *53*, 191–199. [CrossRef]
11. Wright, C.D.; Kucharczuk, J.C.; O'Brien, S.M.; Grab, J.D.; Allen, M.S. Predictors of major morbidity and mortality after esophagectomy for esophageal cancer: A Society of Thoracic Surgeons General Thoracic Surgery Database risk adjustment model. *J. Thorac. Cardiovasc. Surg.* **2009**, *137*, 587–596. [CrossRef]
12. Hirahara, N.; Matsubara, T.; Fujii, Y.; Kaji, S.; Hyakudomi, R.; Yamamoto, T.; Uchida, Y.; Miyazaki, Y.; Ishitobi, K.; Kawabata, Y.; et al. Geriatric nutritional risk index as a prognostic marker of pTNM-stage I and II esophageal squamous cell carcinoma after curative resection. *Oncotarget* **2020**, *11*, 2834–2846. [CrossRef]
13. Pacelli, F.; Bossola, M.; Rosa, F.; Tortorelli, A.P.; Papa, V.; Doglietto, G.B. Is malnutrition still a risk factor of postoperative complications in gastric cancer surgery? *Clin. Nutr.* **2008**, *27*, 398–407. [CrossRef] [PubMed]
14. Menezes, T.M.; Dias, M.O.; Reis, R.; Elias, J.; Lucchesi, F.R.; Araujo, R.L.C. Prognostic value of muscle depletion assessed by computed tomography for surgical outcomes of cancer patients undergoing total esophagectomy and gastrectomy. *J. Surg. Oncol.* **2020**, *121*, 814–822. [CrossRef] [PubMed]
15. Movahed, S.; Norouzy, A.; Ghanbari-Motlagh, A.; Eslami, S.; Khadem-Rezaiyan, M.; Emadzadeh, M.; Nematy, M.; Ghayour-Mobarhan, M.; Tabrizi, F.V.; Bozzetti, F.; et al. Nutritional Status in Patients with Esophageal Cancer Receiving Chemoradiation and Assessing the Efficacy of Usual Care for Nutritional Managements. *Asian Pac. J. Cancer Prev.* **2020**, *21*, 2315–2323. [CrossRef]
16. Hébuterne, X.; Lemarié, E.; Michallet, M.; De Montreuil, C.B.; Schneider, S.M.; Goldwasser, F. Prevalence of malnutrition and current use of nutrition support in patients with cancer. *J. Parenter. Enter. Nutr.* **2014**, *38*, 196–204. [CrossRef] [PubMed]
17. Qiu, Y.; You, J.; Wang, K.; Cao, Y.; Hu, Y.; Zhang, H.; Fu, R.; Sun, Y.; Chen, H.; Yuan, L.; et al. Effect of whole-course nutrition management on patients with esophageal cancer undergoing concurrent chemoradiotherapy: A randomized control trial. *Nutrition* **2020**, *69*, 110558. [CrossRef]

18. Evans, D.C.; Martindale, R.G.; Kiraly, L.N.; Jones, C.M. Nutrition Optimization Prior to Surgery. *Nutr. Clin. Pract.* **2014**, *29*, 10–21. [CrossRef]
19. Gillis, C.; Carli, F. Promoting perioperative metabolic and nutritional care. *Anesthesiology* **2015**, *123*, 1455–1472. [CrossRef]
20. Arends, J.; Bachmann, P.; Baracos, V.; Barthelemy, N.; Bertz, H.; Bozzetti, F.; Fearon, K.; Hütterer, E.; Isenring, E.; Kaasa, S.; et al. ESPEN guidelines on nutrition in cancer patients. *Clin. Nutr.* **2017**, *36*, 11–48. [CrossRef]
21. Galata, C.; Hodapp, J.; Wei, C.; Karampinis, I.; Vassilev, G.; Reißfelder, C.; Otto, M. Skeletal Muscle Mass Index Predicts Postoperative Complications in Intestinal Surgery for Crohn's Disease. *J. Parenter. Enter. Nutr.* **2020**, *44*, 714–721. [CrossRef]
22. Cruz-Jentoft, A.J.; Baeyens, J.P.; Bauer, J.M.; Boirie, Y.; Cederholm, T.; Landi, F.; Martin, F.C.; Michel, J.P.; Rolland, Y.; Schneider, S.M.; et al. Sarcopenia: European consensus on definition and diagnosis. *Age Ageing* **2010**, *39*, 412–423. [CrossRef]
23. Fujihata, S.; Ogawa, R.; Nakaya, S.; Hayakawa, S.; Okubo, T.; Sagawa, H.; Tanaka, T.; Takahashi, H.; Mutsuo, Y.; Takiguchi, S. The impact of skeletal muscle wasting during neoadjuvant chemotherapy on postoperative anastomotic leakage in patients with esophageal cancer. *Esophagus* **2020**, *1*, 3. [CrossRef] [PubMed]
24. Ishida, T.; Makino, T.; Yamasaki, M.; Tanaka, K.; Miyazaki, Y.; Takahashi, T.; Kurokawa, Y.; Motoori, M.; Kimura, Y.; Nakajima, K.; et al. Impact of measurement of skeletal muscle mass on clinical outcomes in patients with esophageal cancer undergoing esophagectomy after neoadjuvant chemotherapy. *Surgery* **2019**, *166*, 1041–1047. [CrossRef] [PubMed]
25. Elliott, J.A.; Doyle, S.L.; Murphy, C.F.; King, S.; Guinan, E.M.; Beddy, P.; Ravi, N.; Renyolds, J.V. Sarcopenia: Prevalence, and Impact on Operative and Oncologic Outcomes in the Multimodal Management of Locally Advanced Esophageal Cancer. *Ann. Surg.* **2017**, *266*, 822–830. [CrossRef] [PubMed]
26. Deng, H.Y.; Zha, P.; Peng, L.; Hou, L.; Huang, K.L.; Li, X.Y. Preoperative sarcopenia is a predictor of poor prognosis of esophageal cancer after esophagectomy: A comprehensive systematic review and meta-analysis. *Dis. Esophagus* **2019**, *32*, doy115. [CrossRef]
27. Mourtzakis, M.; Prado, C.M.M.; Lieffers, J.R.; Reiman, T.; McCargar, L.J.; Baracos, V.E. A practical and precise approach to quantification of body composition in cancer patients using computed tomography images acquired during routine care. *Appl. Physiol. Nutr. Metab.* **2008**, *33*, 997–1006. [CrossRef] [PubMed]
28. Portal, D.; Hofstetter, L.; Eshed, I.; Dan-Lantsman, C.; Sella, T.; Urban, D.; Onn, A.; Bar, J.; Segal, G. L3 skeletal muscle index (L3SMI) is a surrogate marker of sarcopenia and frailty in non-small cell lung cancer patients. *Cancer Manag. Res.* **2019**, *11*, 2579–2588. [CrossRef]
29. Martin, L.; Birdsell, L.; MacDonald, N.; Reiman, T.; Clandinin, M.T.; McCargar, L.J.; Murphy, R.; Ghosh, S.; Sawyer, M.B.; Baracos, V.E. Cancer cachexia in the age of obesity: Skeletal muscle depletion is a powerful prognostic factor, independent of body mass index. *J. Clin. Oncol.* **2013**, *31*, 1539–1547. [CrossRef]
30. Kehlet, H.; Wilmore, D.W. Multimodal strategies to improve surgical outcome. *Am. J. Surg.* **2002**, *183*, 630–641. [CrossRef]
31. Low, D.E.; Allum, W.; De Manzoni, G.; Ferri, L.; Immanuel, A.; Kuppusamy, M.K.; Law, S.; Lindblad, M.; Maynard, N.; Neal, J.; et al. Guidelines for Perioperative Care in Esophagectomy: Enhanced Recovery After Surgery (ERAS®) Society Recommendations. *World J. Surg.* **2019**, *43*, 299–330. [CrossRef]
32. Fransen, L.F.C.; Luyer, M.D.P. Effects of improving outcomes after esophagectomy on the short- and long-term: A review of literature. *J. Thorac. Dis.* **2019**, *11*, S845–S850. [CrossRef]
33. Bhutiani, N.; Quinn, S.A.; Jones, J.M.; Mercer, M.K.; Philips, P.; McMasters, K.M.; Scoggins, C.R.; Martin, R.C.G. The impact of enhanced recovery pathways on cost of care and perioperative outcomes in patients undergoing gastroesophageal and hepatopancreatobiliary surgery. *Surgery* **2018**, *164*, 719–725. [CrossRef] [PubMed]
34. Prado, C.M.; Cushen, S.J.; Orsso, C.E.; Ryan, A.M. Sarcopenia and cachexia in the era of obesity: Clinical and nutritional impact. *Proc. Nutr. Soc.* **2016**, *75*, 188–198. [CrossRef] [PubMed]
35. Järvinen, T.; Ilonen, I.; Kauppi, J.; Salo, J.; Räsänen, J. Loss of skeletal muscle mass during neoadjuvant treatments correlates with worse prognosis in esophageal cancer: A retrospective cohort study. *World J. Surg. Oncol.* **2018**, *16*, 27. [CrossRef] [PubMed]

36. Grotenhuis, B.A.; Shapiro, J.; van Adrichem, S.; de Vries, M.; Koek, M.; Wijnhoven, B.P.L.; van Lanschot, J.J.B. Sarcopenia/Muscle Mass is not a Prognostic Factor for Short- and Long-Term Outcome After Esophagectomy for Cancer. *World J. Surg.* **2016**, *40*, 2698–2704. [CrossRef]
37. Siegal, S.R.; Dolan, J.P.; Dewey, E.N.; Guimaraes, A.R.; Tieu, B.H.; Schipper, P.H.; Hunter, J.G. Sarcopenia is not associated with morbidity, mortality, or recurrence after esophagectomy for cancer. *Am. J. Surg.* **2018**, *215*, 813–817. [CrossRef]
38. Argilés, J.M.; Busquets, S.; Stemmler, B.; López-Soriano, F.J. Cancer cachexia: Understanding the molecular basis. *Nat. Rev. Cancer* **2014**, *14*, 754–762. [CrossRef]
39. Nishigori, T.; Okabe, H.; Tanaka, E.; Tsunoda, S.; Hisamori, S.; Sakai, Y. Sarcopenia as a predictor of pulmonary complications after esophagectomy for thoracic esophageal cancer. *J. Surg. Oncol.* **2016**, *113*, 678–684. [CrossRef]
40. Saeki, H.; Nakashima, Y.; Kudou, K.; Sasaki, S.; Jogo, T.; Hirose, K.; Edahiro, K.; Korehisa, S.; Taniguchi, D.; Nakanishi, R.; et al. Neoadjuvant Chemoradiotherapy for Patients with cT3/Nearly T4 Esophageal Cancer: Is Sarcopenia Correlated with Postoperative Complications and Prognosis? *World J. Surg.* **2018**, *42*, 2894–2901. [CrossRef]
41. Soma, D.; Kawamura, Y.I.; Yamashita, S.; Wake, H.; Nohara, K.; Yamada, K.; Kokudo, N. Sarcopenia, the depletion of muscle mass, an independent predictor of respiratory complications after oncological esophagectomy. *Dis. Esophagus* **2019**, *32*, doy092. [CrossRef]
42. Nakashima, Y.; Saeki, H.; Nakanishi, R.; Sugiyama, M.; Kurashige, J.; Oki, E.; Maehara, Y. Assessment of Sarcopenia as a Predictor of Poor Outcomes after Esophagectomy in Elderly Patients with Esophageal Cancer. *Ann. Surg.* **2018**, *267*, 1100–1104. [CrossRef]
43. Boshier, P.R.; Heneghan, R.; Markar, S.R.; Baracos, V.E.; Low, D.E. Assessment of body composition and sarcopenia in patients with esophageal cancer: A systematic review and meta-analysis. *Dis. Esophagus* **2018**, *31*. [CrossRef]
44. Papaconstantinou, D.; Vretakakou, K.; Paspala, A.; Misiakos, E.P.; Charalampopoulos, A.; Nastos, C.; Patapis, P.; Pikoulis, E. The impact of preoperative sarcopenia on postoperative complications following esophagectomy for esophageal neoplasia: A systematic review and meta-analysis. *Dis. Esophagus* **2020**, *33*, doaa002. [CrossRef] [PubMed]
45. Barberan-Garcia, A.; Ubré, M.; Roca, J.; Lacy, A.M.; Burgos, F.; Risco, R.; Momblán, D.; Balust, J.; Blanco, I.; Martínez-Pallí, G. Personalised Prehabilitation in High-risk Patients Undergoing Elective Major Abdominal Surgery. *Ann. Surg.* **2018**, *267*, 50–56. [CrossRef] [PubMed]
46. Gillis, C.; Buhler, K.; Bresee, L.; Carli, F.; Gramlich, L.; Culos-Reed, N.; Sajobi, T.T.; Fenton, T.R. Effects of Nutritional Prehabilitation, with and without Exercise, on Outcomes of Patients Who Undergo Colorectal Surgery: A Systematic Review and Meta-analysis. *Gastroenterology* **2018**, *155*, 391–410. [CrossRef]
47. Steenhagen, E. Preoperative nutritional optimization of esophageal cancer patients. *J. Thorac. Dis.* **2019**, *11*, S645–S653. [CrossRef]
48. Steenhagen, E.; Van Vulpen, J.K.; Van Hillegersberg, R.; May, A.M.; Siersema, P.D. Nutrition in peri-operative esophageal cancer management Nutrition in peri-operative esophageal cancer management. *Expert Rev. Gastroenterol. Hepatol.* **2017**, *11*, 663–672. [CrossRef]
49. Minnella, E.M.; Awasthi, R.; Loiselle, S.E.; Agnihotram, R.V.; Ferri, L.E.; Carli, F. Effect of Exercise and Nutrition Prehabilitation on Functional Capacity in Esophagogastric Cancer Surgery: A Randomized Clinical Trial. *JAMA Surg.* **2018**, *153*, 1081–1089. [CrossRef]
50. Williams, J.D.; Wischmeyer, P.E. Assessment of perioperative nutrition practices and attitudes—A national survey of colorectal and GI surgical oncology programs. *Am. J. Surg.* **2017**, *213*, 1010–1018. [CrossRef]
51. Visioni, A.; Shah, R.; Gabriel, E.; Attwood, K.; Kukar, M.; Nurkin, S. Enhanced Recovery after Surgery for Noncolorectal Surgery? *Ann. Surg.* **2018**, *267*, 57–65. [CrossRef]
52. Al-Batran, S.E.; Homann, N.; Pauligk, C.; Goetze, T.O.; Meiler, J.; Kasper, S.; Kopp, H.G.; Mayer, F.; Haag, G.M.; Luley, K.; et al. Perioperative chemotherapy with fluorouracil plus leucovorin, oxaliplatin, and docetaxel versus fluorouracil or capecitabine plus cisplatin and epirubicin for locally advanced, resectable gastric or gastro-oesophageal junction adenocarcinoma (FLOT4): A randomised, phase 2/3 trial. *Lancet* **2019**, *393*, 1948–1957.

53. Dindo, D.; Demartines, N.; Clavien, P.A. Classification of surgical complications: A new proposal with evaluation in a cohort of 6336 patients and results of a survey. *Ann. Surg.* **2004**, *240*, 205–213. [CrossRef] [PubMed]
54. Slankamenac, K.; Graf, R.; Barkun, J.; Puhan, M.A.; Clavien, P.A. The comprehensive complication index: A novel continuous scale to measure surgical morbidity. *Ann. Surg.* **2013**, *258*, 1–7. [CrossRef] [PubMed]
55. Le Roy, B.; Pereira, B.; Bouteloup, C.; Costes, F.; Richard, R.; Selvy, M.; Pétorin, C.; Gagnière, J.; Futier, E.; Slim, K.; et al. Effect of prehabilitation in gastro-oesophageal adenocarcinoma: Study protocol of a multicentric, randomised, control trial-the PREHAB study. *BMJ Open* **2016**, *6*, e012876. [CrossRef] [PubMed]

Publisher's Note: MDPI stays neutral with regard to jurisdictional claims in published maps and institutional affiliations.

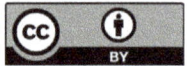

© 2020 by the authors. Licensee MDPI, Basel, Switzerland. This article is an open access article distributed under the terms and conditions of the Creative Commons Attribution (CC BY) license (http://creativecommons.org/licenses/by/4.0/).

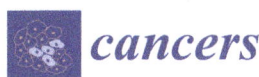

Article

Postoperative Morbidity and Failure to Rescue in Surgery for Gastric Cancer: A Single Center Retrospective Cohort Study of 1107 Patients from 1972 to 2014

Christian Galata [1], Ulrich Ronellenfitsch [2], Susanne Blank [1], Christoph Reißfelder [1,*] and Julia Hardt [1]

[1] Department of Surgery, Universitätsmedizin Mannheim, Medical Faculty Mannheim, Heidelberg University, D-68167 Mannheim, Germany; christian.galata@umm.de (C.G.); susanne.blank@umm.de (S.B.); julia.hardt@umm.de (J.H.)
[2] Department of Visceral, Vascular and Endocrine Surgery, University Hospital Halle (Saale), Martin-Luther-University Halle-Wittenberg, D-06120 Halle (Saale), Germany; ulrich.ronellenfitsch@uk-halle.de
* Correspondence: christoph.reissfelder@umm.de; Tel.:+49-621-383-2555

Received: 19 June 2020; Accepted: 16 July 2020; Published: 18 July 2020

Abstract: Background: The aim of this study was to evaluate postoperative morbidity, mortality, and failure to rescue following complications after radical resection for gastric cancer. Methods: A retrospective analysis of the surgical database of patients with gastroesophageal malignancies at our institution was performed. All consecutive patients undergoing R0 gastrectomy for pT1–4 M0 gastric adenocarcinoma between October 1972 and February 2014 were eligible for this analysis. Patients were divided into two groups according to the date of surgery: an early cohort operated on from 1972–1992 and a late cohort operated on from 1993–2014. Both groups were compared regarding patient characteristics and surgical outcomes. Results: A total of 1107 patients were included. Postoperative mortality was more than twice as high in patients operated on from 1972–1992 compared to patients operated on from 1993–2014 (6.8% vs. 3.2%, $p = 0.017$). Between both groups, no significant difference in failure to rescue after major surgical complications was observed (20.8% vs. 20.5%, $p = 1.000$). Failure to rescue after other surgical and non-surgical complications was 37.8% in the early cohort compared to 3.2% in the late cohort ($p < 0.001$). Non-surgical complications accounted for 71.2% of lethal complications between 1972 and 1992, but only for 18.2% of lethal complications between 1993 and 2014 ($p = 0.002$). Conclusion: In the course of four decades, postoperative mortality after radical resection for gastric cancer has more than halved. In this cohort, the reason for this decrease was reduced mortality due to non-surgical complications. Major surgical morbidity after gastrectomy remains challenging.

Keywords: gastric cancer; gastrectomy; complications; mortality; failure to rescue

---

1. Introduction

Resection for gastric cancer is regarded as a high-risk surgery with significant morbidity and mortality [1,2]. Failure to rescue, defined as the mortality among patients with postoperative complications, has recently been of interest in this context. Patients with gastric cancer have been reported to have even higher failure to rescue rates than patients undergoing esophageal resections [3]. In recent years, the focus of large-scale multicenter studies has been to examine variations in surgical outcomes among patients undergoing surgery for gastric cancer between different institutions [4,5]. Current evidence suggests that high-volume surgical centers might have lower mortality rates [6,7].

A significant reduction in postoperative mortality and failure to rescue from 2011 to 2014 has been reported in a recent study from the Netherlands, where the authors concluded that these effects were at least in part due to increased centralization and newly introduced minimum volume requirements [3]. In 2019, a register-based study from Germany evaluated postoperative mortality in non-bariatric gastric resections among patients operated on between 2010 and 2015 [8]. All these studies compared surgical outcomes of high-volume and low-volume centers over short periods of time. However, changes in surgical outcomes over longer periods of time are rarely reported. Developments in surgical techniques and perioperative management over recent decades are likely to impact patient outcomes. However, relevant results are very often not available due to a lack of long-term data. Therefore, the rationale for this study was to evaluate patients undergoing radical resection for gastric cancer from 1972 to 2014 regarding changes in postoperative morbidity, mortality, and failure to rescue. The same patient collective has recently been investigated regarding the impact of postoperative complications on overall survival. The results showed that postoperative complications are a significant risk factor for poor overall survival, an effect which was mainly caused by complication-associated early mortality [9]. A further objective of the present study was to examine whether—as expected in view of the medical progress—postoperative complications and failure to rescue after gastric cancer surgery were reduced over the course of the four decades studied. In order to examine this hypothesis in more detail, the total study time period was divided in two equally long periods (early versus late) and the outcomes of the two periods were compared.

2. Results

2.1. Patients' Characteristics

Between October 1972 and February 2014, a total of 1107 consecutive patients underwent R0 resection for pT1–4 M0 gastric adenocarcinoma at our institution and were included in the analysis. The standard approach for these patients at our institution was open total or subtotal (4/5) gastrectomy with D2 lymphadenectomy (LAD). To investigate changes in postoperative morbidity and mortality, patients were stratified into two cohorts according to the date of operation, 1972–1992 and 1993–2014. During the early period, 761 patients underwent surgery as compared to 346 patients during the late period.

Patients' characteristics are shown in Table 1. In both cohorts, there were more males than females, 55.1% and 54.6%, respectively. Median patient age was significantly higher in the 1993–2014 group (67 vs. 65 years, $p < 0.001$). After the year 1992, total gastrectomy was more frequently performed than subtotal gastrectomy (56.6% vs. 42.7%, $p < 0.001$). The rate of multivisceral resections was not significantly different (47.0% in the late cohort vs. 45.3% in the early cohort, $p = 0.645$). However, splenectomies were performed significantly more often from 1972 to 1992 (40.2% vs. 20.5%, $p < 0.001$), whereas cholecystectomies were more commonly performed from 1993 to 2014 (23.5% vs. 5.4%, $p < 0.001$).

2.2. Tumor Characteristics

Tumor characteristics are shown in Table 2. Tumor characteristics were comparable between both periods, with no significant differences in tumor location ($p = 0.163$), pT ($p = 0.359$), pN ($p = 0.119$), or American Joint Committee on Cancer/Union Internationale Contre le Cancer (AJCC/UICC) stages ($p = 0.343$) observed. Only for the histological classification based on Laurén's criteria were significantly more cancers of the diffuse type observed in the later years ($p < 0.001$).

Table 1. Patient and procedure characteristics.

Parameter	1972–1992 (n = 761)		1993–2014 (n = 346)		p
	n or median	% or IQR	n or median	% or IQR	
Gender					0.897
Female	342	44.9	157	45.4	
Male	419	55.1	189	54.6	
Age	65	56–71	67	57–74	0.001
Gastrectomy					<0.001
Total	325	42.7	196	56.6	
Subtotal	436	57.3	150	43.4	
Multivisceral resection	345	45.3	158	47.0	0.645
Splenectomy	306	40.2	69	20.5	<0.001
Cholecystectomy	41	5.4	79	23.5	<0.001
Intestinal resection	17	2.2	12	3.6	0.222
Hepatic procedure	9	1.2	11	3.3	0.025
Pancreatic procedure	21	2.8	8	2.4	0.840
Missing data	0		10		

p values in bold type indicate statistical significance.

Table 2. Tumor characteristics.

Parameter	1972–1992 (n = 761)		1993–2014 (n = 346)		p
	n	%	n	%	
Tumor location					0.163
Non-antropyloric	474	62.3	200	57.8	
Antropyloric	287	37.7	146	42.2	
Laurén classification					0.001
Non-diffuse	473	62.2	165	51.6	
Diffuse	287	37.8	155	48.4	
Missing data	1		26		
pT category					0.359
T1–T2	588	77.3	258	74.6	
T3–T4	173	22.7	88	25.4	
pN category					0.119
pN0	377	49.5	153	44.3	
pN1–3	384	50.5	192	55.7	
Missing data	0		1		
AJCC/UICC stage					0.343
IA–IB	358	47.0	157	45.5	
II	183	24.0	80	23.2	
IIIA–IIIB	180	23.7	83	24.1	
IV	40	5.3	25	7.2	
Missing data	0		1		

p values in bold type indicate statistical significance. AJCC: American Joint Committee on Cancer; UICC: Union Internationale Contre le Cancer.

2.3. Postoperative Outcomes

Postoperative outcomes are shown in Table 3. The median length of hospital stay was significantly shorter in the period from 1993 to 2014 compared to the period from 1972 to 1992 ($p < 0.001$). The overall postoperative complication rate was higher in the later cohort (31.9% vs. 22.3%, $p = 0.001$). However, when the rate of major surgical complications (defined as anastomotic leak, postoperative abdominal abscess, fascial dehiscence, peritonitis, sepsis, secondary hemorrhage, or relaparotomy for any reason) was investigated, no statistically significant differences were observed between both groups ($p = 0.071$). Similarly, the anastomotic leak (including duodenal stump leaks) rates did not differ significantly (6.3% in the late cohort vs. 3.8% in the early cohort, $p = 0.084$).

Table 3. Postoperative outcomes.

Outcome	1972–1992 (n = 761)		1993–2014 (n = 346)		p
	n	% or IQR	n	% or IQR	
Postoperative morbidity					
Overall complications	170	22.3	107	31.9	**0.001**
Major surgical complications	72	9.5	44	13.1	0.071
Anastomotic leak	29	3.8	21	6.3	0.084
Other surgical/non-surgical complications	98	12.9	63	18.8	**0.012**
Missing data	0		11		
Postoperative mortality					
30-day mortality	46	6.0	6	1.7	**0.001**
In-hospital mortality	52	6.8	11	3.2	**0.017**
Missing data	0		2		
Failure to rescue					
Overall complications	52/170 *	30.6	11/107 *	10.3	**<0.001**
Major surgical complications	15/72 *	20.8	9/44 *	20.5	1.000
All other complications	37/98 *	37.8	2/63 *	3.2	**<0.001**
Hospital stay (days)	15	13–19	14	11–18	**<0.001**
Missing data	3		3		

* The denominator indicates the total number of patients with each respective complication. p values in bold type indicate statistical significance.

Both 30-day mortality (6.0% vs. 1.7%) and in-hospital mortality (6.8% vs. 3.2%) were significantly higher in the 1972 to 1992 cohort as compared to the 1993 to 2014 cohort. No statistically significant difference in the failure to rescue rate after major surgical complications was observed between both time periods (20.5% in the late cohort vs. 20.8% in the early cohort, $p = 1.000$). In contrast, failure to rescue after non-major surgical complications and non-surgical complications was significantly more common from 1972 to 1992 as compared to the period from 1993 to 2014 (37.8% vs. 3.2%, $p < 0.001$). Mortality-associated complications are shown in Table 4. In the early cohort, non-surgical complications accounted for 71.2% of all lethal complications as compared to 18.2% in the late cohort, whereas major surgical morbidity accounted for 28.8% of complication-related deaths from 1972 to 1992 as compared to 81.8% from 1993 to 2014 ($p = 0.002$). For patients who underwent splenectomy (Table 5), a higher rate of major surgical ($p = 0.016$) and overall complications ($p = 0.005$) was observed in the late cohort (major morbidity 22.7%, overall morbidity 40.9%) compared to the early cohort (major morbidity 11.1%, overall morbidity 23.5%). However, patients who underwent splenectomy in the late cohort had significantly higher T-stages ($p = 0.049$), higher N-stages ($p < 0.001$), and higher UICC stages ($p = 0.001$).

Table 4. Mortality-associated complications.

Type of Lethal Complication	1972–1992 Total Cases: n = 761 Postoperative Mortality: n = 52		1993–2014 Total Cases: n = 346 Postoperative Mortality: n = 11	
	n	% of mortality	n	% of mortality
Major surgical complications	15	28.8	9	81.8
Anastomotic leak	10	19.2	8	72.7
Relaparotomy(other reason/not specified)	4	7.7	0	0
General sepsis	1	1.9	1	9.1
Non-surgical complications	37	71.2	2	18.2
Cardiovascular	13	25.0	0	0
Cardiorespiratory	11	21.2	1	9.1
Respiratory	11	21.2	0	0
Other	2	3.8	1	9.1

Table 5. Patients with splenectomy.

Variable	1972–1992 ($n = 306$)		1993–2014 ($n = 69$)		p
	n	%	n	%	
Overall complications	34	11.1	15	22.7	**0.005**
Major surgical complications	72	23.5	27	40.9	**0.016**
Anastomotic leak	17	5.6	6	9.1	0.267
Missing data	0		3		

p values in bold type indicate statistical significance.

2.4. Risk Factors for Postoperative Mortality

Univariable and multivariable analyses were performed to identify potential risk factors for postoperative mortality. In the entire cohort (1972–2014), patient age and the occurrence of overall postoperative complications, major surgical complications, and anastomotic leak were factors significantly associated with postoperative death in univariable analysis (Table 6). When multivariable analysis was performed, major surgical complications, anastomotic leak, and older patient age remained in the statistical model as factors associated with postoperative in-hospital mortality (Table 7). Subgroup analyses of patients operated on from 1972 to 1992 and from 1993 to 2014 returned similar results (Tables 6 and 7).

Table 6. Variables associated with postoperative mortality in univariable analysis.

Variable	Overall Cohort (1972–2014)		p	Early Group (1972–1992)		p	Late Group (1993–2014)		p
	OR	95% CI		OR	95% CI		OR	95% CI	
Overall complications			**<0.001**			**<0.001**			**<0.001**
Major surgical complications	6.294	3.625–10.928	**<0.001**	4.637	2.401–8.956	**<0.001**	37.157	7.717–178.926	**<0.001**
Anastomotic leak	12.513	6.531–23.971	**<0.001**	8.647	3.783–19.763	**<0.001**	63.795	15.141–268.784	**<0.001**
Age			**0.020**			0.185			**0.001**
Gender	1.197	0.720–1.992	0.516	1.351	0.769–2.374	0.314	0.689	0.198–2.397	0.760
Type of gastrectomy	1.586	0.936–2.687	0.092	1.443	0.799–2.603	0.247	1.594	0.477–5.328	0.541
Multivisceral resection	0.773	0.434–1.240	0.294	0.738	0.414–1.316	0.317	0.745	0.206–2.690	0.775
Tumor location	0.848	0.507–1.418	0.595	0.976	0.542–1.724	1.000	0.404	0.116–1.408	0.214
Laurén classification	1.316	0.772–2.241	0.356	0.969	0.543–1.728	1.000	4.471	0.950–21.031	0.062
pT category			0.116			0.086			0.971
pN category			0.377			0.174			0.729
AJCC/UICC stage			0.122			0.061			0.931

p values in bold type indicate statistical significance. OR: odds ratio; CI: confidence interval.

Table 7. Variables associated with postoperative mortality in multivariable analysis.

Variable	Overall Cohort (1972–2014)			Early Group (1972–1992)			Late Group (1993–2014)		
	OR	95% CI	p	OR	95% CI	p	OR	95% CI	p
Major surgical complications	2.550	1.034–6.292	**0.042**	2.319	0.862–6.237	0.096	9.774	0.712–134.246	0.088
Anastomotic leak	5.550	1.987–15.507	**0.001**	4.000	1.197–13.367	**0.024**	20.391	1.561–266.289	**0.021**
Age	1.030	1.005–1.055	**0.017**				1.191	1.060–1.339	**0.033**

p values in bold type indicate statistical significance. OR: odds ratio; CI: confidence interval.

3. Discussion

This study presents one of the rare reports on the results of surgery for gastric cancer in a large cohort of 1107 consecutive patients (1972 to 1992: $n = 761$ and 1993 to 2014: $n = 346$), over a time period of more than four decades at a European university hospital.

The main finding of the study was that 30-day and in-hospital mortality were significantly lower in the later period. Major surgical complications, anastomotic leak, and older patient age were independent risk factors for postoperative in-hospital mortality in multivariable analysis. However, it is not unlikely that age would have dropped out as a risk factor for postoperative mortality if other known risk factors, such as serum albumin level, Eastern Cooperative Oncology Group (ECOG) performance status, and American Society of Anesthesiologists (ASA) physical status, which were not available in our data set, had been included in the analysis.

Analysis of mortality-associated complications revealed that non-surgical complications accounted for the large majority (71.2%) of all lethal complications in patients with surgery between 1972 and 1992, as compared to only 18.2% of lethal complications in patients with surgery between 1993 and 2014 ($p = 0.002$). Correspondingly, failure to rescue rates for major surgical complications did not differ between the two time periods, while failure to rescue occurred significantly more frequently among patients with non-major surgical and non-surgical complications in the cohort operated on between 1972 and 1992 (37.8% vs. 3.2%). This retrospective study cannot provide further details on the reasons for this shift regarding the type of complications associated with a lethal course. The main driver is most likely the fact that the treatment of acute medical complications, such as pulmonary embolism or myocardial infarction that frequently led to death in former times, has tremendously improved over recent decades.

An analysis of the register data of the Dutch Upper GI Cancer Audit showed similar rates: postoperative mortality after gastric cancer surgery ranged from 7.7% in 2011 to 3.8% in 2014 and failure to rescue occurred in 38.0% of patients with a complication in 2011 and in 19.0% in 2014 [3]. The authors attribute this to quality improvement measures, such as multidisciplinary therapy standards and minimum surgical volume requirements. A recently published large observational study from Germany, using national hospital discharge data (72,528 cases of non-bariatric gastric surgery), revealed that the prevention of mortality after complex gastric surgery mainly depends on the ability to rescue patients with complications. Failure to rescue rates were 28.1% in very low-volume hospitals versus 22.7% in very high-volume hospitals [8]. According to most definitions, institutions with an average of about 50 gastroesophageal resections for malignant indications per year are regarded as high-volume centers [10]. The reported mortality rates of our patients operated on between 1972 and 1992 were consistent with the findings of a recent retrospective cohort study based on American College of Surgeons National Surgery Quality Improvement Program (ACS NSQIP) data: 30-day mortality was 5.2% [11]. This also compares well to the results from a large US cohort study analyzing the National Inpatient Sample (NIS) data of 13,354 patients undergoing gastric resection for malignancy with an in-hospital mortality rate of 6.0% [12]. A much lower short-term mortality was reported by the authors of a Cochrane systematic review investigating the outcomes of laparoscopic versus open gastrectomy for gastric cancer; the pooled short-term mortality of eleven randomized controlled trials (RCTs) was only 0.4% (11/2635) [13].

Further comparison of the two time periods revealed a few more statistically significant differences. Not surprisingly, the length of hospital stay has decreased in the more recent decades, which is most likely the result of the implementation of a modern and evidence-based clinical pathway for gastric resections that follows the principles of the enhanced recovery after surgery (ERAS®) and "fast track" concepts. Moreover, significantly older patients were operated on, which speaks for the advances of modern perioperative medicine that has made it possible to offer curative surgery even to elderly patients. The fact that the number of cases in the early time period was more than twice as high as in the later time period (761 vs. 346) reflects the decline in the incidence of "true" gastric cancer and a shift towards more proximal tumor locations, such as the cardia and distal esophagus, in Europe during recent decades [14]. In general, the clinicopathologic features of the patients in our analysis were consistent with other long-term analyses of patients with surgery for gastric cancer [15].

Interestingly, there were more overall complications (31.9% vs. 22.3%, $p = 0.001$) in the later time period (1993–2014), which may have multifactorial etiology. First, in the later time period, there were significantly more total gastrectomies, which are known to be associated with a higher risk for postoperative morbidity than subtotal gastrectomies. The most plausible explanation for the increase in total gastrectomies is the significantly higher number of cancers of the diffuse type according to Laurén's criteria in the late cohort. Furthermore, the fact that significantly older, and thus potentially frailer and more comorbid patients, were operated on in the 1990s and 2000s could also have resulted in a higher overall complication rate. Besides, the latter may partly explain why we did not find a decrease in major surgical morbidity despite the far-reaching technical and medical advances that took place during the four decades included in our analysis. Nevertheless, the actual clinical relevance of the age difference between the two cohorts remains to be discussed. Life expectancy has also increased during the observation period of more than four decades, and so it may be that the median age difference of 2 years is clinically irrelevant, because the older patients of the late cohort were not biologically older than the chronologically younger patients of the early cohort. We did not evaluate the impact of the extent of LAD on postoperative morbidity and mortality, as the extent of LAD was not thoroughly documented in the early decades of the database. However, the trend towards a more radical LAD (D2 or D3 vs. D1) over time may have contributed to an increase in the overall complication rate in our later cohort, which has been reported in several RCTs from Western countries [16,17]. In this regard, one could also argue that, despite more radical operations (more total gastrectomies and more extensive LAD), a rise in major complications did not occur, which could be the result of advances in surgical techniques and perioperative management. Neoadjuvant treatment of gastric cancer patients was only introduced in the years 2005 to 2006 and thus administered only to the absolute minority of patients included in our study. Therefore, we chose not to include this parameter in our analyses. Yet, most studies on this found no increase in postoperative morbidity or mortality after neoadjuvant treatment [18,19].

There are some limitations to our study. First, the retrospective nature and the inherent potential for misclassification may limit the validity of our data. Second, there may be confounding variables not recorded in our database. Therefore, we cannot exclude the possibility that factors not tracked in the database may have contributed to our findings. Third, missing data and changes in coding and classifications over such a long period as forty-two years may limit the validity of our results. Fourth, the exclusion of R1 resections, because of the aim to exclusively investigate patients in a curative situation and to generate a study population as homogeneous as possible regarding their risk profile for complications, may be called into question in the context of analyzing short-term outcomes after gastric cancer surgery. Thus, the exclusion of R1 resections may be interpreted as a potential limitation of our study because it could have biased the results. Fifth, the use of the Clavien Dindo Classification would have been desirable to increase the comparability of the results. However, the Clavien Dindo Classification was first described in 2004, whereas our institutional database collected cases from 1972 to 2014. Thus, in most cases, complications were not documented according to the Clavien Dindo Classification and a retrospective classification would have been error-prone and unreasonable. Sixth, data on the extent of lymphadenectomy and 90-day mortality would have been of interest in the context of the present study but were not available in sufficient continuity and quality over the long observation period for inclusion into the analyses. The strengths of this study lie in its large sample size, the consecutive, homogenous cohort (only gastric adenocarcinomas, only patients operated on with curative intent, one center), and the long time period covered. Most cohort studies based on data from registers or institutional databases which investigated similar research study objectives included rather heterogeneous patient populations, sometimes even patients who underwent gastric surgery for benign disease. With the aim to reduce bias and confounding factors due to heterogeneity among the included cases, we defined very precise inclusion and exclusion criteria. Nevertheless, the included patient cohort and the setting are still representative in the context of the investigated study objective. Therefore, we assume that the study results have a high external validity and generalizability.

4. Materials and Methods

4.1. Ethics Approval

Ethics board approval was obtained from the Medical Ethics Commission II of the Medical Faculty Mannheim, Heidelberg University, Mannheim, Germany (2019-849R). The study was performed according to the Declaration of Helsinki.

4.2. Study Design

The present study is a single-center retrospective cohort study using data from a prospectively run institutional database.

4.3. Setting and Participants

Medical records from 2252 consecutive patients operated on at the Department of Surgery, University Medical Centre Mannheim, Heidelberg University, Mannheim, Germany between October 1972 and February 2014 were examined, and patients with pT1–4 M0 adenocarcinomas of the stomach who underwent R0 resections were identified. Patients with Barrett's carcinoma and gastric remnant cancer were excluded, as were patients with atypical gastric or esophageal resections. Tumors of the subcardial stomach (Siewert type III) were included, whereas esophagogastric junctional adenocarcinomas (Siewert types I and II) were excluded, as these are classified and staged according to the esophageal scheme in the current AJCC/UICC staging system. Finally, 1107 of the 2252 patients met the inclusion criteria and could be further analyzed. For the present analyses, no follow-up of patients was required.

4.4. Variables, Data Sources, and Risk of Bias

Data on patient, procedure, and tumor characteristics were taken from the institutional database for gastroesophageal malignancies. Patient and procedure characteristics included gender, age, type of gastrectomy (total versus subtotal), and the extent of resection in the case of multivisceral resection. Tumor characteristics comprised tumor location (non-antropyloric versus antropyloric), Laurén's classification, histological type, and pT and pN categories, as well as the AJCC/UICC stages. The latter were available according to the 5th edition for all gastric cancers operated on between 1972 and 2001. The 6th and 7th editions of the AJCC/UICC classification were used on cases from 2002 until 2009 and from 2010 until 2014, respectively. Before analysis, all patients included in this study were restaged according to the 6th edition of the AJCC/UICC staging system for gastric cancer, which was the most recent edition based on which the restaging of all patients was possible, in order to achieve a uniform classification. Data on surgical and non-surgical complications were extracted from the database. Major surgical complications were defined as the documentation of at least one of the following events during the postoperative course: anastomotic leak (including duodenal stump leak), postoperative (abdominal) abscess, fascial dehiscence, peritonitis, sepsis, secondary hemorrhage, and relaparotomy for any reason. When multiple complications occurred, the most severe complication was recorded in the database. In cases where multiple complications were recorded, the most severe complication was used in this analysis. Complication-related postoperative mortality was recorded and presented as early postoperative (30-day) and general in-hospital mortality. Failure to rescue, defined as the mortality among patients with postoperative complications, was calculated as the ratio of the number of patients who died due to certain complications (numerator) to the number of all patients who suffered these complications (denominator).

The options to minimize the risk for bias were limited due to the retrospective nature of the study. As with any other retrospective database review, bias cannot be excluded from the present study. Nevertheless, by using strict inclusion and exclusion criteria, we tried to obtain a study cohort that was as homogeneous as possible, thus minimizing the risk of bias and confounding. Moreover, the data collection was the same in both study periods.

4.5. Statistical Analysis

The median, together with the interquartile range (IQR), was presented for skewed variables. Qualitative variables were quoted as absolute and relative frequencies. Quantitative variables, like age, hospital stay, and number of postoperative complications, were treated as such in the statistical analyses. The variable "date of surgery" was dichotomized into an early (1972–1992) and a late

(1993–2014) group. The Mann–Whitney U test was used to compare continuous variables that were not normally distributed. For dichotomous variables, Fisher's exact test was used. The Cochran–Armitage test for trend was used to assess associations between a dichotomous variable and an ordinal variable with more than two categories. All statistical tests for the comparison of two groups were two-tailed. A test result was considered statistically significant if $p < 0.05$. For the binary outcome "postoperative mortality", a multiple logistic regression analysis was done. Odds ratios are presented together with their 95% confidence intervals (CI). Variables that were statistically significant in the univariable analyses were entered in the multivariable analysis. In the multivariable analysis, a backward stepwise selection based on the probability of the Wald statistic was used and a significance level of $\alpha = 0.10$ was chosen to detect several parameters that might have influenced the outcome. Statistical analyses were performed using IBM SPSS Statistics (version 25, IBM Corp., Armonk, NY, USA).

5. Conclusions

In conclusion, major surgical morbidity after gastrectomy remains a major challenge despite advances in perioperative care and surgical techniques. Over the course of four decades, postoperative mortality after radical resection for gastric cancer has more than halved, which was mainly caused by a reduction in mortality-associated non-surgical complications and an improved ability to rescue patients with complications. Therefore, alertness and adequate infrastructure in order to avoid failure to rescue are paramount for achieving acceptable outcomes after gastrectomy.

Author Contributions: Conceptualization, C.G., U.R., S.B., C.R., and J.H.; Formal analysis, C.G.; Methodology, C.G., U.R., S.B., C.R., and J.H.; Software, C.G.; Supervision, U.R. and C.R.; Writing—original draft, C.G., U.R., S.B., C.R., and J.H.; Writing—review and editing, C.G., U.R., S.B., C.R., and J.H. All authors have read and agreed to the published version of the manuscript.

Funding: This research received no external funding.

Conflicts of Interest: The authors declare no conflicts of interest.

References

1. Ikeguchi, M.; Oka, S.; Gomyo, Y.; Tsujitani, S.; Maeta, M.; Kaibara, N. Postoperative morbidity and mortality after gastrectomy for gastric carcinoma. *Hepato-gastroenterology* **2001**, *48*, 1517–1520. [PubMed]
2. Lepage, C.; Sant, M.; Verdecchia, A.; Forman, D.; Esteve, J.; Faivre, J.; EUROCARE working group. Operative mortality after gastric cancer resection and long-term survival differences across Europe. *Br. J. Surg.* **2010**, *97*, 235–239. [CrossRef] [PubMed]
3. Busweiler, L.A.; Henneman, D.; Dikken, J.L.; Fiocco, M.; van Berge Henegouwen, M.I.; Wijnhoven, B.P.; van Hillegersberg, R.; Rosman, C.; Wouters, M.W.; van Sandick, J.W.; et al. Failure-to-rescue in patients undergoing surgery for esophageal or gastric cancer. *Eur. J. Surg. Oncol.* **2017**, *43*, 1962–1969. [CrossRef] [PubMed]
4. Messager, M.; de Steur, W.O.; van Sandick, J.W.; Reynolds, J.; Pera, M.; Mariette, C.; Hardwick, R.H.; Bastiaannet, E.; Boelens, P.G.; van deVelde, C.J.H.; et al. Variations among 5 European countries for curative treatment of resectable oesophageal and gastric cancer: A survey from the EURECCA Upper GI Group (EUropean REgistration of Cancer CAre). *Eur. J. Surg. Oncol.* **2016**, *42*, 116–122. [CrossRef] [PubMed]
5. Dikken, J.L.; van Sandick, J.W.; Allum, W.H.; Johansson, J.; Jensen, L.S.; Putter, H.; Coupland, V.H.; Wouters, M.W.J.M.; Lemmens, V.E.P.; van de Velde, C.J.H.; et al. Differences in outcomes of oesophageal and gastric cancer surgery across Europe. *Br. J. Surg.* **2013**, *100*, 83–94. [CrossRef] [PubMed]
6. Gruen, R.L.; Pitt, V.; Green, S.; Parkhill, A.; Campbell, D.; Jolley, D. The effect of provider case volume on cancer mortality: Systematic review and meta-analysis. *CA A Cancer J. Clin.* **2009**, *59*, 192–211. [CrossRef] [PubMed]
7. Tol, J.A.M.G.; van Gulik, T.M.; Busch, O.R.C.; Gouma, D.J. Centralization of highly complex low-volume procedures in upper gastrointestinal surgery. A summary of systematic reviews and meta-analyses. *Dig. Surg.* **2012**, *29*, 374–383. [CrossRef] [PubMed]

8. Nimptsch, U.; Haist, T.; Gockel, I.; Mansky, T.; Lorenz, D. Complex gastric surgery in Germany—Is centralization beneficial? Observational study using national hospital discharge data. *Langenbeck's Arch. Surg.* **2019**, *404*, 93–101. [CrossRef] [PubMed]
9. Galata, C.; Blank, S.; Weiss, C.; Ronellenfitsch, U.; Reissfelder, C.; Hardt, J. Role of Postoperative Complications in Overall Survival after Radical Resection for Gastric Cancer: A Retrospective Single-Center Analysis of 1107 Patients. *Cancers (Basel)* **2019**, *11*, 1890. [CrossRef] [PubMed]
10. Mukai, Y.; Kurokawa, Y.; Takiguchi, S.; Mori, M.; Doki, Y. Are treatment outcomes in gastric cancer associated with either hospital volume or surgeon volume? *Ann. Gastroenterol. Surg.* **2017**, *1*, 186–192. [CrossRef] [PubMed]
11. Martin, A.N.; Das, D.; Turrentine, F.E.; Bauer, T.W.; Adams, R.B.; Zaydfudim, V.M. Morbidity and Mortality After Gastrectomy: Identification of Modifiable Risk Factors. *J. Gastrointest. Surg.* **2016**, *20*, 1554–1564. [CrossRef] [PubMed]
12. Smith, J.K. National Outcomes After Gastric Resection for Neoplasm. *Arch. Surg.* **2007**, *142*, 387–393. [CrossRef] [PubMed]
13. Best, L.M.J.; Mughal, M.; Gurusamy, K.S. Laparoscopic versus open gastrectomy for gastric cancer. *Cochrane Database Syst. Rev.* **2016**, *3*, CD011389. [CrossRef] [PubMed]
14. Guggenheim, D.E.; Shah, M.A. Gastric cancer epidemiology and risk factors. *J. Surg. Oncol.* **2013**, *107*, 230–236. [CrossRef]
15. Rosa, F.; Alfieri, S.; Tortorelli, A.; Fiorillo, C.; Costamagna, G.; Doglietto, G. Trends in clinical features, postoperative outcomes, and long-term survival for gastric cancer: A Western experience with 1,278 patients over 30 years. *World J. Surg. Oncol.* **2014**, *12*, 217. [CrossRef]
16. Bonenkamp, J.J.; Hermans, J.; Sasako, M.; Welvaart, K.; Songun, I.; Meyer, S.; Plukker, J.T.M.; Van Elk, P.; Obertop, H.; Gouma, D.J.; et al. Extended Lymph-Node Dissection for Gastric Cancer. *N. Engl. J. Med.* **1999**, *340*, 908–914. [CrossRef] [PubMed]
17. Cuschieri, A.; Joypaul, V.; Fayers, P.; Cook, P.; Fielding, J.; Craven, J.; Bancewicz, J. Postoperative morbidity and mortality after D1 and D2 resections for gastric cancer: Preliminary results of the MRC randomised controlled surgical trial. *Lancet* **1996**, *347*, 995–999. [CrossRef]
18. Marcus, S.G.; Cohen, D.; Lin, K.; Wong, K.; Thompson, S.; Rothberger, A.; Potmesil, M.; Hiotis, S.; Newman, E. Complications of gastrectomy following CPT-11 based neoadjuvant chemotherapy for gastric cancer. *J. Gastrointest. Surg.* **2003**, *7*, 1015–1023. [CrossRef] [PubMed]
19. Luo, H.; Wu, L.; Huang, M.; Jin, Q.; Qin, Y.; Chen, J. Postoperative morbidity and mortality in patients receiving neoadjuvant chemotherapy for locally advanced gastric cancers. *Medicine* **2018**, *97*, e12932. [CrossRef] [PubMed]

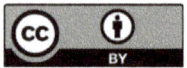

© 2020 by the authors. Licensee MDPI, Basel, Switzerland. This article is an open access article distributed under the terms and conditions of the Creative Commons Attribution (CC BY) license (http://creativecommons.org/licenses/by/4.0/).

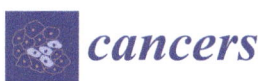

Article

Does Circular Stapler Size in Surgical Management of Esophageal Cancer Affect Anastomotic Leak Rate? 4-Year Experience of a European High-Volume Center

Dolores T. Müller, Benjamin Babic, Veronika Herbst, Florian Gebauer, Hans Schlößer, Lars Schiffmann, Seung-Hun Chon, Wolfgang Schröder, Christiane J. Bruns and Hans F Fuchs *

Department of General, Visceral, Cancer and Transplant Surgery, University of Cologne, Kerpener Str. 62, D-50937 Cologne, Germany; dolores.mueller@uk-koeln.de (D.T.M.); benjamin.babic@uk-koeln.de (B.B.); veronika.herbst3@gmail.com (V.H.); florian.gebauer@uk-koeln.de (F.G.); hans.schloesser@uk-koeln.de (H.S.); lars.schiffmann@uk-koeln.de (L.S.); seung-hun.chon@uk-koeln.de (S.-H.C.); wolfgang.schroeder@uk-koeln.de (W.S.); christiane.bruns@uk-koeln.de (C.J.B.)
* Correspondence: hans.fuchs@uk-koeln.de

Received: 28 October 2020; Accepted: 19 November 2020; Published: 22 November 2020

Simple Summary: One of the most severe postoperative complications after a transthoracic esophagectomy for esophageal cancer is a leakage of the anastomosis created between the remnant esophagus and the stomach. There is substantial debate on which surgical technique and which stapler are the best. The aim of this study was to retrospectively analyze whether the stapler diameter had an impact on postoperative anastomotic leak rates during a 4-year time frame from 2016 to 2020. A total of 632 patients (open, hybrid, and totally minimally invasive esophagectomy) met the inclusion criteria. A total of 214 patients underwent an anastomosis with a 25 mm stapler vs. 418 patients with a 28 mm stapler. Anastomotic leak rates were 15.4% vs. 10.8%, respectively. Stapler size should be chosen according to the individual anatomical situation of the patient and may be of higher relevance in patients undergoing totally minimally invasive reconstruction.

Abstract: Anastomotic leak is one of the most severe postoperative complications and is therefore considered a benchmark for the quality of surgery for esophageal cancer. There is substantial debate on which anastomotic technique is the best for patients undergoing Ivor Lewis esophagectomy. Our standardized technique is a circular stapled anastomosis with either a 25 or 28 mm anvil. The aim of this study was to retrospectively analyze whether the stapler diameter had an impact on postoperative anastomotic leak rates during a 4-year time frame from 2016 to 2020. A total of 632 patients (open, hybrid, and totally minimally invasive esophagectomy) met the inclusion criteria. A total of 214 patients underwent an anastomosis with a 25 mm stapler vs. 418 patients with a 28 mm stapler. Anastomotic leak rates were 15.4% vs. 10.8%, respectively ($p = 0.0925$). Stapler size should be chosen according to the individual anatomical situation of the patient. Stapler size may be of higher relevance in patients undergoing totally minimally invasive reconstruction.

Keywords: esophagectomy; esophageal anastomosis; minimally invasive surgery

1. Introduction

Due to its increasing incidence, a curative treatment of esophageal carcinoma has gained more importance than ever in recent years. For locally advanced but resectable carcinomas, a transthoracic esophagectomy with reconstruction using a gastric conduit and a high intrathoracic anastomosis (Ivor Lewis esophagectomy) depicts the current curative treatment of choice, mostly in a multimodal setting [1]. Despite improvements of perioperative care and surgical technique, this surgical procedure is still related to specific risks, such as anastomotic leak, conduit necrosis, chylothorax, and recurrent nerve injury. In particular, anastomotic leak, as one of the most severe and early postoperative complications, is considered a benchmark for the quality of the esophagectomy and is known to increase postoperative mortality and morbidity, leading to a decreased long-term survival [2–4]. Many surgical factors, including procedure type, localization of the anastomosis, and operative technique, are known to affect the integrity and quality of the anastomosis, and there is substantial debate on which anastomotic technique is the best for patients undergoing Ivor Lewis esophagectomy [5,6]. Our standardized technique and the most common technique in minimally invasive surgery is a circular stapled end-to-side anastomosis with purse string using either a 25 or 28 mm anvil. The current literature has shown this technique to be safe and efficient, leading to a comparatively low anastomotic leak rate of 14% in the EsoBench database [4]. The aim of this study was to retrospectively analyze whether the stapler diameter had an impact on postoperative anastomotic leak rates according to Esophagectomy Complications Consensus Group (ECCG) criteria during a 4-year time frame from 2016 to 2020 at our certified center of excellence for surgery of upper gastrointestinal cancer.

2. Results

A total of 632 patients met the inclusion criteria. In 214 patients (34%), a 25 mm circular stapler was used for the construction of a transthoracic esophagogastric anastomosis, and in 418 patients (66%), a size of 28 mm. For further analysis of results, the patients were grouped according to stapler size (25 mm—small; 28 mm—large). Demographic and oncological data of both patient cohorts are shown in Table 1. In addition, a statistical comparison of the baseline characteristics of both groups was performed, and the p-values are shown.

Table 1. Demographic characteristics and oncological data of the patients undergoing an Ivor Lewis esophagectomy for esophageal cancer with either a 25 or 28 mm circular stapler. The p-values for statistical comparison of the baseline characteristics of both groups were calculated.

	25 mm		28 mm		
	Total/Mean	(%)/Range	Total/Mean	(%)/Range	p-Value
Patients	214	34	418	66	<0.0001
Male/female	150/64	(70.1)/(29.9)	377/41	(90.2)/(9.8)	<0.0001
Age (years)	63	29–91	63	34–85	0.8431
BMI (kg/m^2)	25.68	15–46.71	26.87	14.13–48.44	0.0037
Pathology					
Adenocarcinoma	157	(73.4)	345	(82.5)	0.0092
Squamous cell carcinoma	57	(26.6)	70	(16.8)	0.0045
Other	0	(0)	3	(0.7)	0.5546
Neoadjuvant Chemotherapy					
None	32	(15)	54	(12.9)	0.54
CROSS	137	(64)	240	(57.4)	0.1231
FLOT	40	(18.7)	113	(27.1)	0.0238
Other	5	(2.3)	11	(2.6)	1

BMI: body mass index; CROSS and FLOT are well defined neoadjuvant treatments.

Furthermore, the operative approach was analyzed for both groups and compared with each other. Figure 1 shows the distribution of open, hybrid, and totally minimally invasive procedures among patient cohorts.

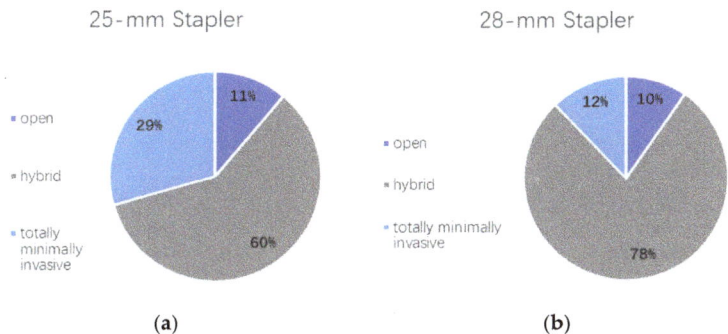

Figure 1. (a) Distribution of surgical approach in the 25 mm stapler patient group. Percentages of patients undergoing an Ivor Lewis esophagectomy using an open, hybrid, or totally minimally invasive approach are shown. (b) Distribution of surgical approach in the 28 mm stapler patient group. Percentages of patients undergoing an Ivor Lewis esophagectomy using an open, hybrid, or totally minimally invasive approach are shown.

While an open approach was used equally often in both cohorts ($p = 0.6809$), a hybrid approach was more often performed in the 28 mm group ($p < 0.0001$), compared with a totally minimally invasive approach, which was more frequently performed in the 25 mm group ($p < 0.0001$). In line with these findings, a two-stage procedure was more often used in the 28 mm stapler size group (6.5% vs. 11.5%; $p = 0.0490$).

A total of 72 patients in the given time frame were operated on using an either completely robotic or hybrid robotic approach. Thirty-one (14.5%) of the patients in the 25 mm stapler group were operated on using a robotic technique compared with 41 (9.8%) in the 28 mm stapler group. No statistically significant difference was shown for the utilization of a robotic technique between both groups ($p = 0.0863$).

A total of 114 patients in the given time frame were operated on using a totally minimally invasive approach (laparoscopic or robotic gastrolysis/thoracoscopic or robotic esophagectomy). Sixty-three (29.4%) of the patients in the 25 mm stapler group were operated on using a totally minimally invasive technique, compared with 51 (12.2%) in the 28 mm stapler group. A totally minimally invasive technique was significantly more often used in the smaller stapler group ($p < 0.0001$).

Postoperative Complications

Table 2 shows the severity of postoperative complications classified according to Clavien–Dindo (CD) of our patient groups. In addition, p-values were obtained to analyze whether statistically significant differences between postoperative outcomes of both cohorts were present.

The median length of stay (LOS) was 15 days in both groups with a range of 9–112 days (standard deviation (SD) 12) in the small stapler group and a range of 7–99 days (SD 11) in the large stapler group with no statistically significant difference between the groups ($p = 0.3993$).

An anastomotic leak was detected in a total of 78 patients (12.3%), 33 in the small stapler group and 45 in the large stapler group. Figure 2 depicts the anastomotic leak rates among patient cohorts. No statistical significance was noted between the groups ($p = 0.09878$); however, a trend approaching statistical significance shows that anastomotic leaks were more frequent in the small stapler size group.

Table 2. Severity of postoperative complications among patient cohorts. The Clavien–Dindo classification was used to objectify the severity of postoperative complications among both patient cohorts. *p*-Values were calculated to analyze whether statistically significant difference between both stapler sizes was present. In addition, further analysis of patients with severe postoperative complications, here classified as CD ≥ IIIa, was performed.

	25 mm Stapler		28 mm Stapler		
	n	(%)	*n*	(%)	*p*-Value
CD 0	66	(30.8)	151	(36.1)	0.2152
CD I	10	(4.7)	21	(5.1)	1
CD II	19	(8.9)	31	(7.4)	0.5354
CD IIIa	79	(36.9)	140	(33.5)	0.4268
CD IIIb	15	(7.1)	26	(6.2)	0.7340
CD IVa	14	(6.5)	24	(5.7)	0.7248
CD IVb	8	(3.7)	13	(3.1)	0.6474
CD V	3	(1.4)	12	(2.9)	0.4075
CD ≥ IIIa	119	(55.6)	215	(51.4)	0.3545

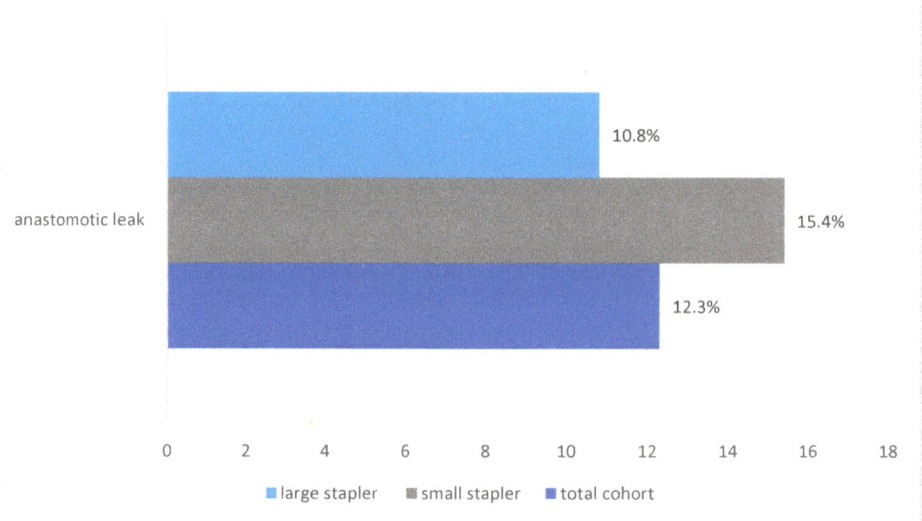

Figure 2. Anastomotic leak rates for the small stapler size (25 mm), the large stapler size (28 mm), and the overall cohort shown as percentages.

Further details on demographic information, preoperative comorbidities, and risk factors of patients who developed an anastomotic leak are shown in Table 3.

Table 3. Demographic information, comorbidities, and risk factors of patients who developed an anastomotic leak. Data are shown for both subgroups (25 mm and 28 mm circular staplers), and percentages of patients from the respective subgroups were calculated.

	Anastomotic Leak				
	25 mm Stapler Size		28 mm Stapler Size		
	Total	(%)	Total	(%)	p-Value
Patients	33	(100)	45	(100)	-
Obesity (BMI > 30 kg/m^2)	6	(18.2)	8	(17.8)	1
Tobacco					
Ex-smoker	17	(51.5)	15	(33.3)	0.1617
Smoker	7	(21.2)	12	(26.7)	0.6068
Alcohol consumption *					
None	18	(54.5)	27	(60)	0.6502
1–3 ×/week	10	(30.3)	10	(22.2)	0.4432
Daily	5	(15.2)	5	(11.1)	0.7351
Cardiac comorbidities					
Coronary artery disease	8	(24.2)	7	(21.2)	0.3911
Arterial hypertension	22	(66.7)	33	(73.3)	0.6176
Atrial fibrillation	4	(12.1)	5	(11.1)	1
Pulmonary comorbidities					
COPD	2	(6.1)	3	(6.7)	1
FEV1 < 80%	5	(15.2)	11	(24.4)	0.4004
VCmax < 80%	6	(18.2)	9	(20)	1
Other comorbidities					
Liver disease	3	(9.1)	3	(6.7)	0.6937
Renal failure (GFR < 60 mL/min)	3	(9.1)	4	(8.9)	1
Diabetes	4	(12.1)	6	(13.3)	1

* Information was given voluntarily; therefore, not all patients answered this question. COPD: chronic obstructive pulmonary disease, FEV1: forced expiratory pressure.

In addition, independent predictors of anastomotic leak were identified by a multivariate logistic regression analysis adjusting for stapler size, operative technique, gender, type of cancer, neoadjuvant therapy, tobacco, alcohol consumption, BMI, and cardiac comorbidities. Besides operative approach (open, hybrid, totally minimally invasive) and gender, no other independent predictors for anastomotic leak were found ($p > 0.05$). With totally minimally invasive approach set as a reference, both other approaches had a significantly higher leak rate when adjusted for all factors mentioned above ($p < 0.05$).

Table 4 shows further details about the distribution of the type of anastomotic leaks as well as the severity of complications using the Clavien–Dindo classification among patients that developed an anastomotic leak. The anastomotic leak rate for a Type II leak was 11.2% in the 25 mm group vs. 8.4% in the 28 mm group and 4.2% vs. 2.2% for Type III leaks, respectively. In addition, the percentage of patients with a certain CD class from the total of anastomotic leaks among the respective stapler sizes is shown. No patient with an anastomotic leak was classified as CD I or II. To investigate how many patients with an anastomotic leak developed organ failure, we included a subgroup analysis of patients classified as CD ≥ IV.

Table 4. Anastomotic leak types and severity of postoperative complications among patients that developed an anastomotic leak. Stapler sizes of 25 and 28 mm were analyzed separately, and p-values for statistical comparison of both groups were calculated. Percentages were calculated as percentage from the cohort that developed an anastomotic leak.

	25 mm Stapler		28 mm Stapler		
	n/Median	(%)/Range	n/Median	(%)/Range	p-Value
Total	33	(100)	45	(100)	-
Type I	0	(0)	1	(2.2)	1
Type II	24	(72.7)	35	(77.8)	0.79
Type III	9	(27.3)	9	(20)	0.5876
Clavien–Dindo Classification					
CD IIIa	14	(42.4)	21	(46.7)	0.8188
CD IIIb	4	(12.1)	6	(13.3)	1
CD IVa	9	(27.3)	9	(20)	0.5876
CD IVb	3	(9.1)	6	(13.3)	0.7259
CD V	3	(9.1)	3	(6.7)	0.6937
CD ≥ IV	15	(45.5)	18	(40)	0.6502
Length of Stay					
LOS	36	16–112	30	13–99	0.3118

3. Discussion

Anastomotic leakage is among the most feared complications in surgery due to its consequences, especially in esophageal cancer surgery. Many technical variations in performing the esophagogastric anastomosis are still used without expert consensus. Our institution has contributed significantly in the past to find innovative and new ways using minimally invasive technology to treat these complications with an interventional approach and mostly without redo surgery, leading to more ECCG Type II anastomotic leaks in recent years [7,8]. Schröder et al. have published in their recent multicenter analysis of high-volume centers from 2011 to 2016 a leakage rate of 13.9% for an intrathoracic circular stapled anastomosis. Our own data from 2016 to 2020 in this present study show an overall leakage rate of 12.3%, meeting the benchmarks in Schröder's and Schmidt's studies [2,4]. When looking into more detail as presented above, we were able to show that in addition to the technology and technique used, even the stapler size may play an essential role in developing an anastomotic leak. In this context, it is important to note that anatomical reasons may play an essential role when choosing the stapler size, and sometimes both options are technically not possible.

Interestingly, we were able to show that a 28 mm stapler was overall significantly more often used at our institution. This result may be biased by the fact that more hybrid than totally minimally invasive procedures were performed in this collective, as the 25 mm stapler was the more commonly chosen technology in the totally minimally invasive subgroup. Also, patients with squamous cell carcinoma more often underwent a 25 mm anastomosis, a fact that can be attributed to the usually higher mediastinal location of the tumors and anatomical reasons not to perform a 28 mm stapled anastomosis.

Few previous studies have focused on the technical factor of the stapler diameter itself, but more often evaluated general technical options, such as circular, linear, and handsewn (technical factors), and anatomical options, such as intrathoracic vs. cervical (anatomical factors) [4,5]. Whereas Markar et al. published a meta-analysis in 2013 showing no significant differences among the technical factors, they were able to show significant differences and an almost fivefold increased leakage rate for cervical vs. intrathoracic anastomosis. In contrast, Schröder's analysis of the EsoBenchmark database showed no difference among the anatomical factors. Even if the difference in leakage rate in our patient collective (10.8% vs. 15.4%) is in favor of the 28 mm stapler group, this technical factor was only nearing statistical significance ($p = 0.0925$).

In our analysis of complications, focusing on the patients with an anastomotic leak (Table 4), we looked at the severity of the leaks according to the ECCG group [9]. No significant difference was found between the two analyzed stapler groups. Nevertheless, there was again a trend of less severe leaks in favor of the 28 mm staplers. No clear differences could be shown for the Clavien–Dindo score between the groups.

In our study, we found a relatively high number of CD ≥ IIIa complications, namely, 51.4% (28 mm) and 55.6% (25 mm). This exceeds the benchmarks set by Schmidt et al. with 30.8%, defined as the "best possible outcome" [2]. Truly, our collective does not comprise a selection of patients with low comorbidities, and esophagectomy was performed both by experts and by trainees under expert supervision at our institution, meaning that our results represent an unbiased, unselected analysis of a prospective cohort. In addition, complications at our institution are thoroughly recorded according to ECCG guidelines, meaning that postoperative interventions such as chest tube placement or postoperative EGD are automatically classified as a IIIa complication. As postoperative endoscopic interventions are considered a "standard of care" in some other centers, these might not be classified in the same way everywhere.

4. Materials and Methods

4.1. Patients

Our academic center is a certified center of excellence for surgery of the upper gastrointestinal tract with more than 250 upper gastrointestinal cancer surgeries being performed annually. All patients undergoing esophagectomy for esophageal cancer in our high-volume center are entered into an IRB-approved prospective database. A retrospective chart review was performed for all patients undergoing an Ivor Lewis esophagectomy for esophageal cancer from May 2016 to May 2020. Patients were included in the analysis if a 25 or 28 mm circular stapler was used for the esophagogastric transthoracic anastomosis. An intraoperative subjective assessment of the patient's anatomy was used to choose the appropriate stapler size. Patients with handsewn anastomoses or other stapler diameters were excluded from the analysis. Retrospective analysis of our prospectively collected data was conducted with approval from the ethical committee at the University of Cologne (IRB reference 13-091). Demographics, endoscopic findings, and biopsies at different follow-up time points, as well as tumor histology and stage, were recorded in our prospective database.

4.2. Assessment of Postoperative Complications

The Clavien–Dindo classification was used to classify the severity of postoperative complications [10]. In addition, our institution contributes to the well-established database of the Esophagectomy Complications Consensus Group (ECCG), which provides a standardized and international assessment of complications following esophagectomy [9]. Therefore, definitions established by the ECCG are used at our clinic to ensure precise documentation. An anastomotic leak was defined as a "full thickness GI defect involving esophagus, anastomosis, staple line, or conduit irrespective of presentation or method of identification." Further subgrouping into three types was applied with Type I being a local defect requiring no change in therapy or being treated medically or with dietary modification, Type II being a localized defect requiring interventional but not surgical therapy, and Type III being a localized defect requiring surgical therapy. Length of hospital stay was calculated in days from the day of the surgical procedure to discharge of the patient.

4.3. Treatment Pathway of Patients with Resectable Esophageal Cancer

Treatment of patients with esophageal cancer at our National Center of Excellence follows a standardized protocol in line with national and international guidelines [1,11–13]. Following restaging, usually 4–6 weeks after neoadjuvant therapy, either a standardized Ivor Lewis esophagectomy with reconstruction using a gastric conduit and a high thoracic esophagogastric anastomosis is performed at our institution, or if suitable, patients with an adenocarcinoma of the gastroesophageal junction Siewert Type II are enrolled into the CARDIA trial, which aims to compare the oncological and surgical outcome after transthoracic esophagectomy and transhiatal extended gastrectomy [14,15]. For a transthoracic esophagectomy, a hybrid procedure (abdominal part—laparoscopically/thoracic part—open) depicts the current standard at our institution. Whenever possible, however, dependent on the patient's anatomy and whether the patient is classified as low risk, a totally minimally invasive approach is chosen (abdominal part—laparoscopically/thoracic part—thoracoscopically). Our thorough risk assessment preoperatively includes a standardized and validated risk scoring system [16]. In addition, the DaVinci Xi robotic surgical system (Intuitive Surgical, Inc., Sunnyvale, CA, USA) is available at our clinic since February 2017. A robotic approach is often especially used for the thoracic part, as the great advantage of the system becomes evident during the thoracic dissection [17]. Furthermore, complete robotic and minimally invasive Ivor Lewis esophagectomies are increasingly performed at our institution.

4.4. Surgical Technique—Abdominal Part

The following steps for preparation of the gastric conduit are performed in a standardized fashion using either a robotic or a laparoscopic approach. Our standardized steps of the operation are the same for the robotic and the laparoscopic procedure: The patient is placed in a French and anti-Trendelenburg position. For the robotic approach, an 8 mm DaVinci trocar is inserted through a supraumbilical median incision using the open technique, and a pneumoperitoneum is established. Four additional trocars are then placed, one 5 mm trocar on the right and one 12 mm trocar on the left edge of the costal arch, a 12 mm trocar in the right upper abdomen and an 8 mm trocar in the left upper abdomen depicting the standard for a minimally invasive robotic DaVinci gastrolysis. If performed laparoscopically, one 5 mm and four 11 mm abdominal ports are used. A 45-degree angled scope (5 mm Stryker indocyanine green (ICG) or robotic 8 mm Intuitive ICG) is inserted through the subxiphoidal trocar. The hiatus is then exposed by elevating the liver with a Cuschieri retractor through the right 5 mm trocar. From here, the peritoneum on the right diaphragmatic crus is incised, and the lower mediastinum outside the hernia sac is dissected and circumferentially mobilized up to the left diaphragmatic crus to dissect the lower esophagus. Opening the right and the left pleura is avoided at any time during the hiatal dissection. Dissection of the lymph nodes along the lesser curvature of the stomach onto the stomach wall follows. The upper margin of the retroperitoneal pancreas is now exposed and can be inspected. A D2 lymphadenectomy following the hepatic ligament, the common hepatic artery, along the celiac trunk continuing along the splenic artery and of the retroperitoneum is performed. The left gastric artery and the left gastric vein are ligated, clipped, and divided. The right gastric artery is preserved. Subsequently, lymph nodes along the retroperitoneum via the crus of the diaphragm up to the lower mediastinum are mobilized, and the lymphadenectomy is completed above the splenic artery all the way up to the hilum of the spleen. Opening the gastrocolic omentum access to the omental bursa is gained, and the greater curvature of the stomach is mobilized starting from the corpus region beyond the epiploic vessels toward the left crus of the diaphragm, while the gastroepiploic arcade is preserved, and the short gastric vessels are divided until visualization of the left diaphragmatic crus is achieved. To later create an omentum wrap covering the anastomosis, a part of the greater omentum just below the spleen is preserved. Mobilization is completed by separating the colon all the way until the splenic flexure, confirming sufficient blood supply for the greater curvature. Dissection at the gastric crow's foot region is performed followed by the construction of the gastric conduit. A tristapler (Endo Gia (Covidien), violet, 45 mm) is applied for the first bite of the construction of the gastric sleeve. Using at least two additional Endo Gia 60 mm violet stapling magazines, construction of the gastric conduit is completed. Intraoperative angiography using indocyanine green (ICG) can, in combination with the robotic DaVinci Xi system of the laparoscopic Stryker system, demonstrate sufficient blood supply of the fundus by showing the gastroepiploic vessels via fluorescence.

4.5. Surgical Technique—Thoracic Part

The following steps for completion of the esophagectomy and reconstruction of the gastrointestinal passage using a gastric conduit are performed in a standardized fashion using either a minimally invasive thoracoscopic, robotic, or open approach: The patient is placed in a left lateral semiprone position for a robotic procedure or in a left lateral decubitus position for an open procedure. Using a double-lumen intubation, artificial atelectasis of the right lung is achieved. Our standardized steps of the operation are the same for the robotic or the open procedure. For a robotic approach, three DaVinci ports and two assistance ports are placed on the right according to the standard, and the robot is docked from the patient's right side, creating a view from the left for the operating surgeon. A right-sided transthoracic approach is used for an open procedure. Using the robotic monopolar cautery hook, the pulmonary ligament is dissected with the lymph nodes adhering to the esophagus upward toward the pericardial layer and the azygos vein. Using a tristapler (Endo Gia (Covidien), gold, 45 mm), the azygos arch is divided. The thoracic duct is identified and clipped with two polymer clips (Grena Click'aV®). Dissection of the periesophageal fat tissue along the aorta dividing small aortic branches and along the pericardium is performed. Especially when using the robotic technique, a radical but controlled dissection of the carinal, retrotracheal, and paratracheal tissue can be performed. Vagal and recurrent nerves are preserved during this step. Opening the hiatus, a connection to the abdominal surgical field is made. A monofilament purse string suture is performed, and the gastric conduit is pulled into the right thoracic cavity. If a minimally invasive approach is chosen, a minithoracotomy of 7 cm length is then created from the incision of the 12 mm upper assistance trocar, and an Alexis S wound protector/retractor (Alexis Laparoscopic System, Applied Medical) is inserted.

4.6. Surgical Technique—The Esophagogastric Anastomosis

Either a 25 or 28 mm stapler head depending on the patient's anatomy is inserted and guided into the esophagus. The prepared purse string suture is used to suture the stapler head into the esophageal remnant. If necessary, a second purse string suture may be placed. Figure 3 shows the setup for the creation of the esophagogastric anastomosis. The gastric conduit is then gently pulled upward into the chest. We always ensure that the fundus lies alongside with the esophageal stump without tension, which further proofs a sufficient length of the conduit. Intraoperative angiography using ICG can be again used with the robotic system to demonstrate sufficient blood supply of the graft. If a robotic approach is chosen, the DaVinci is then disconnected, and the assistant surgeon holds the camera similar to a thoracoscopic approach. Using a variable number of loads of the Endo GIA stapler (Covidien), preparation of the gastric conduit is completed. The specimen is removed and preserved for histopathologic evaluation. A 25 or 28 mm stapler is inserted through the minor curvature of the stomach, and an esophagogastric anastomosis is made, retrieving two complete donuts. Another Endo GIA stapler load is used to staple off the open end of the stomach. The previously prepared omentum wrap is then used to cover the anastomosis. In addition, final control of blood perfusion using ICG fluorescence can be used.

4.7. Data Analysis and Statistical Evaluation

For analysis of data, patients were divided into two groups based on CS (circular stapler) size ("small" = 25 mm circular stapler and "large" = 28 mm circular stapler). In addition, a subgroup analysis of patients who underwent a totally minimally invasive and a robotic esophagectomy was performed. Continuous variables are presented as means and range. Categorical data are presented as numbers and percentages. Student's t-test (for continuous variables) and Fisher's exact test (for nominal or categorical variables) were used for all bivariate analyses. Independent predictors of anastomotic leak were identified by a multivariate logistic regression analysis. All tests were two-sided, with statistical significance set at $p \leq 0.05$. Data were analyzed by GraphPad Software (San Diego, CA, USA) and SPSS Statistics for Mac (version 21, SPSS).

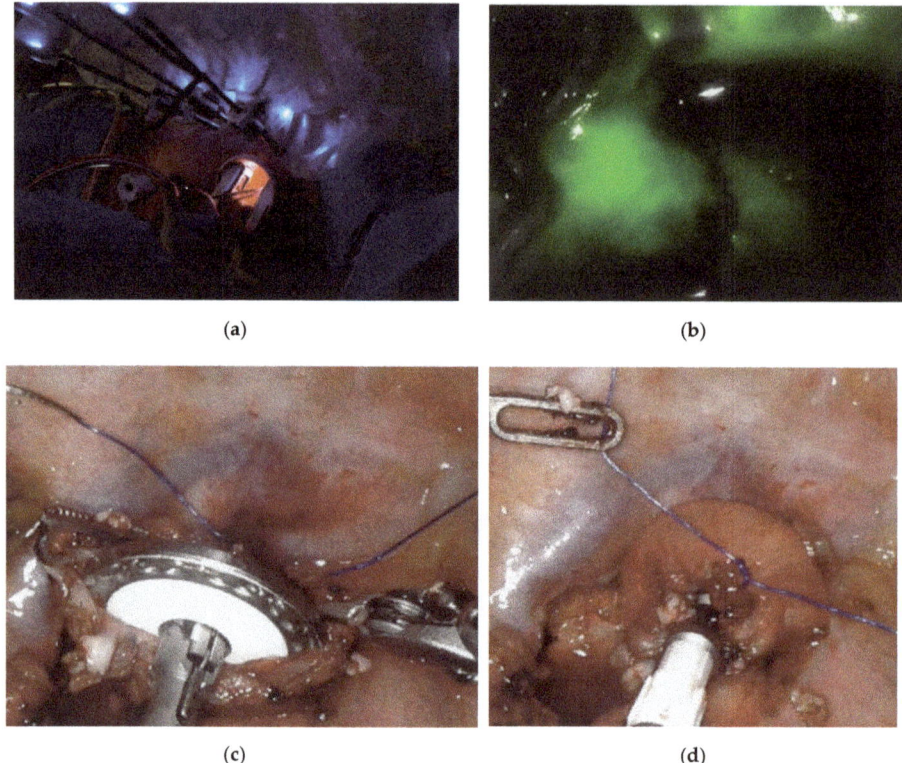

Figure 3. Robotic-assisted minimally invasive esophagectomy. The top left picture (**a**) shows a minithoracotomy of 7 cm length created from the incision of the 12 mm upper assistance trocar and secured with an Alexis S wound protector/retractor. The top right picture (**b**) shows intraoperative angiography using indocyanine green (ICG). The bottom pictures display how the prepared purse string suture is used to suture the stapler head into the esophageal remnant (**c**,**d**).

5. Conclusions

This large single-center analysis clearly defines anastomotic leak rates of a standardized, unselected consecutive patient cohort in a high-volume center. We highly recommend that stapler size be always chosen according to the individual anatomical situation of the patient, but when in doubt, we suggest choosing the larger diameter. This suggestion may be of even higher relevance to patients undergoing minimally invasive thoracic reconstruction.

Author Contributions: Conceptualization, D.T.M., B.B., W.S., C.J.B., H.F.F.; methodology, D.T.M., H.F.F.; formal analysis, D.T.M., H.F.F., V.H.; data curation, V.H., D.T.M.; writing—original draft preparation, D.T.M., H.F.F.; writing—review and editing, D.T.M., B.B., F.G., H.S., L.S., S.-H.C., W.S., C.J.B., H.F.F.; supervision, H.F.F., C.J.B. All authors have read and agreed to the published version of the manuscript.

Funding: This research received no external funding.

Conflicts of Interest: The authors declare no conflict of interest.

References

1. Moehler, M.; Al-Batran, S.-E.; Andus, T.; Anthuber, M.; Arends, J.; Arnold, D.; Aust, D.; Baier, P.; Baretton, G.; Bernhardt, J.; et al. German S3-guideline Diagnosis and treatment of esophagogastric cancer. *Z. Gastroenterol.* **2011**, *49*, 461–531. [CrossRef] [PubMed]
2. Schmidt, H.M.; Gisbertz, S.S.; Moons, J.; Rouvelas, I.; Kauppi, J.; Brown, A.; Asti, E.; Luyer, M.; Lagarde, S.M.; Berlth, F.; et al. Defining Benchmarks for Transthoracic Esophagectomy: A Multicenter Analysis of Total Minimally Invasive Esophagectomy in Low Risk Patients. *Ann. Surg.* **2017**, *266*, 814–821. [CrossRef] [PubMed]
3. Booka, E.; Takeuchi, H.; Suda, K.; Fukuda, K.; Nakamura, R.; Wada, N.; Kawakubo, H.; Kitagawa, Y. Meta-analysis of the impact of postoperative complications on survival after oesophagectomy for cancer. *BJS Open* **2018**, *2*, 276–284. [CrossRef] [PubMed]
4. Schröder, W.; Raptis, D.A.; Schmidt, H.M.; Gisbertz, S.S.; Moons, J.; Asti, E.; Luyer, M.D.P.; Hölscher, A.H.; Schneider, P.M.; Henegouwen, M.I.V.B.; et al. Anastomotic Techniques and Associated Morbidity in Total Minimally Invasive Transthoracic Esophagectomy: Results From the EsoBenchmark Database. *Ann. Surg.* **2019**, *270*, 820–826. [CrossRef] [PubMed]
5. Markar, S.R.; Arya, S.; Karthikesalingam, A.; Hanna, G.B. Technical Factors that Affect Anastomotic Integrity Following Esophagectomy: Systematic Review and Meta-analysis. *Ann. Surg. Oncol.* **2013**, *20*, 4274–4281. [CrossRef] [PubMed]
6. Markar, S.R.; Karthikesalingam, A.; Vyas, S.; Hashemi, M.; Winslet, M. Hand-Sewn Versus Stapled Oesophago-gastric Anastomosis: Systematic Review and Meta-analysis. *J. Gastrointest. Surg.* **2011**, *15*, 876–884. [CrossRef] [PubMed]
7. Bludau, M.; Fuchs, H.F.; Herbold, T.; Maus, M.K.H.; Alakus, H.; Popp, F.C.; Leers, J.M.; Bruns, C.J.; Hölscher, A.H.; Schröder, W.; et al. Results of endoscopic vacuum-assisted closure device for treatment of upper GI leaks. *Surg. Endosc.* **2018**, *32*, 1906–1914. [CrossRef] [PubMed]
8. Chon, S.-H.; Bartella, I.; Bürger, M.; Rieck, I.; Goeser, T.; Schröder, W.; Bruns, C.J. VACStent: A new option for endoscopic vacuum therapy in patients with esophageal anastomotic leaks after upper gastrointestinal surgery. *Endoscopy* **2019**, *52*, E166–E167. [CrossRef] [PubMed]
9. Low, D.E.; Alderson, D.; Cecconello, I.; Chang, A.C.; Darling, G.E.; D'journo, X.B.; Griffin, S.M.; Hölscher, A.H.; Hofstetter, W.L.; Jobe, B.A.; et al. International Consensus on Standardization of Data Collection for Complications Associated With Esophagectomy: Esophagectomy Complications Consensus Group (ECCG). *Ann. Surg.* **2015**, *262*, 286–294. [CrossRef] [PubMed]
10. Dindo, D.; Demartines, N.; Clavien, P.-A. Classification of Surgical Complications: A new proposal with evaluation in a cohort of 6336 patients and results of a survey. *Ann. Surg.* **2004**, *240*, 205–213. [CrossRef] [PubMed]
11. Fuchs, H.; Hölscher, A. Therapeutic decisions in patients with operable, non-metastatic oesophageal cancer. *Zent. Chir.* **2014**, *139*, 32–36. [CrossRef]
12. Moehler, M.; Baltin, C.T.H.; Ebert, M.; Fischbach, W.; Gockel, I.; Grenacher, L.; Hölscher, A.H.; Lordick, F.; Malfertheiner, P.; Messmann, H.; et al. International comparison of the German evidence-based S3-guidelines on the diagnosis and multimodal treatment of early and locally advanced gastric cancer, including adenocarcinoma of the lower esophagus. *Gastric Cancer* **2014**, *18*, 550–563. [CrossRef] [PubMed]
13. Hölscher, A.H.; Stahl, M.; Messmann, H.; Stuschke, M.; Meyer, H.-J.; Porschen, R. New S3 guideline for esophageal cancer: Important surgical aspects. *Der Chirurg.* **2016**, *87*, 865–872. [CrossRef] [PubMed]
14. Lewis, I. The surgical treatment of carcinoma of the oesophagus with special reference to a new operation for growths of the middle third. *Br. J. Surg.* **1946**, *34*, 18–31. [CrossRef] [PubMed]
15. Leers, J.M.; Knepper, L.; Van Der Veen, A.; Schröder, W.; Fuchs, H.; Schiller, P.; Hellmich, M.; Zettelmeyer, U.; Brosens, L.A.A.; Quaas, A.; et al. The CARDIA-trial protocol: A multinational, prospective, randomized, clinical trial comparing transthoracic esophagectomy with transhiatal extended gastrectomy in adenocarcinoma of the gastroesophageal junction (GEJ) type II. *BMC Cancer* **2020**, *20*, 781. [CrossRef] [PubMed]

16. Fuchs, H.; Harnsberger, C.R.; Broderick, R.C.; Chang, D.C.; Sandler, B.J.; Jacobsen, G.R.; Bouvet, M.; Horgan, S. Simple preoperative risk scale accurately predicts perioperative mortality following esophagectomy for malignancy. *Dis. Esophagus* **2016**, *30*, 1–6. [CrossRef] [PubMed]
17. Fuchs, H.; Müller, D.T.; Leers, J.M.; Schröder, W.; Bruns, C.J. Modular step-up approach to robot-assisted transthoracic esophagectomy—Experience of a German high volume center. *Transl. Gastroenterol. Hepatol.* **2019**, *4*, 62. [CrossRef] [PubMed]

Publisher's Note: MDPI stays neutral with regard to jurisdictional claims in published maps and institutional affiliations.

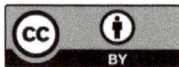 © 2020 by the authors. Licensee MDPI, Basel, Switzerland. This article is an open access article distributed under the terms and conditions of the Creative Commons Attribution (CC BY) license (http://creativecommons.org/licenses/by/4.0/).

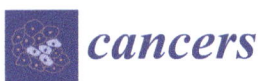

Article

Outcomes of Radiotherapy for Mesenchymal and Non-Mesenchymal Subtypes of Gastric Cancer

Jeong Il Yu [1], Hee Chul Park [1,2,*], Jeeyun Lee [3,*], Changhoon Choi [1], Won Ki Kang [3], Se Hoon Park [3], Seung Tae Kim [3], Tae Sung Sohn [4], Jun Ho Lee [4], Ji Yeong An [4], Min Gew Choi [4], Jae Moon Bae [4], Kyoung-Mee Kim [5], Heewon Han [6], Kyunga Kim [6], Sung Kim [7] and Do Hoon Lim [1]

1. Departments of Radiation Oncology, Samsung Medical Center, Sungkyunkwan University School of Medicine, 81 Irwon-ro, Gangnam-gu, Seoul 06351, Korea; ro.yuji651@gmail.com (J.I.Y.); changhoon1.choi@samsung.com (C.C.); dh8.lim@samsung.com (D.H.L.)
2. Department of Medical Device Management and Research, Samsung Advanced Institute for Health Sciences and Technology, Sungkyunkwan University, Seoul 06351, Korea
3. Division of Hematology-Oncology, Department of Medicine, Samsung Medical Center, Sungkyunkwan University School of Medicine, 81 Irwon-ro, Gangnam-gu, Seoul 06351, Korea; wonki.kang@samsung.com (W.K.K.); sh1767.park@samsung.com (S.H.P.); seungtae1.kim@samsung.com (S.T.K.)
4. Departments of Surgery, Samsung Medical Center, Sungkyunkwan University School of Medicine, Seoul 06351, Korea; ts.sohn@samsung.com (T.S.S.); junho3371.lee@samsung.com (J.H.L.); jar319.an@samsung.com (J.Y.A.); mingew.choi@samsung.com (M.G.C.); jmoon.bae@samsung.com (J.M.B.)
5. Departments of Pathology, Samsung Medical Center, Sungkyunkwan University School of Medicine, Seoul 06351, Korea; km7353.kim@samsung.com
6. Statistics and Data Center, Research Institute for Future Medicine, Samsung Medical Center, Seoul 03181, Korea; heewon818@gmail.com (H.H.); kyunga.j.kim@samsung.com (K.K.)
7. Department of Surgery, Samsung Changwon Hospital, Sungkyunkwan University School of Medicine, Changwon 06351, Korea; sungkimm@skku.edu
* Correspondence: hee.ro.park@gmail.com (H.C.P.); jyun.lee@samsung.com (J.L.); Tel.: +82-2-3410-2612 (H.C.P. & J.L.); Fax: +82-2-3410-2619 (H.C.P. & J.L.)

Received: 25 March 2020; Accepted: 9 April 2020; Published: 10 April 2020

Abstract: *Background:* The purpose of this study was to evaluate the clinical outcomes following postoperative chemotherapy (XP) versus chemoradiotherapy (XP-RT) according to mesenchymal subtype based on RNA sequencing in gastric cancer (GC) in a cohort of the Adjuvant chemoRadioTherapy In Stomach Tumor (ARTIST) trial. Methods: Of the 458 patients enrolled in the ARTIST trial, formalin-fixed, paraffin-embedded (FFPE) specimens were available from 106 (23.1%) patients for RNA analysis. The mesenchymal subtype was classified according to a previously reported 71-gene MSS/EMT signature using the NanoString assay. Results: Of the 106 patients analyzed (50 in XP arm, 56 in XP-RT arm), 36 (34.0%) patients were categorized as mesenchymal subtype by NanoString assay. Recurrence-free survival (RFS, p = 0.009, hazard ratio (HR) = 2.11, 95% confidence interval (CI): 1.21–3.70) and overall survival (OS, p = 0.003, HR = 2.28, 95% CI: 1.31–3.96) were significantly lower in the mesenchymal subtype than in the non-mesenchymal subtype. In terms of post-operative radiotherapy (RT), mesenchymal subtype was not an independent variable to predict RFS or OS regardless to the assigned arm (XP with or without RT) in this patient cohort. However, there was a trend in the adjuvant XP arm, which showed higher OS than the XP-RT arm for the mesenchymal subtype and lower OS than the XP-RT arm for the non-mesenchymal subtype. *Conclusions:* We could not determine any significant differences between the mesenchymal and non-mesenchymal subtypes with respect to the effects of adjuvant XP with or without RT in gastric cancer following curative surgery.

Keywords: adjuvant therapy; gastrointestinal tract; genetic diagnosis; radiosensitivity

1. Introduction

Gastric cancer (GC) remains an unresolved major health problem in the world, ranking fifth among the most common cancers, with an estimated incidence of 951,000 cases in 2012 [1]. Furthermore, it is the third leading cause of cancer-related deaths, with 723,100 patients dying because of it in 2012. Nevertheless, a gradual improvement in GC management has been achieved, based on pathophysiological studies, novel surgical techniques, and/or emerging systemic therapies.

Despite significant improvements in clinical outcomes related to the implementation of screenings, advances in surgical techniques and/or usage of (neo-)adjuvant chemotherapy and/or concurrent chemoradiotherapy, a considerable proportion of patients still experience recurrences and die of GC [2–4].

With the recent development of genetic analysis techniques, the molecular classification of GC and the prognostic value of the different subtypes have been actively studied. The Cancer Genome Atlas Research Network suggested four types of GC molecular classes [5], whereas the Asian Cancer Research Group (ACRG) proposes another classification [6]. In particular, the ACRG suggested prognostic differences according to each molecular subtype and validated the survival differences in an independent cohort. According to this study, the mesenchymal (microsatellite-stable with epithelial-to-mesenchymal transition phenotype, MSS/EMT) tumors showed the worst prognosis with younger age at diagnosis, and higher recurrence rate with first presentation of peritoneal seeding. In addition to these clinical features of the mesenchymal subtype, the association of hypoxia and the increase in poly [adenosine diphosphate-ribose] polymerase-1 (PARP-1), which repairs deoxyribonucleic acid (DNA) damage, has been reported [7–9].

Recently, our group performed a study to predict outcomes in patients with the mesenchymal subtype using a NanoString assay in 70 ACRG specimens [10]. The mesenchymal subtype showed significantly worse survival compared to the non-mesenchymal subtype following curative surgery in GC [11–13]. The impact of mesenchymal subtype which could be clearly related with radioresistance, like hypoxia and increment of PARP-1, in terms of radiotherapy (RT) efficacy has not been defined yet although several studies have demonstrated that mesenchymal subtype predicts poor outcome following chemotherapy in GC [11–13]. It would be appropriate to evaluate the efficacy of RT on mesenchymal subtype of GC through the ARTIST trial which had been conducted to compare postoperative chemotherapy (XP) versus chemoradiotherapy (XP-RT) following complete curative resection with D2 lymph node dissection in GC (clinical trials.gov identifier NCT00323830).

In this study, we investigated the clinical outcomes according to the application of adjuvant XP-RT or XP for mesenchymal and non-mesenchymal subtype cancers in a cohort of the ARTIST trial.

2. Methods

2.1. Patients and Samples

This study was performed on patients who participated in the ARTIST trial who agreed to have their tissue studied, and whose tissue surgical specimens were available and sufficient for ribonucleic acid (RNA) extraction. A total of 458 patients (228 assigned to XP and 230 to XP-RT arm), who had received curative D2 resection without preoperative treatment, were enrolled in the randomized phase III study, ARTIST trial. The XP arm was expected to receive six cycles of XP regimen (capecitabine 1000 mg/m^2 twice daily on days 1 to 14; cisplatin 60 mg/m^2 on day 1 every 3 weeks) and the XP-RT arm would receive 25 fractions of 45 gray (Gy) RT with capecitabine (825 mg/m^2 twice daily) after two cycles of XP (as in the XP arm) followed by two additional cycles of planned XP. The planned treatment was completed in 75.4% of patients in the XP arm and 81.7% in the XP-RT arm [11]. Other details of the ARTIST trial, including chemotherapy and RT protocols, were described in previous reports [8–10]. From the 458 patients enrolled, 106 tissue samples of 359 patients except 99 patients with stage I were available for evaluation in the present study. Of these, 56 patients were in the XP-RT arm and the remaining 50 patients were in the XP arm (Figure 1).

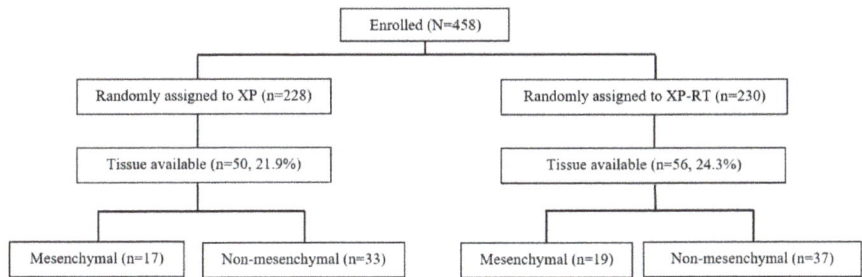

Figure 1. Flow diagram of patient inclusion.

2.2. Mesenchymal Gene Signature

Details about the development of the 71-gene MSS/EMT signature (consisting of 60 upregulated and 11 downregulated genes) using the NanoString assay, and the validation procedure using the conventional Affymetrix method, are described in a previous report [10]. In that study, 73 samples from the ARTIST cohort were tested using the 71-gene MSS/EMT signature to validate their mesenchymal subtype. Twenty out of 73 samples were classified as mesenchymal subtype tumors, which is equivalent to the MSS/EMT subtype in terms of their dismal outcome, typical characteristics of whole stomach involvement, poorly-differentiated or signet ring cell carcinoma, and low microsatellite instability.

In this study, we used the outcomes of previous study evaluating mesenchymal and non-mesenchymal subtype using MSS/EMT gene signature analysis using the NanoString assay in a total of 106 samples, which consisted of 73 samples used as a validation set and 33 additional specimens from patients of the ARTIST trial evaluated through further work after publication of the previous study.

The first site of recurrence was used for the classification and/or analysis of recurrence. Simultaneous recurrence was defined as any recurrence detected within 2 weeks after the first detection of recurrence. Loco-regional recurrence (LRR) was defined as recurrence at one of following sites: anastomosis area, remnant stomach, tumor bed, duodenal stump, or regional lymph nodes (LN) within the RT field in the XP-RT group or the hypothetical RT field in the XP group. All cases of suspected LRR were reviewed and evaluated by dedicated radiation oncologists (JIY and DHL; specialists in gastrointestinal tumors, including stomach cancer) as described in a previous study [13].

2.3. Ethical Approval and Informed Consent Statement

The authors stated that all methods of this study were carried out in accordance with the Declaration of Helsinki, and the protocol for the present study was reviewed and approved by the Samsung Medical Center Institutional Review Board (IRB No. 2010-12-088) and all participants in the ARTIST trial consented to this study after being informed about the purpose and investigational nature.

2.4. Statistical Analysis

Baseline characteristics were compared between the mesenchymal and non-mesenchymal subtypes, using chi-square or Fisher's exact test for categorical variables and Student's t-test or Mann–Whitney U-test for continuous variables, as appropriate. For each survival-related event, such as LRR, recurrence, or death, survival times were calculated from the date of surgery to the date of event detection, or the date of the last follow-up visit. LRR-free survival (LRRFS), recurrence-free survival (RFS) and overall survival (OS) curves were estimated and compared between the XP and XP-RT groups, both for mesenchymal and non-mesenchymal subtypes, with the adjustment for stage, operation type and classification of Lauren based on the multivariate Cox proportional hazards model. Statistical analysis was performed using SAS software version 9.4 (SAS Institute Inc., Cary, NC, USA) and $p < 0.05$ was considered statistically significant.

3. Results

3.1. Patients

Among the 458 patients who participated in the ARTIST trial, a total of 106 (23.1%) formalin-fixed, paraffin-embedded (FFPE) samples that were available for targeted profiling by the NanoString nCounter assay were evaluated and analyzed in the present study. The baseline characteristics of patients enrolled in the present study and all patients in the ARTIST trial are shown in Table S1. Patients enrolled in this study had significantly more metastatic lymph nodes, and lymphovascular invasion (LVI) and perineural invasion (PNI) were more common than those of all the patients in the ARTIST trial. Clinical-Trials.gov identifier: NCT0176146. Trial Registration: clinical trials.gov identifier NCT00323830 (date of registration: May 10, 2006).

Among the 106 patients enrolled in this study, 56 were assigned to the XP-RT group and the remaining 50 patients were assigned to the XP group. When testing molecular subtypes using the developed MSS/EMT signature, 36 out of 106 patients were classified as having the mesenchymal subtype.

Table 1 displays the detailed characteristics of the enrolled patients having mesenchymal or non-mesenchymal subtypes of GC. In the mesenchymal subtype group, the ratio of diffuse-type GC, classified according to Lauren, was significantly higher than that of the non-mesenchymal subtype group (88.9% versus 60.0%, $p = 0.004$). Additionally, the proportion of patients who received total gastrectomy was higher in the mesenchymal subtype group (55.6% versus 40.0%, $p = 0.128$), although no statistical significance was found. No differences in the percentage of patients receiving XP or XP-RT as adjuvant treatment, nor significant differences in the pathologic staging, were found between the two subtypes.

Table 1. Baseline characteristics of patients.

Variables	Mesenchymal (n = 36, %)	Non-Mesenchymal (n = 70, %)	p
Age—yr			
Median	50	57	0.185
Range	36–76	35–75	
Sex			
Male	17 (47.2)	50 (71.4)	0.019
Female	19 (52.8)	20 (28.6)	
Macroscopic type			
0 (superficial)	1 (2.8)	3 (4.3)	
1 (mass)	0 (0.0)	1 (1.4)	
2 (ulcerative)	3 (8.3)	18 (25.7)	0.039
3 (ulceroinfiltrative)	18 (50.0)	39 (55.7)	
4 (diffuse infiltrative)	14 (38.9)	9 (12.9)	
Location of primary tumor			
Proximal	1 (2.8)	3 (4.3)	
Body	23 (63.9)	32 (45.7)	0.161
Antrum	12 (33.3)	29 (41.4)	
Multiple/diffuse	0 (0.0)	6 (8.6)	
Type of operation			
Total gastrectomy	20 (55.6)	28 (40.0)	0.128
Subtotal gastrectomy	16 (44.4)	42 (60.0)	
Lauren classification			
Diffuse	32 (88.9)	42 (60.0)	
Intestinal	2 (5.6)	25 (35.7)	0.004
Unclassified	2 (5.6)	3 (4.3)	
No of dissected LNs			
Median	42	43	0.824
Range	18–92	14–96	

Table 1. Cont.

Variables	Mesenchymal (n = 36, %)	Non-Mesenchymal (n = 70, %)	p
No of positive LNs			
Median	10	8	0.156
Range	0–50	1–38	
AJCC 8th stage (pathologic stage)			
II	0 (0.0)	2 (2.9)	
IIIA	9 (25.0)	23 (32.9)	0.248
IIIB	16 (44.4)	34 (48.6)	
IIIC	11 (30.6)	11 (15.7)	
LVI			
Positive	29 (80.6)	55 (78.6)	
Negative	6 (16.7)	15 (21.4)	0.402
Unknown	1 (2.8)	0 (0.0)	
PNI			
Positive	21 (58.3)	42 (60.0)	
Negative	12 (33.3)	28 (40.0)	0.724
Unknown	3 (8.3)	0 (0.0)	
ARTIST			
XP-RT	19 (52.8)	37 (52.9)	0.994
XP	17 (47.2)	33 (47.1)	

Abbreviations: LN: lymph node, AJCC: American Joint Committee on Cancer, LVI: lymphovascular invasion, PNI: perineural invasion, XP: capecitabine and cisplatin, XP-RT: XP-radiation therapy.

Baseline characteristics of patients randomly assigned to the XP-RT and XP arms of the ARTIST trial are displayed in Table S2. Age was slightly but significantly lower in the XP-RT arm than in the XP arm.

3.2. Patterns of Recurrence

During follow up (median: 43.6 months, range: 1.8–72.0 months), recurrence was identified in 50 patients (47.2%). Among them, 20 (57.1%) recurrences had developed in the mesenchymal subtype group and the remaining 30 (42.3%) recurrences occurred in the non-mesenchymal subtype group. Median time to any recurrence was 12.9 months (range: 3.8–75.1 months) in the mesenchymal subtype group and 18.0 months (range: 4.5–81.3 months) in the non-mesenchymal subtype group. LRR developed in 20 out of 50 patients, and seven of them were classified as mesenchymal subtype. Median time to LRR was 26.9 months (range: 3.8–81.3 months) in the mesenchymal subtype group and 23.7 months (range: 1.77–154.9 months) in the non-mesenchymal subtype group. Detailed patterns of recurrence according to subtype and adjuvant treatment are shown in Table S3. Peritoneal seeding was the major recurrence pattern in the XP-RT arm, especially in the mesenchymal subtype, and LRR was more frequent in the XP arm. Fifty-one deaths were registered during this period (30 in the non-mesenchymal and 21 in the mesenchymal subtype group).

3.3. Prognostic Factors and Survival Outcomes

Table 2 shows the univariate analysis outcomes of LRRFS, RFS and OS according to the variables, including mesenchymal versus non-mesenchymal subtypes. LRRFS was not different for the mesenchymal and non-mesenchymal subtypes ($p = 0.275$); PNI was the only significant prognostic factor for LRRFS ($p = 0.044$, hazard ratio (HR) = 3.57, 95% confidence interval (CI): 1.03–12.20). RFS was significantly lower in the mesenchymal subtype group ($p = 0.009$, HR = 2.11, 95% CI: 1.21–3.70). Other significant prognostic factors for RFS were type IV of the macroscopic type ($p < 0.001$), total gastrectomy ($p = 0.007$), stage IV ($p < 0.001$), PNI ($p = 0.014$), and Lauren classification other than diffuse-type ($p = 0.028$). The RFS was not different according to the adjuvant treatment of XP or XP-RT ($p = 0.500$). OS was also significantly lower in the mesenchymal subtype group ($p = 0.003$, HR = 2.28, 95% CI: 1.31–3.96). Other significant prognostic factors for OS were: type IV of the macroscopic type ($p < 0.001$), PNI ($p = 0.034$), total gastrectomy ($p = 0.002$), and stage IV ($p < 0.001$). Adjuvant treatment of XP or XP-RT did not affect OS.

Table 2. Univariate analysis of loco-regional recurrence-free survival (LRRFS), recurrence-free survival (RFS), and overall survival (OS).

Variable	Factor	Reference	LRRFS			RFS			OS		
			p	HR	95% CI	HR	95% CI	p	HR	95% CI	
Age			0.887	1.00	0.95–1.04	0.99	0.97–1.02	0.950	1.00	0.97–1.03	
Sex	female	male	0.700	0.82	0.31–2.20	1.21	0.68–2.14	0.418	1.26	0.72–2.21	
Macroscopic type	3	0/1/2	0.762	1.20	0.38–2.22	2.52	0.97–6.53	0.082	2.34	0.90–6.09	
	4		0.137	2.94	0.71–12.10	7.35	2.67–20.20	<0.001	6.78	2.50–18.40	
Lauren type	others	diffuse	0.137	0.43	0.14–1.31	0.46	0.23–0.92	0.052	0.52	0.26–1.01	
LVI	positive	negative	0.153	3.02	0.66–13.80	1.09	0.53–2.24	0.851	0.94	0.47–1.87	
PNI	positive	negative	0.044	3.57	1.03–12.20	2.28	1.18–4.40	0.034	2.00	1.05–3.78	
Type of operation	TG	STG	0.504	1.36	0.55–3.36	2.18	1.24–3.82	0.002	2.38	1.36–4.17	
Stage	IIIB	II/IIIA	0.844	1.12	0.35–3.59	0.92	0.81–3.49	0.193	1.62	0.78–3.37	
	IIIC		0.670	1.29	0.40–4.22	2.91	1.55–5.49	<0.001	3.11	1.67–5.80	
Subtype	mesenchymal	non-mesenchymal	0.275	1.71	0.65–4.46	2.11	1.21–3.70	0.003	2.28	1.31–3.96	
ARTIST	XP-RT	XP	0.196	0.52	0.20–1.40	1.21	0.69–2.11	0.393	1.27	0.73–2.21	

Abbreviations: LRRFS: loco-regional recurrence-free survival, RFS: recurrence-free survival, OS: overall survival, HR: hazard ratio, CI: confidence interval, LVI: lymphovascular invasion, PNI: perineural invasion, TG: total gastrectomy, STG: subtotal gastrectomy, XP: capecitabine and cisplatin, XP-RT: XP-radiation therapy.

3.4. Survival Outcomes for Mesenchymal and Non-Mesenchymal Subtypes

To evaluate the different roles of adjuvant XP-RT or XP between mesenchymal and non-mesenchymal subtypes, multivariate analysis in both mesenchymal and non-mesenchymal subtype was performed including the following factors, which were identified as significant factors not only in the present study but also in many other studies: stage, type of operation, and Lauren classification. Table 3 shows the outcomes of multivariate analyses of RFS and OS for mesenchymal and non-mesenchymal subtypes. Additional results of multivariate analyses of RFS and OS for mesenchymal and non-mesenchymal subtypes including another well-known prognostic factor of PNI are presented in Table S4.

Table 3. Multivariate analysis of recurrence-free survival (RFS), and overall survival (OS) in mesenchymal and non-mesenchymal subtypes.

			RFS			OS		
Variable	Factor	Reference	p	HR	95% CI	p	HR	95% CI
Mesenchymal subtype								
Stage	IIIB	II/IIIA	0.013	5.03	1.40–18.05	0.146	2.33	0.73–7.48
	IIIC		0.098	2.41	0.85–6.86	0.079	2.39	0.90–6.34
Type of operation	TG	STG	0.035	2.88	1.08–7.66	0.319	1.53	0.66–3.51
Lauren type	other	diffuse	0.202	0.24	0.03–2.17	0.981	1.02	0.21–5.93
ARTIST	XP-RT	XP	0.878	0.93	0.36–2.39	0.129	2.05	0.81–5.20
Non-mesenchymal subtype								
Stage	IIIB	II/IIIA	0.305	1.67	0.63–4.43	0.257	1.77	0.66–4.74
	IIIC		<0.001	6.08	2.28–16.19	<0.001	7.61	2.68–21.61
Type of operation	TG	STG	0.055	2.11	0.98–4.54	0.007	2.99	1.35–6.59
Lauren type	other	diffuse	0.031	0.36	0.15–0.91	0.029	0.34	0.13–0.89
ARTIST	XP-RT	XP	0.928	0.96	0.44–2.14	0.541	0.78	0.34–1.76

Abbreviations: RFS: recurrence-free survival, OS: overall survival, HR: hazard ratio, CI: confidence interval, TG: total gastrectomy, STG: subtotal gastrectomy, XP: capecitabine and cisplatin, XP-RT: XP-radiation therapy.

In the multivariate analysis of RFS for the mesenchymal subtype, stage and total gastrectomy were significant prognostic factors, compared to the non-mesenchymal subtype, which was significantly affected by stage, and type of Lauren classification. As displayed in Figure 2A,B, adjusted RFS was not significantly different according to the adjuvant treatment of XP or XP-RT, either for the mesenchymal or non-mesenchymal subtype. Forest plots were used to represent adjusted RFS with HR and 95% CI for the mesenchymal and non-mesenchymal subtypes (Figure 3).

No significant prognostic factors were found in the multivariate analysis of OS for the mesenchymal subtype. On the contrary, stage, total gastrectomy, and type of Lauren classification were significant prognostic factors of OS for the non-mesenchymal subtype. OS was not significantly different according to the adjuvant treatment of XP or XP-RT, either for the mesenchymal or non-mesenchymal subtype. As displayed in Figure 2C,D, however, there was a minor difference in OS between mesenchymal and non-mesenchymal subtypes according to the adjuvant treatment group. The adjuvant XP group showed slightly higher adjusted OS than the XP-RT group for the mesenchymal subtype, and lower adjusted OS than the XP-RT group for the non-mesenchymal subtype. Forest plots were used to represent adjusted OS with HR and 95% CI for the mesenchymal and non-mesenchymal subtypes (Figure 3).

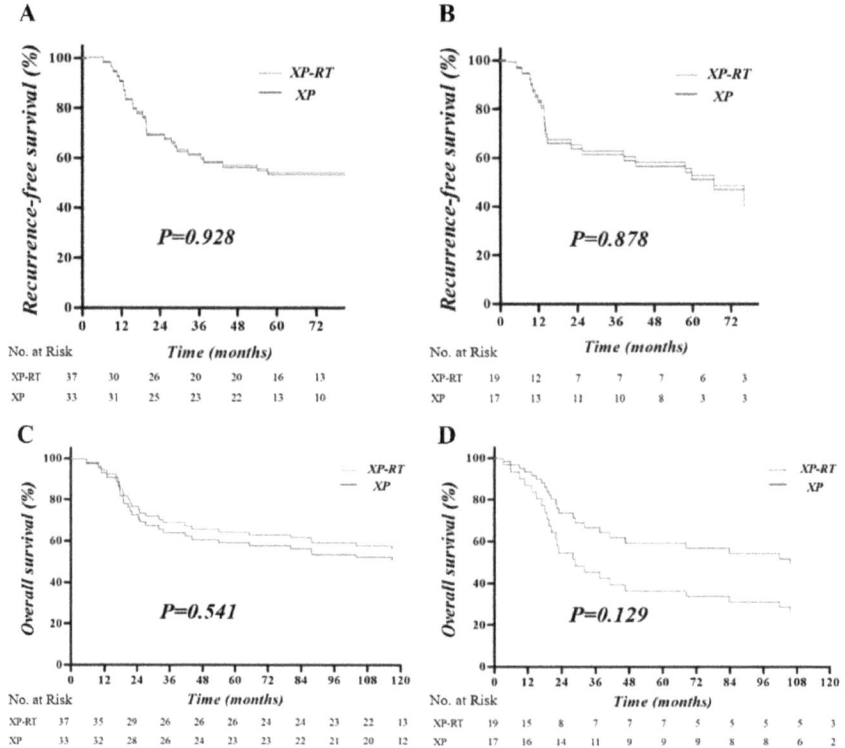

Figure 2. Adjusted curve of recurrence-free survival (RFS, **A,B**) and overall survival (OS, **C,D**) according to the use of adjuvant XP-RT or XP for the mesenchymal (**B,D**) and non-mesenchymal subtypes (**A,C**). In these curves which were displayed for the average value of the covariates in the study population, no significant differences related to the use of adjuvant XP-RT or XP were detected, although OS curves were inverted depending on adjuvant modality for the mesenchymal and non-mesenchymal subtypes (The presented p-values were based on HR test in the Cox proportional hazards model.).

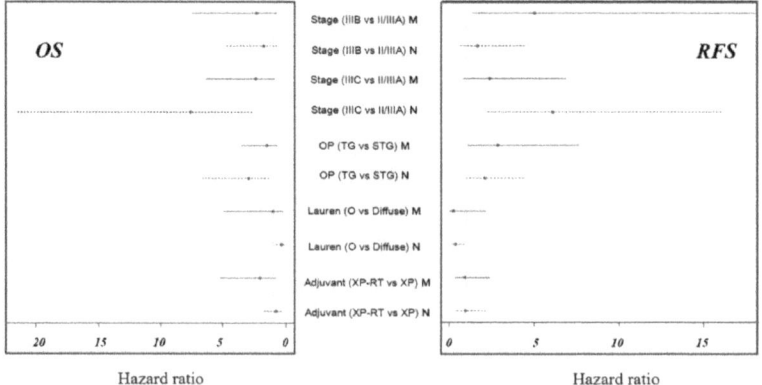

Figure 3. Forest plot for adjusted RFS and OS. No significant differences in RFS related to the use of adjuvant XP-RT or XP for the mesenchymal and non-mesenchymal subtypes were detected (OP, operation; TG, total gastrectomy; STG, subtotal gastrectomy; O, others, M, mesenchymal subtype; N, non-mesenchymal subtype).

4. Discussion

In the present study we evaluated the clinical outcomes according to the adjuvant treatment (XP-RT or XP) for mesenchymal and non-mesenchymal subtypes of GC in a cohort of the ARTIST trial. The mesenchymal subtype showed worse prognostic factors, such as frequent recurrence and lower OS, than the non-mesenchymal subtype, as shown in other reports. However, we could not find any differences between the mesenchymal and non-mesenchymal subtypes in terms of OS as well as RFS.

Beyond the previous histologic and/or anatomic classification of cancer [14–16], there is a growing body of research and evidence supporting the use of molecular analysis for precise classification and tailored management [5,6,17,18]. Although many advances have been made in the management of GC, it still has a poor prognosis in advanced tumors, becoming one of the areas where molecular classification is being actively attempted. Our group, which is the third referral institution of Korea, proposed four subtypes of molecular classification linked to recurrence patterns and prognosis, as well as to distinct patterns of genomic alterations based on ACRG data which have been validated in institutional cohorts [6].

Among the four subtypes of our molecular classification, the mesenchymal-like type, which showed loss of expression of the *CDH1* which encodes the protein E-cadherin. It is known that loss of E-cadherin function decreases the power of cell-to-cell adhesion and increases the cellular motility [19]. It is suggested that the efficacy of local treatment including RT could be limited, because of high metastatic potential originated from these characteristics of the mesenchymal-like type. Actually, it is associated with a younger age of occurrence and is diagnosed as diffuse-type at stage III/IV, showed a significantly higher recurrence rate, higher probability of developing peritoneal seeding at the first site of recurrence, and extremely poor survival compared to other subtypes. Furthermore, it has been reported that PARP-1, which is involved in the mechanism of radiation induced DNA damage repair, is increased in the mesenchymal phenotype, and it could reduce the cell killing effects of RT in prostate cancer [7,8]. In addition, hypoxia, which is a hallmark of tumor and the most important cause of radioresistance, was reported to be associated with the loss of E-cadherin [9].

Our group also proposed the classification of certain GC as mesenchymal type by means of a targeted NanoString gene expression profile [10]. This unique subtype classification may positively impact the standard management of GC, promoting modifications on current treatment protocols which would improve their clinical outcomes.

RT is one of the main therapeutic modalities in the oncology fields. Though adjuvant RT combined with chemotherapy showed survival advantages over surgery alone in the Intergroup trial 0116 [20,21], there is still controversy as to the real efficacy of RT as an adjuvant modality in complete D2-resection GC [22]. The ARTIST trial was a randomized phase III trial designed to evaluate the advantages of adjuvant XP-RT over adjuvant XP after complete D2-resection in GC [11–13]. Superiority of adjuvant XP-RT over XP was not detected in these patients, except for those with LN metastasis.

Although the optimal indications of adjuvant XP-RT remain controversial, RT is still one of the most valuable and important treatment modalities in the management of GC, especially in the neoadjuvant or palliative setting. Furthermore, there is a rapid development of RT technology [23], also accompanied by an increased understanding of radiation biology [24,25]. In this respect, evaluating and comparing the effects of RT on GC of the mesenchymal subtype is of paramount importance, considering its heterogeneity and difficult therapeutic management.

The mesenchymal subtype is known to be closely related to younger age of occurrence and diffuse type of the Lauren classification, showing a worse prognosis and higher recurrence rate compared with other subtypes [6,17,18]. Those characteristics of the mesenchymal subtype were observed in the present study as well. Our group has continued to conduct studies to screen out which GC patients might benefit from adjuvant XP-RT over XP [4,11–13,22]. We found and reported that the benefit of adjuvant XP-RT over XP in GC is reduced to patients with diffuse-type GC and younger age, which correspond to characteristics of the mesenchymal type [12].

The effect of adjuvant XP-RT in mesenchymal subtype of GC in the present study was not significantly different than that of non-mesenchymal subtype in terms of RFS, in contrast to the possibility that the effect of RT might be reduced when considering the characteristics of this subtype. On the other hand, the adjuvant XP-RT group showed a lower OS curve than the XP group for the mesenchymal subtype, although without statistical significance. Although we failed to detect significant difference of RFS between the subtypes according to the adjuvant XP-RT and XP, this marginal difference of OS might be related to the different patterns of recurrence between the subtypes, especially LRR and/or peritoneal seeding. Therefore, the possibility of poorer outcomes after adjuvant XP-RT than after XP for the mesenchymal subtype with complete D2-resection cannot be ruled out. Further research on this issue is needed.

The present study has some important limitations. First, this study was evaluated in a fraction of the participants in the ARTIST trial, mainly because of availability of tissue specimens. Therefore, it is not possible to avoid selection bias in the XP-RT and XP groups, which is minimized by the random allocation nature of phase III. Second, the patients enrolled in this study have characteristics that differ from those of all patients in the ARTIST trial. Third, there could be problems originating from variation in outcomes due to ethnic differences, since the ARTIST trial was conducted at a single Korean institution. Further similar studies are essential for validation in other ethnicities in order to generalize present outcomes, because it is well-known that the characteristics and/or clinical outcomes of gastric cancer are quite distinct according to ethnicity [26–28].

5. Conclusions

We could not determine any significant differences on the effect of adjuvant XP-RT on RFS between mesenchymal and non-mesenchymal subtypes in this cohort of the ARTIST trial. There was a minor difference, however, in the adjuvant XP-RT group showing lower OS than the XP group for the mesenchymal subtype and higher OS for the non-mesenchymal subtype.

Supplementary Materials: The following are available online at http://www.mdpi.com/2072-6694/12/4/943/s1, Table S1. Baseline characteristics of enrolled patients of present study and all patients of ARTIST trial; Table S2. Baseline characteristics of patients according to adjuvant treatment; Table S3. Detailed patterns of recurrence according to subtype and adjuvant treatment; Table S4. Multivariate analysis of recurrence-free survival (RFS), and overall survival (OS) in mesenchymal and non-mesenchymal subtypes including perineural invasion.

Author Contributions: Conceptualization and design: J.I.Y., H.C.P., and J.L.; Development of methodology: J.I.Y., H.C.P., J.L., C.C., K.-M.K., D.H.L., H.H., and K.K.; Acquisition of data: J.I.Y., H.C.P., J.L., C.C., W.K.K., S.H.P., S.T.K., S.K., T.S.S., J.H.L., J.Y.A., M.G.C., J.M.B., K.-M.K., and D.H.L.; Analysis and interpretation of data: J.I.Y., H.C.P., J.L., K.-M.K., H.H., and K.K.; Writing, review, and/or revision of the manuscript: all authors. All authors have read and agreed to the published version of the manuscript.

Funding: This research was partly supported by a Basic Science Research Program through the National Research Foundation of Korea (NRF) funded by the Ministry of Education (NRF-2017R1D1A1B03031275).

Conflicts of Interest: The authors declare no conflict of interest.

References

1. Ferlay, J.; Soerjomataram, I.; Dikshit, R.; Eser, S.; Mathers, C.; Rebelo, M.; Parkin, D.M.; Forman, D.; Bray, F. Cancer incidence and mortality worldwide: Sources, methods and major patterns in GLOBOCAN 2012. *Int. J. Cancer* **2015**, *136*, E359–E386. [CrossRef]
2. Jung, K.W.; Won, Y.J.; Kong, H.J.; Lee, E.S. Community of Population-Based Regional Cancer Registries. Cancer Statistics in Korea: Incidence, Mortality, Survival, and Prevalence in 2015. *Cancer Res. Treat.* **2018**, *50*, 303–316. [CrossRef]
3. Ock, M.; Choi, W.J.; Jo, M.W. Trend analysis of major cancer statistics according to sex and severity levels in Korea. *PLoS ONE* **2018**, *13*, e0203110. [CrossRef]

4. Yu, J.I.; Lim, D.H.; Lee, J.; Kang, W.K.; Park, S.H.; Park, J.O.; Park, Y.S.; Lim, H.Y.; Kim, S.T.; Lee, S.J.; et al. Comparison of the 7th and the 8th AJCC Staging System for Non-metastatic D2-Resected Lymph Node-Positive Gastric Cancer Treated with Different Adjuvant Protocols. *Cancer Res. Treat.* **2019**, *51*, 876–885. [CrossRef]
5. Cancer Genome Atlas Research Network. Comprehensive molecular characterization of gastric adenocarcinoma. *Nature* **2014**, *513*, 202–209. [CrossRef]
6. Cristescu, R.; Lee, J.; Nebozhyn, M.; Kim, K.M.; Ting, J.C.; Wong, S.S.; Liu, J.; Yue, Y.G.; Wang, J.; Yu, K.; et al. Molecular analysis of gastric cancer identifies subtypes associated with distinct clinical outcomes. *Nat. Med.* **2015**, *21*, 449–456. [CrossRef]
7. Pu, H.; Horbinski, C.; Hensley, P.J.; Matuszak, E.A.; Atkinson, T.; Kyprianou, N. PARP-1 regulates epithelial-mesenchymal transition (EMT) in prostate tumorigenesis. *Carcinogenesis* **2014**, *35*, 2592–2601. [CrossRef]
8. Stark, T.W.; Hensley, P.J.; Spear, A.; Pu, H.; Strup, S.S.; Kyprianou, N. Predictive value of epithelial-mesenchymal-transition (EMT) signature and PARP-1 in prostate cancer radioresistance. *Prostate* **2017**, *77*, 1583–1591. [CrossRef]
9. Theys, J.; Jutten, B.; Habets, R.; Paesmans, K.; Groot, A.J.; Lambin, P.; Wouters, B.G.; Lammering, G.; Vooijs, M. E-Cadherin loss associated with EMT promotes radioresistance in human tumor cells. *Radiother. Oncol.* **2011**, *99*, 392–397. [CrossRef]
10. Lee, J.; Cristescu, R.; Kim, K.M.; Kim, K.; Kim, S.T.; Park, S.H.; Kang, W.K. Development of mesenchymal subtype gene signature for clinical application in gastric cancer. *Oncotarget* **2017**, *8*, 66305–66315. [CrossRef]
11. Lee, J.; Lim, D.H.; Kim, S.; Park, S.H.; Park, J.O.; Park, Y.S.; Lim, H.Y.; Choi, M.G.; Sohn, T.S.; Noh, J.H.; et al. Phase III trial comparing capecitabine plus cisplatin versus capecitabine plus cisplatin with concurrent capecitabine radiotherapy in completely resected gastric cancer with D2 lymph node dissection: The ARTIST trial. *J. Clin. Oncol.* **2012**, *30*, 268–273. [CrossRef]
12. Park, S.H.; Sohn, T.S.; Lee, J.; Lim, D.H.; Hong, M.E.; Kim, K.M.; Sohn, I.; Jung, S.H.; Choi, M.G.; Lee, J.H.; et al. Phase III Trial to Compare Adjuvant Chemotherapy With Capecitabine and Cisplatin Versus Concurrent Chemoradiotherapy in Gastric Cancer: Final Report of the Adjuvant Chemoradiotherapy in Stomach Tumors Trial, Including Survival and Subset Analyses. *J. Clin. Oncol.* **2015**, *33*, 3130–3136. [CrossRef]
13. Yu, J.I.; Lim, D.H.; Ahn, Y.C.; Lee, J.; Kang, W.K.; Park, S.H.; Park, J.O.; Park, Y.S.; Lim, H.Y.; Kim, S.T.; et al. Effects of adjuvant radiotherapy on completely resected gastric cancer: A radiation oncologist's view of the ARTIST randomized phase III trial. *Radiother. Oncol.* **2015**, *117*, 171–177. [CrossRef]
14. Japanese Gastric Cancer Association. Japanese classification of gastric carcinoma: 3rd English edition. *Gastric Cancer* **2011**, *14*, 101–112. [CrossRef]
15. Chen, Y.C.; Fang, W.L.; Wang, R.F.; Liu, C.A.; Yang, M.H.; Lo, S.S.; Wu, C.W.; Li, A.F.; Shyr, Y.M.; Huang, K.H. Clinicopathological Variation of Lauren Classification in Gastric Cancer. *Pathol. Oncol. Res.* **2016**, *22*, 197–202. [CrossRef]
16. Hu, B.; El Hajj, N.; Sittler, S.; Lammert, N.; Barnes, R.; Meloni-Ehrig, A. Gastric cancer: Classification, histology and application of molecular pathology. *J. Gastrointest. Oncol.* **2012**, *3*, 251–261.
17. Alessandrini, L.; Manchi, M.; De Re, V.; Dolcetti, R.; Canzonieri, V. Proposed Molecular and miRNA Classification of Gastric Cancer. *Int. J. Mol. Sci.* **2018**, *19*, 1683. [CrossRef]
18. Chia, N.Y.; Tan, P. Molecular classification of gastric cancer. *Ann. Oncol.* **2016**, *27*, 763–769. [CrossRef]
19. van Roy, F. Beyond E-cadherin: Roles of other cadherin superfamily members in cancer. *Nat. Rev. Cancer* **2014**, *14*, 121–134. [CrossRef]
20. Macdonald, J.S.; Smalley, S.R.; Benedetti, J.; Hundahl, S.A.; Estes, N.C.; Stemmermann, G.N.; Haller, D.G.; Ajani, J.A.; Gunderson, L.L.; Jessup, J.M.; et al. Chemoradiotherapy after surgery compared with surgery alone for adenocarcinoma of the stomach or gastroesophageal junction. *N. Engl. J. Med.* **2001**, *345*, 725–730. [CrossRef]
21. Smalley, S.R.; Benedetti, J.K.; Haller, D.G.; Hundahl, S.A.; Estes, N.C.; Ajani, J.A.; Gunderson, L.L.; Goldman, B.; Martenson, J.A.; Jessup, J.M.; et al. Updated analysis of SWOG-directed intergroup study 0116: A phase III trial of adjuvant radiochemotherapy versus observation after curative gastric cancer resection. *J. Clin. Oncol.* **2012**, *30*, 2327–2333. [CrossRef]

22. Yu, J.I.; Lim, D.H.; Lee, J.; Kang, W.K.; Park, S.H.; Park, J.O.; Park, Y.S.; Lim, H.Y.; Kim, S.T.; Lee, S.J.; et al. Necessity of adjuvant concurrent chemo-radiotherapy in D2-resected LN-positive gastric cancer. *Radiother. Oncol.* **2018**, *129*, 306–312. [CrossRef]
23. Cho, B. Correction: Intensity-modulated radiation therapy: A review with a physics perspective. *Radiat. Oncol. J.* **2018**, *36*, 171. [CrossRef]
24. Kim, J.H.; Jenrow, K.A.; Brown, S.L. Novel biological strategies to enhance the radiation therapeutic ratio. *Radiat. Oncol. J.* **2018**, *36*, 172–181. [CrossRef]
25. Nicosia, L.; Gentile, G.; Reverberi, C.; Minniti, G.; Valeriani, M.; de Sanctis, V.; Marinelli, L.; Cipolla, F.; de Luca, O.; Simmaco, M.; et al. Single nucleotide polymorphism of GSTP1 and pathological complete response in locally advanced rectal cancer patients treated with neoadjuvant concomitant radiochemotherapy. *Radiat. Oncol. J.* **2018**, *36*, 218–226. [CrossRef]
26. Kim, J.; Mailey, B.; Senthil, M.; Artinyan, A.; Sun, C.L.; Bhatia, S. Disparities in gastric cancer outcomes among Asian ethnicities in the USA. *Ann. Surg. Oncol.* **2009**, *16*, 2433–2441. [CrossRef]
27. Kim, J.; Sun, C.L.; Mailey, B.; Prendergast, C.; Artinyan, A.; Bhatia, S.; Pigazzi, A.; Ellenhorn, J.D. Race and ethnicity correlate with survival in patients with gastric adenocarcinoma. *Ann. Oncol.* **2010**, *21*, 152–160. [CrossRef]
28. Rhome, R.M.; Ru, M.; Moshier, E.; Mazumdar, M.; Buckstein, M.H. Stage-matched survival differences by ethnicity among gastric cancer patients of Asian ancestry treated in the United States. *J. Surg. Oncol.* **2019**, *119*, 737–748. [CrossRef]

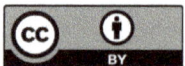 © 2020 by the authors. Licensee MDPI, Basel, Switzerland. This article is an open access article distributed under the terms and conditions of the Creative Commons Attribution (CC BY) license (http://creativecommons.org/licenses/by/4.0/).

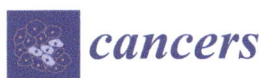

Article

Conversion Surgery in Metastatic Gastric Cancer and Cancer Dormancy as a Prognostic Biomarker

Hun Jee Choe [1], Jin Won Kim [1,*,†], Song-Hee Han [2,3], Ju Hyun Lee [1], Sang-Hoon Ahn [4], Do Joong Park [4,5], Ji-Won Kim [1], Yu Jung Kim [1], Hye Seung Lee [2,*,†], Jee Hyun Kim [1], Hyung-Ho Kim [4] and Keun-Wook Lee [1]

1. Department of Internal Medicine, Seoul National University Bundang Hospital, Seoul National University College of Medicine, Seongnam 13620, Korea; hunjeechoe@snu.ac.kr (H.J.C.); r1219@snubh.org (J.H.L.); jiwonkim@snubh.org (J.-W.K.); cong1005@snubh.org (Y.J.K.); jhkimmd@snubh.org (J.H.K.); hmodoctor@snubh.org (K.-W.L.)
2. Department of Pathology, Seoul National University Bundang Hospital, Seoul National University College of Medicine, Seongnam 13620, Korea; pshsh625@gmail.com
3. Department of Pathology, Dong-A University Hospital, Dong-A University College of Medicine, Busan 49201, Korea
4. Department of Surgery, Seoul National University Bundang Hospital, Seoul National University College of Medicine, Seongnam 13620, Korea; viscaria@snubh.org (S.-H.A.); djparkmd@snu.ac.kr (D.J.P.); hhkim@snubh.org (H.-H.K.)
5. Department of Surgery, Seoul National University Hospital, Seoul National University College of Medicine, Seoul 03080, Korea
* Correspondence: jwkim@snubh.org (J.W.K.); mw9195@snubh.org (H.S.L.); Tel.: +82-31-787-7053 (J.W.K.); +82-31-787-7714 (H.S.L.)
† These authors contributed equally to this work.

Received: 4 November 2019; Accepted: 24 December 2019; Published: 30 December 2019

Abstract: The role of conversion surgery in metastatic gastric cancer remains unclear. Cancer dormancy markers might have a role in predicting the survival in patients with conversion surgery. We identified 26 patients who went through conversion surgery, i.e., a curative-intent gastrectomy with metastasectomy after chemotherapy in initially metastatic gastric cancer. As controls, 114 potential candidates for conversion surgery who only received chemotherapy were included for the propensity score matching. Conversion surgery showed a significantly longer overall survival (OS) compared with only palliative chemotherapy (median—43.6 vs. 14.0 months, respectively, $p < 0.001$). This better survival in the conversion surgery group persisted even after propensity matching ($p < 0.001$), and also when compared to patients with tumor response over 5.1 months in the chemotherapy only group ($p = 0.005$). In the conversion surgery group, OS was longer in patients with R0 resection (22/26, 84.6%) than without R0 resection (4/26, 15.4%) (median—not reached vs 22.1 months, respectively, $p = 0.005$). Although it should be interpreted with caution due to the primitive analysis in a small population, the positive expression of NR2F1 showed a longer duration of disease-free survival (DFS) after conversion surgery ($p = 0.016$). In conclusion, conversion surgery showed a durable OS even in patients with initially metastatic gastric cancer when R0 resection was achieved after chemotherapy.

Keywords: gastric cancer; conversion surgery; cancer dormancy; nuclear receptor NR2F1

1. Introduction

The incidence of gastric cancer is widely varied geographically. Despite the trend of steady decline and country-specific disparity, it remains to be the fifth most prevalent cancer and the third cause of death worldwide [1,2]. Curative operation is the treatment of choice for resectable diseases. As for metastatic gastric cancer, systemic chemotherapy is the standard treatment modality. However, the prognosis remains poor with a median survival of about 12 months, despite recent advancements made in chemotherapeutics, including molecular targeting agents and cancer immunotherapy [3].

Conversion surgery is a term for operative resection of primary or metastatic lesions with a curative intent, after confirming either a complete response (CR) or partial response (PR), following several cycles of palliative chemotherapy. Although addition of gastrectomy (without metastasectomy) to palliative chemotherapy in metastatic gastric cancer did not show survival benefit when compared with chemotherapy only in the previous REGATTA trial [4], there have been recent attempts to conduct surgery in selected patients with a good initial response to palliative chemotherapy [5–12]. It has been shown to improve the prognosis in a few retrospective studies. However, whether this improvement of survival is attributed to conversion surgery or good tumor biology in patients undergoing conversion surgery remains unclear. The characteristics of patients that might benefit from conversion surgery also remain unknown.

Cancer dormancy is a clinical phenomenon in which the metastatic disease develops years or even decades after successful treatment with curative surgery and adjuvant treatment [13]. Dormant tumor cells might stay in the quiescent state for many years as solitary tumor cells or micrometastases that are not clinically apparent. Cancer dormancy could be associated with early or late recurrence after conversion surgery in patients with initial systemic metastasis.

In this study, we compared the outcomes of patients with metastatic gastric cancer who subsequently underwent conversion surgery after palliative chemotherapy, with patients who only received palliative chemotherapy using propensity score analysis. We also investigated whether the expression of cancer dormancy markers might play a role in predicting survival in patients receiving conversion surgery as a pilot study.

2. Results

2.1. Patients' Demographic Data

Patient characteristics and the clinicopathologic findings are shown in Table 1. In the conversion surgery group, 6 patients (23.1%) were ≥70 years old, and 10 patients (38.5%) had macroscopic peritoneal dissemination. Of these, the favorable response of CR or PR to palliative chemotherapy was seen in 17 patients (65.4%). In the chemotherapy only (the control) group, 31 patients (27.2%) were ≥70 years old. A slightly higher portion of patients had macroscopic peritoneal dissemination (50.9%), as compared to the conversion surgery group (38.5%). CR or PR was achieved in the lower proportion of patients with palliative chemotherapy (51.8%). Both groups were balanced after propensity score matching (1:2) in terms of baseline characteristics.

All patients received a fluoropyrimidine in combination with a platinum analogue as a first-line palliative chemotherapy in both groups. Those who showed an overexpression of HER2 also received trastuzumab. All conversion surgeries were conducted during the first-line chemotherapy, except in one patient who received conversion surgery during the second-line chemotherapy. The median duration of first-line chemotherapy before conversion surgery was 5.1 months. After conversion surgery, the first-line chemotherapy was continued in 13 patients (50%) as a maintenance therapy.

Table 1. Demographics and baseline characteristics of patients.

Variable	Conversion Surgery (n = 26) No. (%)	Chemotherapy Only		p-Value [a]	p-Value [b]
		Before Propensity Score Matching (n = 114) No. (%)	After Propensity Score Matching (n = 52) No. (%)		
Age (Median, Range)	58 (39–78)	61 (52–70)	57 (52–68)	0.855	1.000
<70 years	20 (76.9%)	83 (72.8%)	40 (76.9%)		
≥70 years	6 (23.1%)	31 (27.2%)	12 (23.1%)		
Sex				0.829	0.514
Male	18 (69.2%)	84 (73.7%)	41 (78.8%)		
Female	8 (30.8%)	30 (26.3%)	11 (21.2%)		
Metastatic site				0.355	0.935
Category 1–2	16 (61.5%)	56 (49.1%)	30 (57.7%)		
Category 3–4	10 (38.5%)	58 (50.9%)	22 (42.3%)		
1st line palliative chemotherapy [c]				0.011	0.180
S1/capecitabine + cisplatin/oxaliplatin	14 (53.8%)	67 (58.8%)	31 (59.6%)		
FOLFOX	5 (19.2%)	36 (31.6%)	15 (28.8%)		
Herceptin + capecitabine + cisplatin	7 (26.9%)	6 (5.3%)	4 (7.7%)		
5-fluorouracil + cisplatin	0 (0.0%)	4 (3.5%)	1 (1.9%)		
Docetaxel + 5-fluorouracil + cisplatin	0 (0.0%)	1 (0.9%)	1 (1.9%)		
Best tumor response				0.298	1.000
CR, PR	17 (65.4%)	59 (51.8%)	34 (65.4%)		
SD, NE	9 (34.6%)	55 (48.2%)	18 (34.6%)		

[a] Between conversion surgery (n = 26) and chemotherapy only group (n = 114). [b] Between conversion surgery (n = 26) and propensity score matched chemotherapy only group (n = 52). [c] Two of 26 patients in conversion surgery group and 8 of 114 patients in chemotherapy only group were under clinical trial and received combination therapy with an additional investigational agent including cetuximab, axitinib, and sunitinib. FOLFOX: oxaliplatin, 5-fluorouracil, leucovorin; CR, complete response; PR, partial response; SD, stable disease; NE, not evaluable for response.

In the conversion surgery group, R0 resection was achieved in 22 patients (84.6%). Pathologic CR was shown in 2 patients (7.7%). Subtotal gastrectomy, total gastrectomy, and extended total gastrectomy were performed in 42.3%, 30.8% and 26.9%, respectively. Lymphatic invasion, vascular invasion, and perineural invasion were present in 80.8%, 42.3% and 65.4%, respectively (Table 2). At the first diagnosis before palliative chemotherapy, category 2 was the most prevalent biological disease status (42.3%), followed by category 4 (23.1%), category 1 (19.2%), and category 3 (15.4%). At the time of conversion surgery, CR, PR, stable disease (SD), and not evaluable (NE) had been established with chemotherapy in 2 (7.7%), 15 (57.7%), 3 (11.5%) and 6 (23.1%) patients, respectively.

Table 2. Clinicopathological characteristics of tumor in conversion surgery patients.

Variable	N (%)
Initial biological disease category before palliative chemotherapy	
Category 1	5 (19.2)
Category 2	11 (42.3)
Category 3	4 (15.4)
Category 4	6 (23.1)
Best tumor response before conversion surgery	
Complete response	2 (7.7)
Partial response	15 (57.7)
Stable disease	3 (11.5)
Not evaluable	6 (23.1)
Type of resection	
Subtotal gastrectomy	11 (42.3)
Total gastrectomy	8 (30.8)
Extended total gastrectomy	7 (26.9)
R0 resection	
R0	22 (84.6)
R2	4 (15.4)
Lymphatic invasion	
Not identified	5 (19.2)
Present	21 (80.8)
Vascular invasion	
Not identified	15 (57.7)
Present	11 (42.3)
Perineural invasion	
Not identified	9 (34.6)
Present	17 (65.4)
Lauren classification	
Intestinal	13 (50.0)
Diffuse	10 (38.5)
Indeterminate	1 (3.8)
Others	2 (7.7)
Histologic differentiation	
Tubular adenocarcionma	16 (61.5)
Poorly cohesive carcinoma	5 (16.2)
Papillary adenocarcinoma	3 (11.5)
No tumor	2 (7.7)

Table 2. Cont.

Variable	N (%)
TNM [a]	
ypT	
0	1 (3.8)
1	2 (7.7)
2	3 (11.5)
3	12 (46.2)
4	7 (26.9)
ypN	
0	8 (30.8)
1	2 (7.7)
2	6 (23.1)
3	10 (38.5)
Postoperative stage	
0	2 (7.7)
I	2 (7.7)
II	3 (11.5)
III	10 (38.5)
IV	9 (34.6)

[a] AJCC, American Joint Committee on Cancer 8th edition. One case was diagnosed as poorly differentiated adenocarcinoma at initial preoperative endoscopic biopsy, but the immunostaining of the resected tumor revealed a large cell neuroendocrine carcinoma component.

2.2. Survival Outcomes of Conversion Surgery and Palliative Chemotherapy Only Group

The median follow-up duration was 36.1 months in the conversion surgery group and 13.0 months in the palliative chemotherapy only group. Overall survival (OS) was significantly longer for patients who received conversion surgery compared to those who only received palliative chemotherapy (Median OS: 43.6 months, 95% confidence interval [CI], 31.6–not reached [NR]; 14.0 months, 95% CI 11.0–15.0, respectively, $p < 0.001$, Figure 1a). The median duration of palliative chemotherapy before conversion surgery was 5.1 months, whereas 53 of 114 patients (46.5%) who only received chemotherapy had tumor progression before 5.1 months, while on chemotherapy. Thus, to avoid a potential selection bias, additional comparison was made between all patients in the conversion surgery group and the subgroup of patients in the chemotherapy only group whose tumor responded to or were stabilized with chemotherapy for greater than 5.1 months. This latter group of patients demonstrated a median OS of 21.0 months (95% CI 15.0–32.0), which nevertheless was appreciably shorter than that of the conversion surgery group ($p = 0.005$, Figure 1b).

Out of 26 patients that underwent conversion surgery, 22 patients received R0 resection. Cancer recurred in 15 of 22 patients (68.2%) that underwent conversion surgery with R0 resection. In those who underwent successful R0 resection, disease-free survival (DFS) from conversion surgery was 15.1 months (95% CI 7.5–NR). OS was longer in the R0 resection group (median value—NR, 95% CI 34.8–NR) compared with those without successful resection (21.1 months, 95% CI 12.2–NR, $p = 0.005$, Figure 1c, Table S1). There was no statistical difference in OS from the initial palliative chemotherapy between the group who received noncurative resection (21.1 months, 95% CI 12.2–NR) and the group who only received chemotherapy (14.0 months, 95% CI 11.0–15.0) ($p = 0.642$, Figure 1d).

Patients who received R0 resection in conversion surgery were further analyzed according to the initial biological disease status before palliative chemotherapy, chemotherapy duration before conversion surgery, tumor response to chemotherapy at conversion surgery, and postoperative pathological staging. A shorter duration of chemotherapy before conversion surgery was associated with a longer duration of DFS ($p < 0.001$) from conversion surgery. A less advanced pathological stage was also associated with DFS from conversion surgery ($p = 0.005$). In contrast, the between-group differences in DFS regarding the initial biological disease status before palliative chemotherapy were not clinically significant ($p = 0.071$). Tumor response to chemotherapy was not associated with DFS from conversion surgery in the conversion surgery group ($p = 0.712$), but was a prognostic factor in the chemotherapy only group (OS and progression-free survival (PFS): $p = 0.005$, $p = 0.003$, respectively). The characteristics and clinical course of patients who showed long-term survival (>3 years) among patients with conversion surgery are described in Table 3.

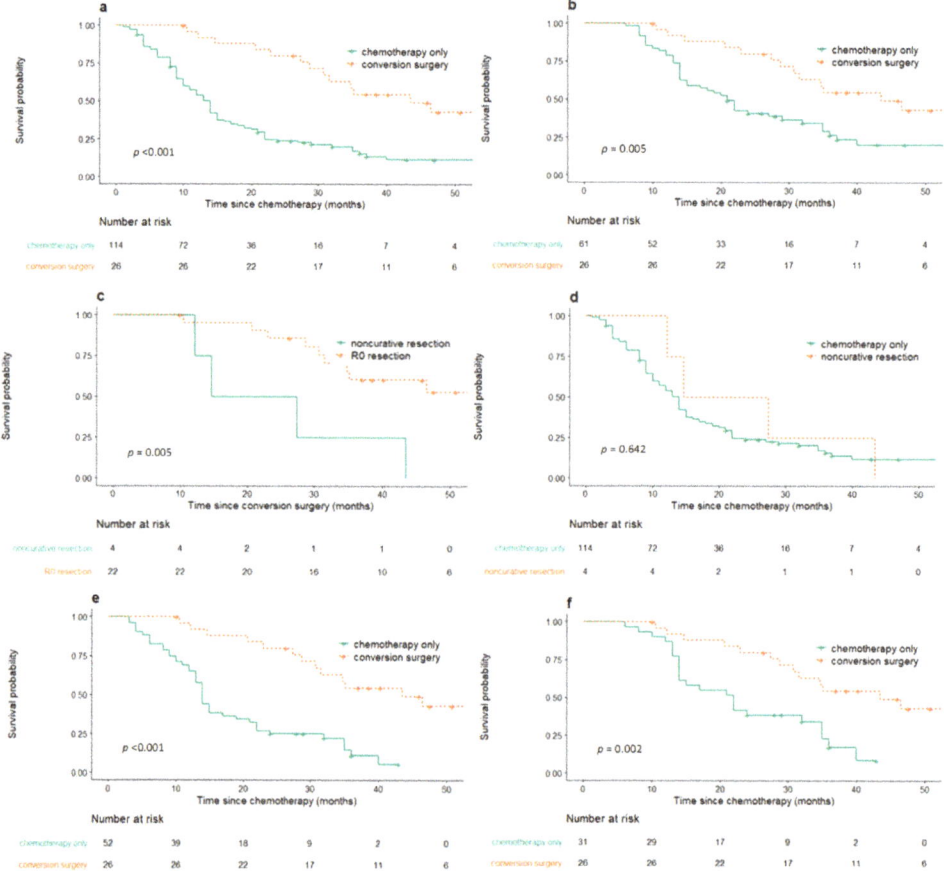

Figure 1. Kaplan–Meier curve for overall survival (OS) in patients who received conversion surgery and only chemotherapy. (**a**) Comparison of OS after chemotherapy in patients who received conversion surgery ($n = 26$) and those that only received chemotherapy ($n = 114$) ($p < 0.001$). (**b**) Comparison of OS after chemotherapy in patients who received conversion surgery ($n = 26$) vs. subgroup of patients in the chemotherapy only group whose tumor responded to or were stabilized with chemotherapy for 5.1 or more months ($n = 61$) ($p = 0.005$). (**c**) Comparison of OS in patients who received R0 resection ($n = 22$) vs. noncurative resection in conversion surgery ($n = 4$) ($p = 0.005$). (**d**) Comparison of OS after chemotherapy in patients who received noncurative resection in conversion surgery ($n = 4$) vs. only chemotherapy ($n = 114$) ($p = 0.642$). (**e**) After propensity score matching, comparison of OS after chemotherapy in patients who received conversion surgery ($n = 26$) vs. only chemotherapy ($n = 52$) after propensity score matching ($p < 0.001$). (**f**) After propensity score matching, comparison of OS after chemotherapy in patients who received conversion surgery ($n = 26$) vs. subgroup of patients with tumor response of 5.1 or more months after propensity score matching ($n = 31$) ($p = 0.002$).

Table 3. The characteristics and clinical course of patients who showed long-term survival (> 3 years) among patients with conversion surgery.

Case No.	Age (Years)	Sex	Initial Metastatic Sites	Initial Biological Category Before Palliative Chemotherapy	Initial Chemotherapy	Chemotherapy Duration Before Conversion Surgery (Months)	Chemotherapy Response	Operation	Curativity	TNM Stage	Maintenance Chemotherapy	Recur	Survival Status	Overall Survival (Months)
1	64	M	Liver	2	FOLFOX	4.0	PR	TG + D2 + intraoperative radiofrequency ablation (scar change)	R0	pT2N1	Yes	No	alive	142.2
2	65	F	Liver and pancreas invasion	2	FOLFOX	3.8	CR	STG + D2	R0	pT0N0	No	No	alive	91.2
3	45	M	Peritoneal seeding, paraaortic LN	4	XELOX	4.1	PR	extended TG + D3 dissection	R0	pT0N0	Yes	No	alive	66.5
4	46	F	Retroperitoneal LN	2	XP + Herceptin	3.1	PR	STG + D3	R0	pT1N2	No	Yes	alive	61.8
5	56	F	Portocaval LN	2	XELOX	3.8	SD	STG + D3	R0	pT3N3a	Yes	No	alive	56.2
6	47	F	Peritoneal seeding	3	XELOX	4.7	NE	TG + D2	R0	pT2N0	Yes	Yes	alive	50.9
7	43	M	Retroperitoneal LN	1	XP + Herceptin	4.9	PR	STG + D3	R0	pT1N0	Yes	No	alive	47.6
8	51	M	Peritoneal seeding, Retroperitoneal LN	4	TS1 + Cisplatin	10.1	SD	TG + D3	R0	pT4aN3bM1(LN #16b1, #14)	Yes	Yes	expired	46.5
9	73	M	Peritoneal seeding, Colon and pancreas invasion	4	FOLFOX	3.2	CR	STG + D2	R0	pT2N0M1 (LN #13)	No	No	alive	46.0
10	65	M	Retroperitoneal LN	2	XP	11.1	PR	STG + D3	R2	T3N2M1(residual lesion at cardia)	Yes	Yes	expired	43.6
11	57	M	Peritoneal seeding	3	XELOX	13.9	SD	TG + D2	R0	pT3N2	No	Yes	alive	40.3
12	76	M	Pancreas body, and gallbladder invasion	2	XP + Herceptin	4.4	PR	STG + D2 + cholecystectomy + LN dissection (#8)	R0	pT3N2	Yes	No	alive	38.5
13	56	M	Retroperitoneal LN	2	TS1 + Cisplatin	5.0	NE	STG + D2 (no visual retroperitoneal LN)	R0	pT3N0	Yes	No	alive	37.1

LN, lymph nodes; FOLFOX folinic acid, fluorouracil, leucovorin, oxaliplatin; XELOX capecitabine and oxaliplatin; XP capecitabine and cisplatin; TS1, Tegafur/gimeracil/oteracil; CR, complete response; PR, partial response; SD, stable disease; NE, not evaluable for response; STG, subtotal gastrectomy; TG, total gastrectomy; TNM, tumor-node-metastasis.

2.3. Propensity Score Matching Analysis

Propensity score matching analysis was conducted with the purpose of balancing any confounding covariates, including initial biological disease status category before palliative chemotherapy, best response to chemotherapy, age, and sex. OS in patients who received conversion surgery and those that only received chemotherapy was 43.6 months (95% CI 31.6–NR) and 14.0 months (95% CI 13.0–21.0), respectively, after propensity score matching ($p < 0.001$, Figure 1e). Subgroup analysis was performed with the selected group of patients in which continuous tumor response to chemotherapy was obtained for 5.1 months or longer in the matched cohort, to reduce selection bias. The median OS was 22 months in this group (95% CI 14.0–35.0), which was also shorter than that in the conversion surgery group ($p = 0.002$, Figure 1f).

2.4. Mortality and Morbidity of Conversion Surgery

Of the 26 patients who received conversion surgery, there was no treatment-related mortality. Postoperative morbidity was evaluated according to the revised Clavien–Dindo classification of surgical complications [14]. Overall, 19.2% of patients had an adverse event with grade II or III; one pleural effusion (grade IIIa), one serous leakage (grade II), one pulmonary thromboembolism, and deep vein thrombosis (grade II), one ileus (grade II), and one pneumonia (grade II).

2.5. Cancer Dormancy Marker Expression

For the group of patients that went through conversion surgery, tissue microarray (TMA) was performed for the expression of cancer dormancy markers in 18 out of 26 initial biopsy specimens. Although positive expression (moderate to strong) of NR2F1 was identified in only 4 patients, the expression of NR2F1 was correlated with DFS after conversion surgery ($p = 0.016$). No significant differences in DFS were observed as per the expression of NANOG and MIG6 ($p = 0.909$, $p = 0.314$, respectively, Figure S1).

3. Discussion

The prognosis for those undergoing systemic therapies only for gastric cancers who were either initially diagnosed as metastatic or having developed recurrence after initial curative resection was dismal, in spite of recent advancements made in targeted and immune-based therapies [3]. Accordingly, there have been attempts to proceed to conversion surgery in metastatic gastric cancer in an effort to add survival benefit to chemotherapy even when systemic treatment only could at least temporarily control the microscopic disease [4–12].

The strengths of a well-designed randomized trial are indisputable; however, in studies involving surgical cases, such a study is difficult [15]. It is particularly difficult to undertake a randomized controlled study design when involving surgical cases of advanced gastric cancer. This is because surgery is currently the only option for curative treatment in advanced gastric cancer. Consequently, previous reports that studied conversion surgery in metastatic gastric cancer have adopted observational study models [4,6–8,10,15–20]. For this reason, most previous studies have obvious inherent limitations associated with selection bias in patients who received conversion surgery, i.e., better initial response to systemic chemotherapy or a lesser degree of peritoneal seeding, compared with the group who only received palliative chemotherapy. Furthermore, due to the inadequate tumor sample data in previous retrospective studies, there had not been attempts to define specific biological subgroups of patients who might benefit from conversion surgery.

In this study, we have implemented a propensity score modeling, producing a matched cohort based on baseline characteristics, as well as the extent of initial biological disease, before palliative chemotherapy and response to chemotherapy. Our findings were consistent with previous studies that advocated conversion surgery if R0 resection could be achieved, even after adjusting for potential confounding factors [9,10,12,21,22]. It is noteworthy that patients who underwent conversion surgery exhibited a longer survival rate after additionally excluding early disease progression in the chemotherapy only group. In addition, a shorter duration of preoperative chemotherapy was an independent predictor of DFS from conversion surgery, which was contradictory to the previous study [21]. This might in part be attributable to better chemotherapy efficacy in the subgroup of patients with a shorter duration of preoperative chemotherapy, leading to tumor shrinkage that facilitated conversion surgery [23]. Another explanation can be lead-time bias, which indicates that a shorter duration of chemotherapy before conversion surgery leads to a longer DFS after conversion surgery. Although there was no significant interaction between the initial biological disease status category before palliative chemotherapy and OS in the conversion surgery group, OS was significantly longer in patients who had reached less advanced pathological staging, emphasizing the role of systemic chemotherapy in clinical efficacy for tumor control and down-staging of the tumor for the improvement of the R0 resection rate.

In the initial phases of the metastatic disease, which is a candidate of conversion surgery but is very likely to have microscopic metastasis, cancer dormancy could be associated with recurrence after macroscopic curative resection. NR2F1 is an example of a cancer dormancy marker. It was an orphan nuclear receptor that was thought to be linked to longer DFS in breast and prostate cancer, undergoing a prolonged asymptomatic dormancy status before resuming metastatic growth [24,25]. Based on our results, a positive expression of NR2F1 in the initial biopsy specimen conferred a survival benefit in patients that went through conversion surgery, although this analysis was too primitive to provide any evidence, due to the small sample size. The small sample size also limited our ability to demonstrate the statistical significance as prognostic predictors in NANOG, MIG6, and PERK.

The present study has some limitations. First, this study might have some inherent biases due to the retrospective nature. Nevertheless, we tried to compare patients who received conversion surgery objectively by propensity score matching and excluding early disease progression in the control group. Some of the subgroup analyses were novel findings in our study. Second, preoperative staging without staging laparoscopy could have resulted in over-staging, particularly in cases of peritoneal seeding. Diagnostic staging laparoscopy and re-evaluation of peritoneal metastasis with staging laparoscopy might be helpful in improving the diagnostic accuracy and optimizing candidates for conversion surgery [26,27]. Third, the clinical efficacy of cancer dormancy marker expression in conversion surgery cannot be definitively concluded, given the relatively small sample size of this study. Even though the expression of NR2F1 was statistically significant as a good prognostic marker, there were only four patients who expressed NR2F1 among those who received R0 resection in the conversion surgery group. Other cancer dormancy markers that might have also played a role in determining the prognosis had limited power to show a statistically significant difference due to the small number of patients included. The number of patients in the conversion surgery cohort itself, however, was not small as compared to previous studies. Therefore, adopting cancer dormancy markers as a prognostic marker in conversion surgery remains a promising option. Fourth, cancer dormancy markers were evaluated only in the conversion surgery group and those who had only received chemotherapy did not have comparable tumor tissues for tumor dormancy marker staining. In the future, studies with a larger sample size comparing the various aspects of cancer dormancy marker expression in both the conversion surgery group and chemotherapy only group might be warranted for developing a clearer criterion in selecting patients apt for conversion surgery with better outcomes. Nonetheless, to the best of our knowledge, this is the first study to adopt the cancer dormancy concept in patients undergoing gastric conversion surgery, to date.

4. Patients and Methods

4.1. Patients with Conversion Surgery

Forty-nine patients with initially metastatic gastric cancer who underwent gastrectomy after palliative chemotherapy between January 2006 and August 2016 at Seoul National University Bundang

Hospital (SNUBH) were identified from the pathology database. Patients were eligible for inclusion if they had a histological confirmation of adenocarcinoma in the initial biopsy, which was initially metastatic and had curative-intent gastrectomy or metastasectomy, after two or more cycles of chemotherapy. The exclusion criteria were the history of neoadjuvant chemotherapy in initially resectable disease and surgery with palliative intent, i.e., bleeding control. The choice of palliative chemotherapy was based on physicians' preference. Twenty-six patients were finally included in the conversion surgery group (Figure 2).

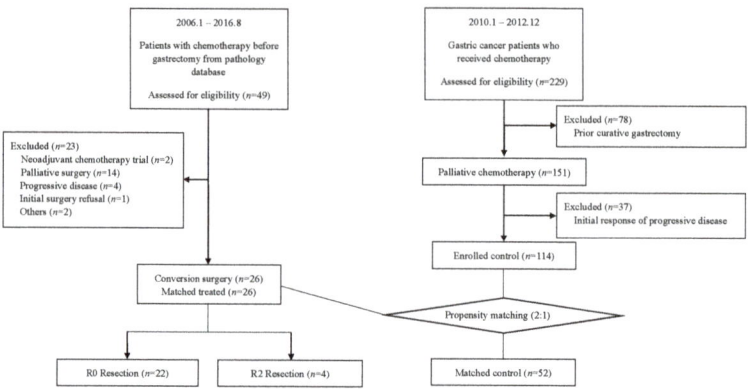

Figure 2. Consort diagram of the study.

4.2. Control Patients for Propensity Score Analysis

As for the control group in the propensity score analysis, 229 patients who received palliative first-line chemotherapy, from January 2010 to December 2012 at SNUBH, were initially screened. Of these, 78 patients who showed a metastatic recurrence after previous curative gastrectomy were excluded. Thirty-seven patients with the disease progression at first response evaluation as a result of primary resistance to palliative chemotherapy were also excluded (Figure 2). After excluding these 115 ineligible patients, 114 patients were considered as the potential candidates for conversion surgery. To mitigate selection bias for conversion surgery and the potential confounding factors, we adjusted for the baseline characteristics of the selected patients by propensity score analysis. Propensity scores were generated with the dependent variables "initial biological disease category before palliative chemotherapy" and "best responses to chemotherapy", which were clinically relevant covariates prior to conversion surgery. Other matched variables included "age" and "sex". Patients were then 1:2 matched without replacement into conversion surgery and palliative chemotherapy only groups. Fifty-two patients were finally matched in the palliative chemotherapy only group.

4.3. Data Collection

Initial patients' disease states before palliative chemotherapy were classified according to the biological categories of classification, based on the classification of stage IV gastric cancer by Yoshida et al. [12]. In brief, patients without macroscopic peritoneal seedings were further classified into category 1 (potentially resectable metastasis, i.e., single liver metastasis, few para-aortic lymph node: 16a2, b1) and category 2 (marginally resectable metastases, i.e., liver metastatic lesion >1, liver tumor size >5 cm, liver lesion close to the hepatic vein or the portal vein, distant lung metastasis, Virchow's node metastasis, or para-aortic lymph nodes: 16a1, b2). Patients with macroscopic peritoneal seeding were classified into category 3 (incurable, no involvement of contiguous organs), and category 4 (incurable metastases, invasion into other organs). CT scans were conducted to measure the extent of the disease and evaluate the response after chemotherapy. Tumor responses were divided into CR, PR, SD, NE, and progressive disease (PD), according to the Response Evaluation Criteria in Solid Tumors version 1.1. All patients and tumor information were retrieved from the electronic medical record.

4.4. Expression of Cancer Dormancy Marker

TMA was used for the analysis of the expression of cancer dormancy markers, including NR2F1, NANOG, MIG6, and PERK. TMAs were generated as described below. Tissue samples from endoscopic biopsy were fixed in 10% buffered formalin for 24–48 h, and then embedded in paraffin. The representative cores (2 mm in diameter) were isolated from the individual paraffin blocks and arranged in new tissue array blocks using a trephine apparatus (Superbiochips Laboratories, Seoul, Korea). Included cases had tumors occupying more than 10% of the core area. The TMA blocks contained up to 60 cores. The 4 μm sections from TMA blocks were stained with the following primary antibodies—rabbit monoclonal anti-NR2F1 (Abcam, Cambridge, MA, USA); rabbit monoclonal anti-NANOG (Abcam, Cambridge, MA, USA); rabbit polyclonal anti-MIG6 (Sigma-Aldrich, St. Louis, MO, USA); and rabbit monoclonal anti-PERK (Cell Signaling Technology, Danvers, MA, USA). Immunostaining was performed using the BenchMark XT platform (Ventana Medical Systems, Tucson, AZ, USA) according to the manufacturer's instructions. The intensity of expression was interpreted as 0, 1+, 2+, and 3+. Intensity of 2+ or 3+ in at least 10% tumor cells was defined as positive expression; that of 0 or 1+ was defined as negative expression (Figure 3).

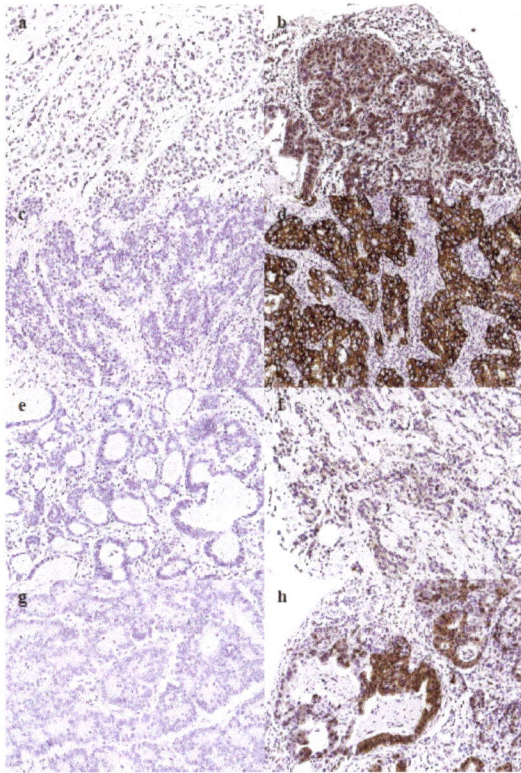

Figure 3. Tissue microarray (TMA) core of the cancer dormancy markers. (**a**) Negative expression of the NR2F1. (**b**) Positive expression of the NR2F1. (**c**) Negative expression of the NANOG. (**d**) Positive expression of the NANOG. (**e**) Negative expression of the MIG6. (**f**) Positive expression of the MIG6. (**g**) Negative expression of the PERK. (**h**) Positive expression of the PERK.

4.5. Statistical Analysis

Patient characteristics were compared in the matched cohorts via chi-square tests. Survival curves were compared using the Kaplan–Meier method by log-rank test. DFS was calculated from the time of conversion surgery to the first evidence of recurrence or death from any cause. We defined PFS as the time elapsed between the initiation of first-line palliative chemotherapy and disease progression or death from any cause. OS was measured from the initiation of first-line palliative chemotherapy to death from any cause or follow-up loss. A two-sided p-value of less than 0.05 was considered statistically significant. All statistical analyses were performed using the R software version 3.5.0.

This study was conducted in accordance with the ethical standards of the Declaration of Helsinki and the national and international guidelines. This study was approved by the institutional review board at SNUBH (B-1708/417-306 and B-1402/240-004).

5. Conclusions

In conclusion, patients with initially metastatic gastric cancer might benefit from conversion surgery and reach durable survival if the R0 resection can be achieved after chemotherapy. Although further studies are warranted for validation, the expression of cancer dormancy markers, i.e., NR2F1, might be predictive in achieving better postoperative survival outcome in patients undergoing conversion surgery.

Supplementary Materials: The following are available online at http://www.mdpi.com/2072-6694/12/1/86/s1, Figure S1: DFS from conversion surgery with R0 resection according to cancer dormancy marker expression, Table S1: The characteristics and clinical course of patients who received noncurative resection with conversion surgery.

Author Contributions: Conceptualization, J.W.K. and H.S.L.; Data curation, H.J.C. and S.-H.H.; Formal analysis, H.J.C., J.W.K. and J.H.L.; Methodology, H.J.C., J.W.K. and J.H.L.; Project administration, J.W.K.; Resources, J.W.K., S.-H.H., S.-H.A., D.J.P., J.-W.K., Y.J.K., H.S.L., J.H.K., H.-H.K. and K.-W.L.; Writing—original draft, H.J.C. and J.W.K.; Writing—review & editing, H.J.C., J.W.K., S.-H.H., J.H.L., S.-H.A., D.J.P., J.-W.K., Y.J.K., H.S.L., J.H.K., H.-H.K. and K.-W.L. All authors have read and agreed to the published version of the manuscript.

Funding: There was no funding received for this study.

Acknowledgments: The authors thank the Division of Statistics in Medical Research Collaborating Center at Seoul National University Bundang Hospital for assistance in statistical analyses.

Conflicts of Interest: There is no conflict of interest to disclose.

References

1. Jung, K.W.; Won, Y.J.; Kong, H.J.; Lee, E.S. Prediction of Cancer Incidence and Mortality in Korea, 2019. *Cancer Res. Treat.* **2019**, *51*, 431–437. [CrossRef] [PubMed]
2. Bray, F.; Ferlay, J.; Soerjomataram, I.; Siegel, R.L.; Torre, L.A.; Jemal, A. Global cancer statistics 2018: GLOBOCAN estimates of incidence and mortality worldwide for 36 cancers in 185 countries. *CA* **2018**, *68*, 394–424. [CrossRef] [PubMed]
3. Guideline Committee of the Korean Gastric Cancer Association (KGCA), Development Working Group & Review Panel. Korean Practice Guideline for Gastric Cancer 2018: An Evidence-based, Multi-disciplinary Approach. *J. Gastric Cancer* **2019**, *19*, 1–48. [CrossRef] [PubMed]
4. Fujitani, K.; Yang, H.K.; Mizusawa, J.; Kim, Y.W.; Terashima, M.; Han, S.U.; Iwasaki, Y.; Hyung, W.J.; Takagane, A.; Park, D.J.; et al. Gastrectomy plus chemotherapy versus chemotherapy alone for advanced gastric cancer with a single non-curable factor (REGATTA): A phase 3, randomised controlled trial. *Lancet Oncol.* **2016**, *17*, 309–318. [CrossRef]
5. Du, R.; Hu, P.; Liu, Q.; Zhang, J. Conversion Surgery for Unresectable Advanced Gastric Cancer: A Systematic Review and Meta-Analysis. *Cancer Investig.* **2019**, *37*, 16–28. [CrossRef]
6. Einama, T.; Abe, H.; Shichi, S.; Matsui, H.; Kanazawa, R.; Shibuya, K.; Suzuki, T.; Matsuzawa, F.; Hashimoto, T.; Kohei, N.; et al. Long-term survival and prognosis associated with conversion surgery in patients with metastatic gastric cancer. *Mol. Clin. Oncol.* **2017**, *6*, 163–166. [CrossRef]

7. Fukuchi, M.; Mochiki, E.; Ishiguro, T.; Kumagai, Y.; Ishibashi, K.; Ishida, H. Prognostic Significance of Conversion Surgery Following First- or Second-line Chemotherapy for Unresectable Gastric Cancer. *Anticancer Res.* **2018**, *38*, 6473–6478. [CrossRef]
8. Fukuchi, M.; Mochiki, E.; Ishiguro, T.; Ogura, T.; Sobajima, J.; Kumagai, Y.; Ishibashi, K.; Ishida, H. Efficacy of Conversion Surgery Following S-1 plus Cisplatin or Oxaliplatin Chemotherapy for Unresectable Gastric Cancer. *Anticancer Res.* **2017**, *37*, 1343–1347.
9. Kim, K.H.; Lee, K.W.; Baek, S.K.; Chang, H.J.; Kim, Y.J.; Park, D.J.; Kim, J.H.; Kim, H.H.; Lee, J.S. Survival benefit of gastrectomy ± metastasectomy in patients with metastatic gastric cancer receiving chemotherapy. *Gastric Cancer* **2011**, *14*, 130–138. [CrossRef]
10. Mieno, H.; Yamashita, K.; Hosoda, K.; Moriya, H.; Higuchi, K.; Azuma, M.; Komori, S.; Yoshida, T.; Tanabe, S.; Koizumi, W.; et al. Conversion surgery after combination chemotherapy of docetaxel, cisplatin and S-1 (DCS) for far-advanced gastric cancer. *Surg. Today* **2017**, *47*, 1249–1258. [CrossRef]
11. Morgagni, P.; Solaini, L.; Framarini, M.; Vittimberga, G.; Gardini, A.; Tringali, D.; Valgiusti, M.; Monti, M.; Ercolani, G. Conversion surgery for gastric cancer: A cohort study from a western center. *Int. J. Surg.* **2018**, *53*, 360–365. [CrossRef] [PubMed]
12. Yoshida, K.; Yamaguchi, K.; Okumura, N.; Tanahashi, T.; Kodera, Y. Is conversion therapy possible in stage IV gastric cancer: The proposal of new biological categories of classification. *Gastric Cancer* **2016**, *19*, 329–338. [CrossRef] [PubMed]
13. Paez, D.; Labonte, M.J.; Bohanes, P.; Zhang, W.; Benhanim, L.; Ning, Y.; Wakatsuki, T.; Loupakis, F.; Lenz, H.J. Cancer dormancy: A model of early dissemination and late cancer recurrence. *Clin. Cancer Res.* **2012**, *18*, 645–653. [CrossRef]
14. Katayama, H.; Kurokawa, Y.; Nakamura, K.; Ito, H.; Kanemitsu, Y.; Masuda, N.; Tsubosa, Y.; Satoh, T.; Yokomizo, A.; Fukuda, H.; et al. Extended Clavien-Dindo classification of surgical complications: Japan Clinical Oncology Group postoperative complications criteria. *Surg. Today* **2016**, *46*, 668–685. [CrossRef]
15. Cook, J.A. The challenges faced in the design, conduct and analysis of surgical randomised controlled trials. *Trials* **2009**, *10*, 9. [CrossRef] [PubMed]
16. Kim, S.W. The result of conversion surgery in gastric cancer patients with peritoneal seeding. *J. Gastric Cancer* **2014**, *14*, 266–270. [CrossRef]
17. Fukuchi, M.; Ishiguro, T.; Ogata, K.; Kimura, A.; Kumagai, Y.; Ishibashi, K.; Ishida, H.; Kuwano, H.; Mochiki, E. Risk Factors for Recurrence After Curative Conversion Surgery for Unresectable Gastric Cancer. *Anticancer Res.* **2015**, *35*, 6183–6187.
18. Fukuchi, M.; Ishiguro, T.; Ogata, K.; Suzuki, O.; Kumagai, Y.; Ishibashi, K.; Ishida, H.; Kuwano, H.; Mochiki, E. Prognostic Role of Conversion Surgery for Unresectable Gastric Cancer. *Ann. Surg. Oncol.* **2015**, *22*, 3618–3624. [CrossRef]
19. Nakamura, M.; Ojima, T.; Nakamori, M.; Katsuda, M.; Tsuji, T.; Hayata, K.; Kato, T.; Yamaue, H. Conversion Surgery for Gastric Cancer with Peritoneal Metastasis Based on the Diagnosis of Second-Look Staging Laparoscopy. *J. Gastrointest. Surg.* **2019**, *23*, 1758–1766. [CrossRef]
20. Beom, S.H.; Choi, Y.Y.; Baek, S.E.; Li, S.X.; Lim, J.S.; Son, T.; Kim, H.I.; Cheong, J.H.; Hyung, W.J.; Choi, S.H.; et al. Multidisciplinary treatment for patients with stage IV gastric cancer: The role of conversion surgery following chemotherapy. *BMC Cancer* **2018**, *18*, 1116. [CrossRef]
21. Yuan, S.Q.; Nie, R.C.; Chen, S.; Chen, X.J.; Chen, Y.M.; Xu, L.P.; Yang, L.F.; Zhou, Z.W.; Peng, J.S.; Chen, Y.B. Selective Gastric Cancer Patients with Peritoneal Seeding Benefit from Gastrectomy after Palliative Chemotherapy: A Propensity Score Matching Analysis. *J. Cancer* **2017**, *8*, 2231–2237. [CrossRef] [PubMed]
22. Zurleni, T.; Gjoni, E.; Altomare, M.; Rausei, S. Conversion surgery for gastric cancer patients: A review. *World J. Gastrointest. Oncol.* **2018**, *10*, 398–409. [CrossRef] [PubMed]
23. Cunningham, D.; Allum, W.H.; Stenning, S.P.; Thompson, J.N.; Van de Velde, C.J.; Nicolson, M.; Scarffe, J.H.; Lofts, F.J.; Falk, S.J.; Iveson, T.J.; et al. Perioperative chemotherapy versus surgery alone for resectable gastroesophageal cancer. *N. Engl. J. Med.* **2006**, *355*, 11–20. [CrossRef] [PubMed]
24. Thompson, V.C.; Day, T.K.; Bianco-Miotto, T.; Selth, L.A.; Han, G.; Thomas, M.; Buchanan, G.; Scher, H.I.; Nelson, C.C.; Greenberg, N.M.; et al. A gene signature identified using a mouse model of androgen receptor-dependent prostate cancer predicts biochemical relapse in human disease. *Int. J. Cancer* **2012**, *131*, 662–672. [CrossRef]

25. Borgen, E.; Rypdal, M.C.; Sosa, M.S.; Renolen, A.; Schlichting, E.; Lonning, P.E.; Synnestvedt, M.; Aguirre-Ghiso, J.A.; Naume, B. NR2F1 stratifies dormant disseminated tumor cells in breast cancer patients. *Breast Cancer Res.* **2018**, *20*, 120. [CrossRef]
26. Miki, Y.; Tokunaga, M.; Tanizawa, Y.; Bando, E.; Kawamura, T.; Terashima, M. Staging Laparoscopy for Patients with cM0, Type 4, and Large Type 3 Gastric Cancer. *World J. Surg.* **2015**, *39*, 2742–2747. [CrossRef]
27. Yasufuku, I.; Nunobe, S.; Ida, S.; Kumagai, K.; Ohashi, M.; Hiki, N.; Sano, T. Conversion therapy for peritoneal lavage cytology-positive type 4 and large type 3 gastric cancer patients selected as candidates for R0 resection by diagnostic staging laparoscopy. *Gastric Cancer* **2019**. Epub ahead of print. [CrossRef]

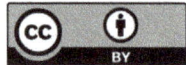

© 2019 by the authors. Licensee MDPI, Basel, Switzerland. This article is an open access article distributed under the terms and conditions of the Creative Commons Attribution (CC BY) license (http://creativecommons.org/licenses/by/4.0/).

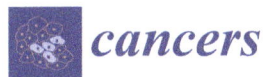

Review

From Interconnection between Genes and Microenvironment to Novel Immunotherapeutic Approaches in Upper Gastro-Intestinal Cancers—A Multidisciplinary Perspective

Giulia Accordino [1], Sara Lettieri [1], Chandra Bortolotto [2], Silvia Benvenuti [3], Anna Gallotti [2], Elisabetta Gattoni [4], Francesco Agustoni [5], Emma Pozzi [5], Pietro Rinaldi [6], Cristiano Primiceri [6], Patrizia Morbini [7], Andrea Lancia [8] and Giulia Maria Stella [1,*]

1. Department of Medical Sciences and Infective Diseases, Unit of Respiratory Diseases, Istituto di Ricovero e Cura a Carattere Scientifico (IRCCS) Policlinico San Matteo Foundation and University of Pavia Medical School, 27000 Pavia, Italy; accordino@gmail.com (G.A.); sara.lettieri01@universitadipavia.it (S.L.)
2. Department of Intensive Medicine, Unit of Radiology, IRCCS Policlinico San Matteo Foundation and University of Pavia Medical School, 27000 Pavia, Italy; c.bortolotto@smatteo.pv.it (C.B.); a.gallotti@smatteo.pv.it (A.G.)
3. Candiolo Cancer Institute, Fondazione del Piemonte per l'Oncologia (FPO)-IRCCS-Str. Prov.le 142, km. 3,95, 10060 Candiolo (TO), Italy; silvia.benvenuti@ircc.it
4. Department of Oncology, Azienda Sanitaria Locale (ASL) AL, 27000 Casale Monferrato (AL), Italy; bettygattoni@gmail.com
5. Department of Medical Sciences and Infective Diseases, Unit of Oncology, IRCCS Policlinico San Matteo Foundation and University of Pavia Medical School, 27000 Pavia, Italy; f.agustoni@smatteo.pv.it (F.A.); e.pozzi@smatteo.pv.it (E.P.)
6. Department of Intensive Medicine, Unit of Thoracic Surgery, IRCCS Policlinico San Matteo Foundation and University of Pavia Medical School, 27000 Pavia, Italy; p.rinaldi@smatteo.pv.it (P.R.); c.primiceri@smatteo.pv.it (C.P.)
7. Department of Diagnostic Medicine, Unit of Pathology, IRCCS Policlinico San Matteo Foundation and University of Pavia Medical School, 27000 Pavia, Italy; p.morbini@smatteo.pv.it
8. Department of Medical Sciences and Infective Diseases, Unit of Radiation Therapy, IRCCS Policlinico San Matteo Foundation and University of Pavia Medical School, 27000 Pavia, Italy; a.lancia@smatteo.pv.it
* Correspondence: g.stella@smatteo.pv.it; Tel.: +39-0382503369; Fax: +39-0382502719

Received: 7 July 2020; Accepted: 25 July 2020; Published: 29 July 2020

Abstract: Despite the progress during the last decade, patients with advanced gastric and esophageal cancers still have poor prognosis. Finding optimal therapeutic strategies represents an unmet need in this field. Several prognostic and predictive factors have been evaluated and may guide clinicians in choosing a tailored treatment. Data from large studies investigating the role of immunotherapy in gastrointestinal cancers are promising but further investigations are necessary to better select those patients who can mostly benefit from these novel therapies. This review will focus on the treatment of metastatic esophageal and gastric cancer. We will review the standard of care and the role of novel therapies such as immunotherapies and CAR-T. Moreover, we will focus on the analysis of potential predictive biomarkers such as Modify as: Microsatellite Instability (MSI) and PD-L1, which may lead to treatment personalization and improved treatment outcomes. A multidisciplinary point of view is mandatory to generate an integrated approach to properly exploit these novel antiproliferative agents.

Keywords: immunotherapy; genetics; gastric cancer; esophageal cancer; multidisciplinary

1. Introduction

The definition of upper gastrointestinal (GI) cancers essentially refers to gastric and esophageal tumors. The latter, including both squamous cell carcinoma and adenocarcinoma histologies represents the nineth cause of cancer death worldwide and nearly 40% of patients present with metastatic disease at diagnosis [1–3]. The median 5-year survival rate is 47% in case of early stage diseases whereas it decreases to 25% in locally advanced and to 5% for metastatic disease, respectively. Gastric cancer (GC) remains one of the most common and deadly cancers worldwide. Over one million cases of GCs are diagnosed every year around the world. It is the 5th most diagnosed cancer in the world [4]. The epidemiology of stomach cancer harbors substantial geographical heterogeneity and the 5-year survival rate is around 20%, with peaks of about 65% in Japan and 71.5% in South Korea, due high number of diagnosis in early stage disease revealed by massive population screening programs [5]. The geographic variations are mainly related to differences in environmental factors such as dietary patterns and salt intake, the prevalence of *Helicobacter pylorii* (H.P) infection and the virulence of strains, as well as host factors [6]. Overall patients affected by resectable cancer can undergo surgery and perioperative therapy with potentially curative purposes. However, most of GC diagnoses are performed in stage III or IV disease and patients are candidates only to palliative chemotherapy. In metastatic diseases, 5-year survival rate is poor with a median overall survival (OS) lower than 12 months [7]. Genomic and proteomic expression profiles of oncogenic signaling pathways unveiled different molecular subtypes of gastric and gastro-esophageal cancers, characterized by specifically targetable markers [8–10]. The most relevant example regards the HER2 inhibitor trastuzumab, a monoclonal antibody that binds to the extracellular domain of the receptor, which is now approved in United States and Europe as the first-line treatment in combination with conventional chemotherapy for HER2-overexpressing locally advanced or metastatic GCs (about 20% of cases [11]) leading to increased overall response rates and survivals [12]. Nevertheless, the introduction of targeted molecules does not result in increased outcome rates and most phase III clinical trials evaluating molecularly designed agents in GC have failed [13]. In this complex landscape, growing evidence supports the routine use of immunotherapy with checkpoint inhibitors in the treatment of upper GI cancers, although their effective role is, still, poorly understood. The main reason is due to the lack of knowledge on how the genetic asset cooperates with the surrounding stroma giving rise to the highly malignant phenotype which defines these tumors. Here we summarize the already available data on the use of checkpoint inhibitors and discuss more recent findings regarding the use of modern immunotherapy, including adoptive cell therapy and vaccines, alone or in combination with conventional drugs. A deep understating of the complex interaction between tumor microenvironment and genetic heterogeneity in this group of tumors, fully requires a multidisciplinary approach that will allow effective and significant clinical results.

2. How to Diagnose and Stage Upper GI Cancers

Primary esophageal cancer (EC) constitutes the majority (more than 95%) of all esophageal malignancies. The two main pathologic subtypes of esophageal cancer are squamous cell (ESCC) carcinoma and adenocarcinoma (EAC). The latter can mimic metastases or direct extension from tumors of lung or breast. Adenocarcinomas (AC) represent more than 90% of gastric cancers; considering tumor localization they are subdivided into true gastric AC and GEJ-AC. Growing evidence documents a shift in the anatomical distribution of gastric cancer, which increasingly originates from the proximal stomach near the junction with the esophagus and in parallel an increase of EAC affecting the lower esophagus [14]. Thus, a significant uncertainty might regard the identification of the primary organ site of adenocarcinomatous transformation. Immunohistochemistry (IHC) is helpful in defining pathologic entities in case of undifferentiated cancers from the upper GI tract [15,16]. The most common secondary malignant lesions are associated to localization of lymphoma and sarcoma; metastatic masses arousing in the esophagus are rare [17]. Table 1 summarizes the main morphological and IHC features of primary upper GI cancers. In the case of esophageal adenocarcinoma lesion, differential diagnosis to establish the putative primary origin takes into consideration the lung, in which cells frequently express the thyroid transcription factor 1 (TTF-1), and breast adenocarcinomas, which are generally positive for estrogen receptor (ER), mammaglobin, gross cystic fluid protein and GATA3. On the other hand, ESCCs carry some of the same features of small cells carcinomas which develop in other organs, particularly in the lung and which differentially express common neuroendocrine markers, namely synaptophysin, chromogranin A and CD56/NCAM. Notably, the TTF-1 expression can be found in a proportion of ESCCs as well; thus it cannot specifically indicate the lung only as site of primary tumor growth.

Table 1. A summary of the morphologic and immunohistochemical profiles of upper GI tumors [18–20]. The most common morphologic and immunohistochemical (IHC) traits distinctive of main neoplastic lesions affecting the upper GI tract.

Tumor Type	IHC Markers			Gross Features	
	+	−	+/−	Macroscopic Appearance	Imaging
ESCC	CK5, CK6, CK10, CK14, p40	CK7, CK20	p53, p16 in cases associated to HPV infection	Early cancer - Plaque-like lesions: Small, sessile polyps or depressed lesions Advanced cancer - Luminal constriction (stricture) with nodular or ulcerated mucosa -Polypoid, ulcerative, varicoid, irregular constricting forms	Double-contrast esophagography: best for detection of early cancer CT: Useful for staging. Mediastinal and abdominal lymphadenopathy and metastases PET/CT: superior to CT in detecting regional and distant metastases Endoscopic ultrasonography (EUS): best technique for determining locoregional extent of tumor
EAC	CK7, CK8, AMACR, weak focal CDX-2	p40, p16, ER, GATA 3, TTF-1	CK20		
Esophageal small cell carcinoma	Chromogranin A, NSE, Synaptophysin, CD56, CK8		p40	TTF-1	
Gastric adenocarcinoma	CK8, CK7	TTF1, p40, ER, p16, MUC1, E-cadherin (Poorly cohesive)	CK20, CDX-2, MUC1, MUC2, MUC5AC	Polypoid or circumferential mass with no peristalsis through lesion (at fluoroscopy)	Best imaging tool: Double-contrast barium study, CT, EUS

SCC = squamous cell cancer ER = estrogen receptor TTF-1 = thyroid transcriptional factor-1 NSE = neuron specific enolase.

Comprehensive description of epidemiologic, clinic and pathologic features of upper GI cancers goes beyond the scope of this work and is already available in many published review papers. All the data summarized in Table 2. Once diagnosis of esophageal/gastric cancer is accurately confirmed, disease pathologic classification and staging are required to address patients to the better therapeutic approach. Siewert classification is a widely used anatomic classification of adenocarcinoma of GEJ and it is based on tumor location with respect to the gastric cardia. Three types are described: Siewert type I tumors are adenocarcinomas of distal esophagus, Siewert type II tumors are adenocarcinomas of gastric cardias and Siewert type III tumors correspond to sub-cardial adenocarcinomas of proximal stomach infiltrating the GEJ. The most recent WHO histopathological classification (WHO Classification of tumors: Digestive system tumors 2019) modified the conventional Lauren's criteria distinguishing gastric cancer into diffuse and intestinal types: diffuse type was reclassified as "poorly cohesive, including signet ring histotype," while intestinal type was split into architectural types papillary and tubular [21,22]. Previous gastrectomy is a known risk factor for the onset of gastric cancer. The so-called Gastric Stump Cancer (GSC), which occurs in the gastric remnant at least 5 years after the surgery for peptic ulcer, identifies a separate subtype of GC (1.1/7% of diagnosis) which mainly affects men [23–25]. The TNM classification represents the most used staging system for upper GI tumors. Details regarding upper GI staging and classification are available as Supplementary Material as Table S1–S7 [26–30].

Table 2. Clinical, anatomic, pathologic and imaging characteristics of upper GI cancers. Main clinically relevant features of esophageal and gastric cancers derived from already available literature data [31–46].

Features	Esophageal Cancer		Gastric Cancer
	Squamous Cell Cancer	Adenocarcinoma	Adenocarcinoma
Geographic distribution	Eastern Asia	United States and certain European countries	East Asia, Eastern Europe, Central, South America
Smoking history	✔	✔	✔
Other associated conditions		- Obesity - Gastroesophageal reflux disease (GERD)	- Obesity - Socioeconomic position (minors, fishermen, machine operators, nurses, cooks, launderers, dry cleaners) - Gastrectomy
Dietary factors	Low apport of fruits and vegetables leading to low antioxidant levels and vitamin deficiencies	- Red meat and processed food items - Protective role of raw fruits and vegetables and dark-green, leafy and cruciferous vegetables, carbohydrates, fiber, iron	- Alcohol - Protective role of fresh fruits and dark green, light green and yellow vegetables rich in B carotene, vitamin C, E and foliate
Histology and Anatomic localization	Squamous lining of middle esophagus	- Glandular differentiation featuring tubular, tubulo-papillary or papillary pattern of growth. - Distal part of esophagus	- Diffuse type: poorly cohesive, including signet ring histotype - Intestinal type: - papillary - tubular - Proximal stomach near the junction - Distal stomach (intestinal type)
Endoscopic features	Polypoid masses, flat or ulcerated	- Mucosal irregularities, which might be associated to ulcerated or infiltrative lesions - Exophytic masses which can obstruct the lumen	Early GC (EGC): - elevated - superficial ➢ superficial elevated, ➢ superficial flat ➢ superficial depressed - depressed. The most common lesions of EGC were usually manifested by erythema and erosion.
Oncogenic viruses	*Human Papilloma Virus* (HPV): role not well established	*Helicobacter pylorii* (HP) infection is inversely correlated	- *Helicobacter pylorii* (HP) - Epstein-Barr virus (EBV) associated to GSC
Chronic inflammation	Achalasia		
Premalignant lesions	Squamous dysplasia	Barrett's esophagus (BE)	- HP-related chronic atrophic gastritis - Intestinal metaplasia and dysplasia - Early GC (10% of diagnosis)
Variants and differentiations	- Basaloid squamous cell carcinoma - Verrucous carcinomas - Spindle cell carcinoma (or carcinosarcoma)	- Mucinous - Signet ring cell	- Mucinous - Mixed

3. Main Mutational Patterns and Regulatory Networks

3.1. Oesophageal Cancer

The genomic landscape of ESCC and EAC have been extensively studied through next generation sequencing (NGS) and computational approaches, even though the understanding of the complex network of its driver genes is far to be fully understood. ESCC and EAC display distinct sets of driver genes, mutational signatures and prognostic biomarkers.

Esophageal squamous cell carcinomas resemble squamous carcinomas of other organs more than they did esophageal adenocarcinomas. The work conducted by Cancer Genome Atlas Research Network revealed that ESCC showed frequent genomic amplifications of *CCND1* and *SOX2* and/or *TP63* genes, whereas *ERBB2*, *VEGFA* and *GATA4* and *GATA6* were more commonly amplified in adenocarcinomas [47]. Inactivation of the tumor suppressor *NOTCH1* gene has been reported in ESCC but not in EAC [48]. Interestingly inactivating mutations clustered in defined geographic areas, being more frequent in those ECSSs which affect North American patients than in those aroused in Chinese population. Moreover, germline mutations in the RHBDF2 gene (17q25) which cause tylosis (focal non-epidermolytic palmoplantar keratoderma) have been reported to be markers of genetic familial susceptibility for the early onset of ESSC [49–51].

On the other hand, EAC derives from progressive accumulation of multiple genetic abnormalities and aneuploidy. Comparative analysis show that most mutations found in EAC could be already detected in the matched BE which, - at least under genetic profile - identifies an early phase of malignant transformation [52]. Mutations in the *PIK3CA* oncogene and in the *CTNNB1* gene that encodes for β-catenin are known to occur in BE and changes in several tumor suppressor genes involved in chromatin remodeling, such as *ARID1A* and *SMARCA4* as well as in *TP53* and *SMAD4* are usually found in tissues with high-grade dysplasia and EAC. Oncogene amplification is typically a late event in EAC progression. Coherently, genomes of BE tissues are relatively stable compared to those of invasive tumors, in which almost 40% of the genome is non-diploid. The only common copy number alteration found in BE is 9p loss of heterozygosity (*CDKN2A*) [53,54]. Advanced tumors have an increased copy numbers of several oncogenes (*GATA4, KLF5, MYB, PRKCI, CCND1, FGF3, FGF4, FGF19* and *VEGFA*) and loss of common fragile sites (*FHIT, WWOX, PDE4D, PTPRD* and *PARK2*) [55,56]. In conclusion, EACs emerge rather than from the gradual accumulation of tumor-suppressor alterations, from a straighter pathway driven by mutations in *TP-53* gene and subsequent acquisition of oncogene amplifications [57]. In this perspective, EACs strongly resemble the chromosomally unstable variant of gastric adenocarcinoma, suggesting that these cancers could be considered as a single disease entity. However, some molecular features, including DNA hypermethylation, occur disproportionally in esophageal adenocarcinomas. Epigenetic modifications are known to contribute significantly to the pathogenesis of the disease and specific methylation signatures are known to be associated to tumor progression processes and thus emerge as novel actionable markers. Among them, the methylation classifier which encompasses the *TRIM15, TACC3, SHANK2, MCC* and *CDKN2A* gene silencing is differentially reported in the progression from BE to transformed areas and not in normal mucosa [58].

3.2. Gastric Cancer

Genetic Features

Gastric cancer is characterized by an extreme molecular heterogeneity, which is defined by the occurrence of multiple genetic and epigenetic alteration in each disease stage. It should be underlined that 3–15% of all diagnosis refer to familial and hereditary gastric cancers, among which hereditary diffuse gastric cancer (HDGC), gastric adenocarcinoma and proximal polyposis of the stomach (GAPPS) and familial intestinal gastric cancer (FIGC). One third of HDGC is attributed to hereditary *CDH1* mutations [59–61]. Other hereditary syndromes, such as Lynch syndrome, familial adenomatous polyposis (FAP), Li-Fraumeni, Muir-Torre and Peutz-Jeghers syndromes can occur with gastric involvement as well [62–64]. In case of genetic diagnosis, prophylactic gastrectomy might be suggested [65,66]. Within respect to the non-hereditary forms of GC, recent molecular profiling studies have allowed the shift from the conventional histological classification systems to four molecularly-based classification groups: (i) EBV-positive cancers (9–10% of gastric AC) harboring high frequency of *PI3KCA* gene changes (80%), high levels of DNA hypermethylation, mutations in *PTEN, SMADA, CDKN2A, ARIDA* (55%) and *BCOR* (23%) and increased copies of *JAK2, ERBB2, PD-L1* and *PD-1* genes, (ii) microsatellite unstable (MSI) tumors, accounting for 22% of diagnosis, which mainly arise in women and older patients and frequently carry hypermethylation MLH1 promoter in association with recurrent mutations in the *PIK3CA, ERBB3, ERBB2* and *EGFR* genes [67–69], (iii) genomically stable (GS) tumors (20% of cases, mainly diffuse-type AC) which mostly affect younger subjects and are enriched with recurrent *CDH1* (37%), *RHOA* (15%) and inactivating *ARID1A* gene changes. Fusions involving the RHO-family GTPase-activating proteins CLDN18 and ARHGAP26, have been reported as well [70]; (iv) chromosomal unstable (CIN) subtypes [71] which account for 50% of GCs and harbor extensive aneuploidy, *TP53* mutations (71%) and increased copy number of several genes encoding for receptor tyrosine kinases and their downstream effectors as *EGFR, ERBB2, ERBB3, VEGFA, FGFR2, MET, NRAS/KRAS, JAK2, CD274, PDCD1LG2* and *PIK3CA* [72]. Overall tyrosine kinase receptors (TKR) are among the most frequently altered oncogenes in GC and identify actionable therapeutic targets. A recent genomic study of gastric cancers identified somatic copy number alterations of seven oncogenes involved in tyrosine kinase/MAP-kinase pathways: *KRAS, EGFR, HER2, FGFR1, FGFR2, MET* and *IGF1R* [73].

3.3. Targeted-Based Therapeutic Strategies

Although a deep analysis of genetic basis of targeted therapy in GCs falls beyond the scope of this review, some relevant issues are discussed due not only to their clinically relevant role but mainly to their interaction with microenvironment and immune response. A first example regards the blockade of HER2 signaling which has significantly improved the outlook for esophagogastric cancer patients and has allowed the approval of trastuzumab in HER2-positive metastatic gastric/gastroesophageal junction cancers, as first line approach in combination with cisplatin and a fluoropyrimidine (capecitabine or 5-fluorouracil) [12,74]. HER2 is activated most frequently by increased gene copy number, whereas somatic mutations rarely occur [75]. *HER2* gene amplification in GC is associated with higher invasive and proliferative tumor cell capacity [76]. HER2-overexpression is associated with male gender, intestinal type and well/moderate cell differentiation [77]. Anti EGFR antibodies, cetuximab and panitumumab, combined with chemotherapy did not show benefit in overall survival in first line treatment in metastatic gastric patients, as reported in two phase III trials, EXPANDED and REAL 3 [78,79]. The angiogenesis is another target in the therapeutic strategy against some solid tumors like breast, colon and lung cancer and in some instances; it resulted as good target of therapy. In upper GI cancer Bevacizumab with chemotherapy obtained in one phase III trial better overall response rate but failed to gain benefit in overall survival (OS), the primary endpoint of that study [80]. Ramucirumab also, another antiangiogenic drug, combined with chemotherapy compared with chemotherapy alone in phase III trial in metastatic GC patient chemotherapy naive, showed better progression free survival (PFS) (5.7 vs. 5.4 months) in absence of significant OS improvement [81]. In metastatic patients progressed after platinum-based chemotherapy, ramucirumab plus paclitaxel gained benefit in OS, as reported in RAINBOW, phase III trial [82]. Also used as single agent, in a phase III double blind study, in metastatic patient progressed after standard first line chemotherapy, ramucirumab obtained benefit in OS and good tolerability (REGARD STUDY) [83]. Inappropriate activation of MET signaling occurs in a several cancer types, including gastric cancer and promotes tumor cell growth, survival, migration and invasion, namely the Invasive growth genetic program which is involved tumor spreading and metastatic growth [84,85]. Amplification/overexpression of the HGF-receptor MET rather than mutated gene can activate receptor tyrosine kinase [86,87]. MET overexpression/amplification is more common in intestinal-type GC and reported in diffuse GC [88]. Notably, a cross talk between amplified MET and EGFR, HER2 and HER3 has been described and can establish a signaling network, allowing constitutive PI3K/AKT cascade activation [89]. This observation suggests robust rationale for combinatorial therapeutic approaches against MET and EGF receptor family, at least in metastatic GCs [90,91]. DNA repair *BRCA1/2* genes mutations are implicated in defective DNA repair processes and are known to be associated to the susceptibility towards hereditary breast and ovarian cancers and can occur in other sporadic cancers, among which gastric cancers. *BRCA1/2* mutations are found in 15% of GCs and are associated with poor patient survival [92]. Overall, *BRCAness*—the phenotypic condition that characterizes some cancers with carry defective caretaker gene functions—is associated to high sensitivity to the antitumor agents which cause double strand breaks of DNA, such as platinum [93]. However this condition suggests that GCs might benefit from either platinum therapy or poly (ADP-ribose) polymerase (PARP) inhibitors, a family of nuclear proteins with enzymatic, scaffolding properties and recruiting ability for DNA repair proteins and have been already tested in gastric cancer. However, the first results with PARP inhibitors did not provide encouraging results in metastatic gastric cancer according to a phase 3 study (GOLD), in which olaparib was used in combination with paclitaxel, since the study did not meet its first endpoint—defined by increase in overall survival—there being some advantage in those cases featuring low expression of ATM telangiectasia mutated) protein measured by IHC [94]. These results confirm that even in a biomarker-enriched population, GC results in a variety and unpredictable pattern of responses in absence of frankly evident drivers.

3.4. miRNAs as Actionable Biomarkers

Strong evidence suggests that alteration in micro-RNA (miRNA) expression acts as important hallmark of cancer [95–97]. Expression profiles of miRNAs can distinguish esophageal tumor histology and can discriminate between normal tissue and the transformed one. Moreover microRNA expression might identify patients with BE at high risk for progression to adenocarcinoma [98–100]. MiRNA signatures have been investigated in GC for both diagnostic, prognostic purposes as well as to differentiate histologic subtypes and other gastrointestinal cancers [101–109]. Thus, miRNA signatures might act as diagnostic and prognostic in upper GI tumors, biomarkers as summarized in Table 3.

Table 3. MiRNA expression in esophageal and gastric cancers. In each case, expression has been associated with its functional (diagnostic and/or prognostic) value based on literature reports (PubMed search according to the following keywords: esophageal/gastric cancer & miRNA).

Cancer Type	Diagnosis	Prognosis
Esophageal Cancer	• Expression in transformed tissues, not in normal areas: miR-21, -34a, -205, -203, -93, -375, -494, -29c, -148, -203 • Role in tumor onset: miR-4286, -502, -374a • Expression in pre-neoplastic lesions: miR-144, -155 • Increased cancer risk: miR-196a2, -146a, -423 • Association with tumor regression: miR-192, -194	• Tumor cell proliferation and invasive phenotype: miR-26a-5p, -195, -338, -200a-3p, -196a, -486-5p, -218, -503, -374a, -183, -150-5p • Inhibition of cell proliferation and migration: miR-652, -124, -485-5p, -139-5p, -203-3p, -21-5p, -155 • ↑ Tumor progression and metastatic capacity: miR-4319, -451, -1207-5p, -143-5p, -3687, -6743-5p, 20b • ↓ Patient survival: miR-1301-3p, -431-5p, -769-5p, -451 • ↓ Metastatic potential: miR-124, -210, -491, -140 • Resistance to chemotherapy: miR-193, -141-3p, -27, -96 • Sensitivity to chemotherapy: miR-218 • Radioresistance: miR-24, -133a, -96 • Radiosensitivity: miR-124
ESCC	• Expression in transformed tissues, not in normal areas: miR-17-, -19a, -7, -1297, -196a, -613, -143, -122, -302b • Role in tumor onset: miR-373, -153-3p, -145-3p, -449a-5p, -483-5p, -455-3p, -100, -181a: • Increased cancer risk: miR-423, -196a2, -499, -219-1	• ↑ Cancer progression and metastatic capacity: miR-124, -130a-5p, -196a, -214, -23b-3p, -370, -129, -31, -548k, -612, -30b, -146a-5p, -92b, -483-3, -425, -1290, -192, -503, -195, -183 • ↓ Tumor progression: miR-33a-5p, -384, -133a-3p, -615-3p, -120-3p, -196a, -126, -30d, -199a-5p, -338-3p, -203 • Tumor cell proliferation and invasive phenotype: miRNA-141, -10b-3p, -365, -424, -1470, -214, -503, -375, -18, -101, -889, -208, -16, -518b • ↓ Tumor cell proliferation: miR-133b, -338-5p, -10a, -6775-3p, -125b, -302a, -1, -99a, -26, -100, -34a, -150, -383, -186, -1291, -106a, -129-2, ↑ survival: miR-30e, miR-124, -874-3p, -502,-335 • ↑ Cell migration and invasion: miR-548-3p, -576-5p,-25,-99b,-375,-106b, -630, -675, -373, -200b,-25, -205,-92a • ↓ Patient survival: miR-145, -191, -138, -1469, -574-3p, -625, -382, -17, -18a, -19a, -150, -486-5p: • ↓ Cell survival, migration and invasion: miR-145, -202, -92b, -328, -204, -520g, let-7g, let-7i, -218, -101, -217, -494, -508, -429 • ↑ Radiosensitivity: miR-27a, -136, -339-5p, -193b,-338-5p,-381, miR-22 • Sensitivity to chemotherapy: miR-145, -125a-5p, -214-3, -449, -218 • Resistance to chemotherapy: miR-24, -455-3p, -483, -214, -141

Table 3. Cont.

Cancer Type	Diagnosis	Prognosis
EAC	• Higher expression in EAC (vs ESCC): miR-148a, -29c • Early tumor onset: miR-92a-3p, -223, -31, -375, -192, -196a, -203a, -130,-663b, -421, -502-5p, -1915-3p, -601, -4286, -630, -575, -494, -320e,-203, -625-3p, -21, -31, -192, -194, -200a, -194 • Low expression in BE evolving to EAC: miR-153, -192, -194, -194-3p, -200a, -215, -133b, -203, -205,-143, -145, -31, -31-3p, -375, -143, -145, -215	• Tumor progression and invasive phenotype: miR-196, -145, -17, -19a/b, -20a, -106a, -330-5p, -99b, -199a-3p, -199a-5p • Tumor recurrence: miR-331-3p • Better prognoses and ↑ patient survival: miR-100-5p, -133b, -302c, -222 • ↓ Patient survival: miR-126, -125a, -15, –375(lower): • Chemoresistance: -221, -187 • Chemosensistivity: mir-330-5p, -148 • Increased expression after chemotherapy: miR-222, -549 • Radiosensitivity: miR-31: • Pathologic response (low expression): miR-505 *, -99b, -451, -145 • ↓ Patient survival: miR-375, -31, -21
Gastric Cancer	• Higher expression in cancer (vs normal tissue and gastritis): miR-19a-3p, -22-3p, -146a-5p, -483-5p, -421, -29b-1-5p, -27b-5, -10b, -21, -93, -107, 124, -20a, -22, -10b, -21, -93, -107, -106 a • High expression in health gastric mucosa (vs cancer): miR-26a, -375, -1260, -26a, -142-3p, -148a, -195, -545 • High expression in gastritis (vs cancer): miR-146a, -155 • Histologic differential expression: miR-200c, intestinal-type: miR-32, -182, -143, 520c, -229-5p; signet ring: miR-99a-5p, Lauren differentiation: 193b • Expression in pre-invasive areas: let-7i-5p, miR-146b-5p, -185-5p, 22-3p • Early cancer onset: miR-101-3p, 106a, -9 17-92, 223, -324-3p • HP-associated cancer: miR-17-3p, -17-5p/3p, -222-3p, -143-3p • Cancer susceptibility: miR-993 • Ectopic expression: miR-143, -145, -4290: significant impact on tumor growth	• ↑ Cancer progression and metastatic capacity: miR-21,-125b, -199a, -100,-34a, -146a, -335, -301a, -224-5p, -92a, -136, -106, -129, -215, 423-5p, iR-181a-5, -28, -26a, -155, -589, -142-3p, -23a, -658, -491-5p, -4284, -200, -634, -196b-5p, -135b-5p, -638, -155, -93-5p, -204, -211, -93-5p, -144,-229-5p,- 425-5p, -221,-222,-497,- 146a, -15b-5p,-182-5p,-425-5p, -1258, -551b, -491-5p,-532,-132-3p,-423-3p, -3622b-5p, -187, -1296-5p, -574-3p, -520b/e, -376c-3p, -330-3p, -187,-501-5p, -107,-125b,-221-3p, -558,-135a, -483-5p,- 224, -214, -222, -218, -224,-363, -935, -371-5p,-183,-500, -181a, -221-3p, -93-5p, -1296-5p, -663, -508-5p, -96-5p, 32-5p,-373, -153, miR-29c, -124, -135a,-148a, -892a, -20b, -451a, -130a, -398,- 192,-215, -23b-3p, -130a-5p -181a, -18a/19a, -429,-34a, -588,- 543,-885-5p, -153, - 452, -216b, -92a, -675, -223-3p, -214, -93-5p, -23a, -761,- 424-5p, -520c, -101, -425-5p, -203, -638, -15b-3p • Tumor recurrence: miR-590-3p • Suppression of malignant development: miRNA-339-5p, -129-5p, -139-5p, -489, -520f-3p, -143, -148a-5p, -539-3p, -129-3p, -197, -410,-345,-100, -2195p, -133b, -378, -204, -338, -141, -663, -449a, -376c-3p,-135a, -223, -371-5p, -214,- 630, -539, -218, -202-3p, -16, -1292-5p,- 5590-3p,-155-5p, -361-5p, -449c, -129-5p, -518, -483, -198, -1236-3p, -338-3p, -337-3p,-107,-551b, -138, -204, -29a-3p, -495, -223-5p, -148b-3p, -338, -125a-5p, -585, -148a, -491-5p, -519d-3p, -122-5p, -188-5p, -708, -122-5p, -429, -100, -630,- 203a, -143, -199a/b-3p,- 454, -204, -152, -200a, -302b, -373, -185, -3174, 582-5p, -377, -216a,-361-5p, 142-5p, 329, -197, -599, -130a-3p, 937, -454, -129, -802, -143,-145, 381, -154, -4317, 519d, -31, -124, -584-3p, -140-5p, -154, -302b-3p, -26a/b, -143, -206, -455, -379, -320a, -613, -30c-5p, -944,-30a-5p, -211, -138, -31, -218, -646, -508-5p, -133b, -455,-429, -2392, -195,- 217, -129-5p, -1228, -181,- 509-3-5P, -584-5p, -135a, 134, -101-3p, -381, -29c, 495, -15a-3p, -16-1-3p, 144-3p, 133a, -1296-5p, -647, -224, -644a, -219-5p, -494, -194, -337-3p, -494, -326, -561, -509-3p, -133b, -218, -208a-3p, -1248, -19b, -520f, -203, -18, -370, -200b, -205, -193b, -524-5p, -203, -448, -144-3p, -133a, -1296-5p, -31, -145, -2392, -143, -206, 302b-3p, -1296-5p, -429, - 577, -129-5p/3p, -330-3p, -524-5p, -3174, -139-5p, -375, -32, -485-5p, 1915-3p, -16, -198, -12129, - 876-5p, 105, -1284, -miR-155-5p, 25-3p, -503, -629, 449c, -125a-5p, 127, -331, 1224, -142-3p, 491-5p, 339-5p, 129-3p, -519d, 944, -206,- 411, -4316, -539-3p, -671-5p, -139-5p183, -503, -551b, -99b-3p, -449a, -505, -129-5p, -93-5p, -429, -132, -874, -493, -124-3p, -135a, -206, -148a, -621, -337-3p, -211, -429, -203a, -761, -19b-3p, -6852, -598, - 884-5p, -520a-3p, 140-5p, -1236-3p, -489, -100-3p, -140-5p, -4268, -618, -1297, -378, -216b, 38 • Increased cell proliferation and motility: miR-425-5p, -330-3p, -99a-5p, -216b, -638, -17, -4513, -374a, -761, -181a, -647, -217,-144, -23a/27a/24-2, -425-5p,-592,- 374b,-208a, -103a-3p, -423-5p, -340, -136, -615-3p, -28, -93, -214, -205, -23a/b, -16a-3p, -130a, -105, -744, -215, -370, - 215, -103, -196a-5p, -224, -186, -17-5p, -490-3p, -23a/27a/24-2-, 96-5p, -638, -1269, -200c, -3619, -421, -320a, -192-5p, -181a, -148a-3p, -145, let-7 • Chemoresistance: -103, -107, -508-5p, -23b-3p, -590-5p, -13147,-5-5p, 195-5p, -17, -20a, 21-5p, -125b, -200, -145, -132, -939, 129, 99a, -491-135a, -424-5p, -1284, -135b, -17-5p, -765,- 522, -106a • Chemosensitivity: miR-223, -200c, ↓-21, -16, - 494, ↓135b-5p, -21-5p, -939, -623, -429, -204, -124 or -3-494, -1, -200, -542-3p, - 320a7, -101, 34a, -33b-5p, -495, -524-5p, -30a, -149, -590-5p, -375, -92a, 375, -362-5p, -7, -192-5p, -613, -590-5p, -218

Table 3. *Cont.*

Cancer Type	Diagnosis	Prognosis
		• Pro-angiogenic effect: miR-574-5p, -616-3p • Anti-angiogenic effect: miR-218, • Radiosensitivity: miR-196b, -190 • ↓ Patient survival: miR -486-5p, -552, -647, -519a, -126, -532-5p, -125b, -204, -539, -22, -141, -31, -185, -1297, -19a-3p, -1298, -375, -338-3p, -203, -490-3p, -144, -302a, -302b, -302c, -204, -485-5p, -29c, -124, -135a, -148a, -198, 92a, -1258, -519a, -141, -3923, -29c-3p, 193b, -155 (inverse correlation with tumor stage)

4. Tumor Inflammatory and Immune Microenvironment

The concept of targeted cancer approach has been centered on the neoplastic cells. This paradigm has been now shifted to a more comprehensive understanding of molecular machinery of cancer development which points out the complex interaction between malignant cells and tumor surrounding stroma, which is essential to support each steps of malignant progression [110,111]. This issue is mainly relevant in upper GI cancers in which, on one hand, detection of actionable genetic drivers is rarely reported and on the other, environmental exposure is known to induce inflammatory responses, which ultimately leads to constitutive activation of cellular pro-proliferative and pro-survival signals.

4.1. Cancer-Related Immunogenic Cascades

Esophageal cancer cells are considered to display high immunogenicity and can induce massive antitumor immune responses already in the early disease stages. Moreover, all the main cancer-associated risk factors, namely smoking and alcohol, are associated with chronic irritation of the esophageal epithelium and to tissue damage mediated by the consequent production of reactive-oxygen-species (ROS) [112,113]. In addition, changes in the microbiome defined by a relevant decrease of Gram-positive bacteria, are associated to both esophagitis and BE [114] and promote production of lipopolysaccharide (LPS) which in turn, induces inflammation via Toll-like receptor 4 and NF-κB activation. Overall, chronic inflammation activates several cancer-associated signaling pathways [115]. Among them, interleukin 6 (IL-6)/signal transducer and activator of transcription 3 (STAT3) cascades are known to play a relevant pathogenic role in EC. Many different cell types, monocytes, fibroblasts and endothelial cells that reside around the tumor mass produce IL-6. Moreover, EC cells produced both IL-6 and its receptor (IL-6R), thus suggesting that an autocrine/paracrine loop might cooperate in tumor progression and invasion [116,117]. The overexpression of NF-κB (nuclear factor kappa-light-chain-enhancer of activated B cells) transcription factor defines a second mechanism that is known to modulate EC-surrounding microenvironment. Notably, NF-κB is emerging as a potentially effective target since it is involved in regulating cellular apoptosis and angiogenesis [118]. Its main downstream transducers are interleukin-1β (IL-1β) and interleukin-8 (IL-8). The latter, also known as CXCL-8 (C-X-C Motif Chemokine Ligand 8), acts as neutrophil chemotactic molecule and is implicated in the progression of several cancer types, among which EC [119]. Similarly, the activation of IL-1β is associated to tumor growth, chemoresistance and poor patient prognosis [120]. STAT3 and NF-κB converge on several transducers: among them, prostaglandin E, produced by cyclooxygenase-2 (COX-2), which is active in promoting upper GI cancer-related inflammatory reactions and, ultimately, in inducing chemo-resistance [121]. Chronic inflammation is also involved in attenuating anti-tumor immunity, which is orchestrated by several cell populations such as myeloid-derived suppressor cells (MDSCs) and regulatory T cells (Tregs). Expansion of MDSC or immature myeloid cells is modulated by inflammatory mediators (IL-1β, IL-6 and PGE2) [122] and growth factors (i.e., VEGF). These cells can directly inhibit T-cell activation and natural killers (NKs) cytotoxicity, while induce Tregs [123]. The latter are also directly recruited by EC cells through CCL-17 (C-C Motif Chemokine Ligand 1) and CCL-22 (C-C Motif Chemokine Ligand 22) production and by macrophages via the CC-R4 (C-C chemokine receptor 4 receptor) [124]. Moreover, they can derive from the conversion of Th-17 cells when stimulated by TGF-β and IL-6 [125]. Other immune cells, such as tumor-associated macrophages

(TAM), display more pro-tumorigenic functions, such as induction of angiogenesis and promotion of malignant cell invasive capacity. TAM expansion with M2 polarization can occur in the presence of Th2-related cytokines. Furthermore, TAMs and malignant cells both express immune checkpoint molecules as PD-L1/2 that can inhibit T cell activation. Indeed, high PD-1/2 expression in EC [126] has been correlated with decreased CD8+ T cell infiltration [127]. The other checkpoint molecule CTLA-4 most often acts as inhibitory receptor on immune cells; however, its expression has been also reported directly in tumor cells [128]. In EAC patients, the upregulation of Th-2 associated cytokine (e.g., IL-4 and IL-13) promotes M2-differentiated macrophage infiltration. In ESCC patients, increased secretion of tumor-derived macrophage chemoattractant protein-1 (MCP-1) results in TAM infiltration [128]. In addition to the above described cells, which overall feature immunosuppressive behavior, another type of stromal element, the cancer associated fibroblasts (CAFs) negatively modulate antitumor immunity in various cancer types, among which EC [129]. CAFs—in EC—can trigger the expression of fibroblast activation protein (FAP) and, in turn, induces the secretion of IL-6 and CCL2 [130] which are involved in creating an immune-suppressive tumor stroma, mainly characterized by M2 polarization of activated macrophages [131].

Esophageal cancer and gastric cancers are known to carry many common molecular features, which are, more frequently, shared by EACs and intestinal type of gastric tumors [132]. They derived from the inflammation-metaplasia cascade that occurs in the esophageal epithelium in OAC and in the gastric epithelium in intestinal-type GC. Barrett esophagus and OAC may thus originate from a unique gastric stem fraction, originated from the cardia. Within respect to GC, by matching two key elements, which define the tumor-associated immune milieu, namely the tumor-infiltrating lymphocytes (TILs) and the PD-L1 expression level, four different neoplastic subgroups, emerge with specific and prognostic score. The type I (TILs+ PD-L1+) is defined by adaptive immune resistance, quite opposite the type II (TILs− PD-L1−)is characterized by immune neutrality; type III (TILs− PD-L1+), shows intrinsic induction whereas in type IV (TILs+ PD-L1−) other suppressors might have a role in initiating immune tolerance. [133]. Overall, high expression of PD-L1 associated to CD8+, CD3+ and CD57+ TILs and low densities of FOXP3+ TILs represent favorable prognostic factors [133]. As reported above, an increase in the M2 macrophage component predicts poor prognosis, except for signet ring cell carcinoma and mucinous adenocarcinoma in which it has been associated to a favorable outcome [134].

4.2. The Role of Extracellular Vesicles

Extracellular vesicles (EV) cooperate in modulating the crosstalk between GC cells and surrounding stroma. They are secreted by several cell types and released to the extracellular space; based on their size they are defined as: exosomes (30–100 nm in diameter), microvesicles (MVs, 100–1000 nm in diameter) and apoptotic bodies (1000–5000 nm in diameter). The smallest type, the exosomes, are nano-sized vesicles, which are enveloped by a lipid bilayer and are, then, secreted from the plasma membrane into the extracellular space. They play an important role in GC onset and progression [14] mainly through overexpression of multiple proteins, miRNAs and LncRNAs [135,136]. Interestingly it has been documented that they actively promote distant growth of neoplastic clones. In detail, Zhang et al. showed that epidermal growth factor receptor (EGFR)-containing exosomes secreted by GC cells can be delivered into the liver, where they were ingested by liver stromal cells. Here, EGFR, by inhibiting miR-26a/b expression, activated hepatocyte growth factor (HGF) [137]. The latter, through a quite paracrine loop, bound its receptor MET expressed on the migrated cancer cells thus triggering the MET-driven invasive growth process [138].

4.3. Modulation of Tumor Microenvironment by Ionizing Radiation

In this complex context, the role of ionizing radiation and its interaction with TME emerges as relevant, both locally and under the perspective of its potential abscopal effect. Indeed radiotherapy (RT) represents one of the main treatment strategies in the therapeutic management of oncologic patients, among which those affected by upper GI cancers. Although primarily addressed to kill cancer cells, ionizing radiation also regulates the expression of the different immune cells normally recruited at the periphery of the tumor [139]. Such interactions are likely to impact on tumor growth/dissemination and the capability of a systemic treatment to be particularly efficacious in tumor control. More specifically, radiation, which can be delivered in different doses and treatment fractions, can from one side act as an in situ vaccine leading to immunogenic tumoral cell death; this event is responsible for the release of specific tumor associated-antigen and other molecules (DAMPS) which activates antigen-presenting cells (APC) which ultimately lead to CD8+ Cells activation. Besides, radiation can not only stimulate intratumoral infiltration of macrophages but can also lead to an overexpression of both FGF2 and its receptors (FGFRs). This signaling pathway can switch macrophage phenotype from M1 to M2, which is typically associated to resistance to radiation [140]. Moreover, in EC and GC, increased PD-L1 expression levels have been associated to worse response to ionizing radiation, at least in neoadjuvant setting. The mechanistic explanation of this finding has been related to the overexpression of PD-L1. The latter is directly promoted by the interferon-gamma produced by the CD8+ lymphocytes, through the Janus kinases-Signal Transducer and Activator of Transcription proteins (JAK-STAT) pathway. Notably, high PD-L1 expression has been associated with the induction of the epithelial-to-mesenchymal transition phenomenon is required to tumor distant spreading [141].

5. Immunotherapies: Novel Insights and Advances

Systemic treatment of advanced upper GI cancers encompasses combination of multiple lines of chemotherapy, in absence of standard of care regimens. Combinatorial schedules include platinum and fluoropyrimidine doublets, cisplatin/5-fluorouracil (5-FU) or cisplatin/capecitabine. Trastuzumab is associated in HER2-positive cases. Other molecules, such as irinotecan and taxanes, can be associated with fluoropyrimidines and/or platinum or monoclonal antibodies as ramucirumab (a fully humanized molecule directed against vascular endothelial growth factor receptor 2-VEGFR2) or used as monotherapy for unfit patients (for detail see https://www.nccn.org, [142–146]).

5.1. Immune Checkpoint Inhibition in Clinical Trials

Immunotherapy with immune checkpoint inhibitors (ICIs) has led to a deep change in therapeutic paradigms of advanced tumors, including that of upper GI cancers. However, until now no validated role for immunotherapy has been approved. About 50% of these tumors express PD-L1 but unlike NSCLC or melanoma, this expression occurs predominantly in the peri-tumor inflammatory stroma while it is minimal on cancer cells [147]. Thus, the specific localization, affects, on one hand, PD-L1 expression as validated biomarker, whereas, on the other, is coherent to the poor responses to ICIs that typically characterize these cancers. Similarly, CTL-4 is considerably expressed in GCs (about 80% of cases but it mostly regards immune stroma cells. Detailed lists of studies evaluating immune checkpoint inhibitors are easily available in literature [148,149]: Table 4 summarizes the first and key clinical trials which evaluate the role of most known ICIs (nivolumab and pembrolizumab) in therapeutic intervention against upper GI tumors. The results from ATTRACTION family trials provide robust evidence for the use of nivolumab in case of first line chemotherapy failure. Overall, they led to the approval of nivolumab as therapeutic option in PD-1-unselected metastatic/recurrent gastric cancer in Asian population (Japan, Taiwan and Korea) [150,151]. The PD-binding monoclonal antibody pembrolizumab has been reported, by the KEYNOTE series trials, to add an advantage in patient outcome when used in advanced disease, mainly in those tumors which overexpress PD-L1. However, in the KEYNOTE061 trial [152], pembrolizumab failed to provide a survival benefit over paclitaxel in advanced GC patients who had progressed after first line treatment with standard chemo. More recently, the novel anti PD-1 antibody, toripalimab, has demonstrated a safe profile and promising antitumor activity in patients with advanced GC alone or in combination with conventional chemotherapy schedules. In this context, the high tumor mutational burden (TMB) emerged as powerful predictive marker of overall survival (OS) [153]. The phase III, randomized

JAVELIN Gastric 300 trial has been the first comparing avelumab, an anti-PD-L1 antibody, with chemotherapy in the third-line setting in advanced GC/GEJ cancers. Avelumab failed in improving OS but demonstrated an anti-tumor activity comparable to that of chemotherapy with a more advantageous safety profile [154]. The combination of two different ICIs (anti PD-1 and PD-L1 or anti CTL4) have shown, until now, controversial results. The association of tremelimumab (anti CTLA-4) to durvalumab (anti PD-L1) did not add significant advantages in chemo-refractory GC and GJE cancers [155], whereas the combination of nivolumab and ipilimumab demonstrated more favorable safety and efficacy profiles [156]. Although further investigations are required, combinatorial approaches are now under investigation even in adjuvant settings [157,158]. Among phase III studies, the KEYNOTE-585 trial (NCT03221426) is evaluating perioperative administration of pembrolizumab plus chemotherapy [159] and the Asian ATTRACTION-05 trial (NCT03006705) is comparing S-1/CAPOX (capecitabine plus oxaliplatin) plus nivolumab vs. S-1/CAPOX plus placebo as postoperative approach. Furthermore, two randomized phase II trials are currently ongoing: the DANTE trial (NCT 03421288) evaluating peri-operative use of atezolizumab (anti-PD-L1 antibody) combined with FLOT (docetaxel, oxaliplatin, leucovorin and 5-fluorouracil) [160] and the IMAGINE NCT04062656 randomized, four-arm, chemotherapy-controlled modular trial in subjects with histologically confirmed, resectable GC or GEJ adenocarcinoma. An increase to 35% is estimated to be clinically relevant when patients are treated with either nivolumab in combination with chemotherapy or nivolumab and another immuno-oncology agent (e.g., ipilimumab or relatlimab) [161,162]. Great interest is now addressed to the combination of ICIs and targeted molecules, which seems to be promising although findings are still afar to be conclusive. The combination of durvalumab, targeting PD-L1 olaparib, a PARP (poly ADP ribose polymerase) inhibitor, seemed to be well tolerated in absence of serious adverse event as demonstrated by the phase II MEDIOLA basket trial, which included advanced GCs [163]. Similar results, in terms of safety and clinical activity, have been obtained by adding durvalumab to targeted VEGFR2 inhibitor ramucirumab [164].

Table 4. Main clinical trials evaluating ICI in upper GI cancers [165–172].

Study	Design and Phase	ICI	Cancer Type	Population	Endpoint	Results
ATTRACTION-1	open-label, single-arm, II	nivolumab	ESCC refractory or intolerant to standard chemotherapies.	65 Japanese pts	Safety, efficacy	Positive
ATTRACTION-2	randomized, double-blind, placebo-controlled, III	nivolumab	unresectable advanced or recurrent G/GEJ cancer refractory to, or intolerant of standard chemotherapy	49 pts (Japan, South Korea, Taiwan)	OS	Nivolumab group median OS: 5.26 months vs. 4.14 months in the placebo group. The 12-month OS was 26.2% with nivolumab and 10.9% with placebo
ATTRACTION-3	multicenter, randomized, open-label, III	nivolumab vs. chemotherapy	unresectable advanced- recurrent ESCC (regardless of PD-L1 expression)	419 pts (210 nivolumab vs. 209 chemotherapy)	OS	increased OS (median OS 10.9 vs. 8.4 months)
ATTRACTION-4	multicenter, randomized, open-label, II	nivolumab + S1 +SOX or capecitabine	unresectable advanced or recurrent HER2-negative G/GEJ cancer	40 randomized pts, 39 (nivolumab plus SOX, 21; nivolumab plus CapeOX, 18) and 38 (21 and 17)	Safety, efficacy	Well tolerated. ORR 57.1% with nivolumab plus SOX and 76.5% with nivolumab plus CapeOX. Median PFS 9.7 months and 10.6 months.
KEYNOTE-012	multicentre, open label, 1b	pembrolizumab	PD-L1–positive advanced G/GEJ adenocarcinoma	39 patients	Safety, objective response	13% pts grade 3/4 treatment-related adverse events. 22% ORR

Table 4. Cont.

Study	Design and Phase	ICI	Cancer Type	Population	Endpoint	Results
KEYNOTE-059	global, open-label, single-arm, multicohort, II	pembrolizumab	previously treated G/GEJ cancers	259 pts	Safety, efficacy	ORR: 11.6% complete response: 2.3% serious adverse events: 0.8%
KEYNOTE-180	open-label, interventional, single-arm, II	pembrolizumab	metastatic ESCC, EAC that progressed after 2 or more lines of therapy	121 pts	ORR	ORR: 9.9% among all patients, median duration of response not reached
KEYNOTE-181	open-label, randomized, III	pembrolizumab vs. investigator's choice chemo as second-line therapy	advanced/metastatic ESCC and EAC or Siewert type I GEJ adenocarcinoma	628 and 123 pts in the global and China cohorts.	OS in the ITT, and PD-L1 CPS ≥10 populations.	Pembro and chemo showed comparable OS. Pembro: showed favorable OS in ESCC and CPS ≥10 groups in the global cohort and in all groups in the China cohort. Pembro showed favorable safety in both cohorts
KEYNOTE-061	randomised, open-label, III	Pembrolizumab vs. paclitaxel	Advanced GCs, progressed after first-line treatment with fluoropyrimidine and platinum	592 pts (30 Countries)	OS, PFS in PD-L1 CPS > 1	Failure. Median OS: 9.1 months with pembro vs. 8.3 months with paclitaxel. Median PFS 1.5 months with pembro and 4.1 months with paclitaxel
KEYNOTE-062	III	Pembrolizumab or pembrolizumab + chemotherapy	advanced gastric or GEJ adenocarcinoma			non-inferior/better to chemotherapy in PD-L1
	II	Tremelimumab	second-line treatment in advanced EAC -GC	18	Safety, clinical efficacy, immunologic activity	Most drug-related toxicity was mild; 1 death due to bowel perforation. Four patients SD with clinical benefit; 1 pt PR after 8 cycles

Overall, there is an extreme heterogeneity regarding the efficacy of immune checkpoint inhibition in upper GI cancers. It should be noted that published data are highly heterogeneous within respect to disease stage, treatment schedules, different methods of evaluation of PD-L1 expression levels (tumor proportion score (TPS), combined positive score (CPS), different antibodies used for PD-L1 immunostaining, heterogeneity of considered cells (tumor, stroma and immune cells), cut-offs for positivity (1–50%). Moreover, results could be biased by the fact most of the trials have been conducted only in Asia. The findings also reflect the heterogeneity of the patients enrolled in the trials, which led to controversial results concerning the prognostic implications of PD-L1-expressing tumors. From published data however, several issues deserve main special attention. A relevant example regards a meta-analysis of 15 studies (the vast majority enrolling Asian patients) performed by Gu et al. Overall the authors analyzed 3291 patients and a tremendous heterogeneity in PD-L1 IHC positive expression was reported (from 14.3% to 69.4%) mainly as a consequence of the cut-off values used in different studies (ranging between >1% and >50%) [173].

5.2. Tumor Mutational Burden as Actionable Targets

As above mentioned, tumor mutational burden (TMB) behaves as effective biomarker for response to anti-PD-L1 treatment in diverse tumor types and in chemo-refractory GCs [157,174]. Accurate TMB measure requires next generation sequencing techniques (NGS), thus surrogate markers are under investigation for routine sample management. Among them, the TGFB family members (TGFB1, TGFB2 and TGFB3) are active transducers in the epithelial-to-mesenchymal transition (EMT) process.

Overexpression of TGFB2 has been reported to be positively associated with EMT status and negatively with TMB levels in GC. It affects TMB levels by regulating the DNA damage repair pathways and immune infiltrates, thus suggesting that detection of TGFB2 expression may predict response to ICIs in GC patients [175]. Furthermore, immune checkpoint inhibitors have been used to treat advanced GCs carrying high-frequency microsatellite instability (MSI-H) or mismatch repair defects (dMMR). Microsatellites are short tandem repeats of DNA, which are mostly located in the non-coding genetic or near the chromosome telomeres and their instability defines hyper-mutable phenotype likely caused by defects in mismatch repair (MMR) [176]. The presence of defective MMR genes, which affect about 17–21% of GCs [177] increases the occurrence of somatic mutation to a mean value of more than 1780 compared to 70 changes that can be found in non-defective lesions [178]. It might predict response to anti PD-L1 agents since the occurrence of genetic changes can potentially allow to encode for not-self immunogenic neoantigens.

5.3. Active Immunization Strategies

The above-described results provide a solid rationale for identifying GC patients who may benefit from ICI therapy based on specific tumor genetic asset [179]. In addition, more recent progresses have been reached in the field of tumor immunotherapy. During the past decade, the definition of a strategy to molecularly identify tumor antigens (TA) recognized by immune cells in patients with cancer lead to dramatic progress in tumor immunology. Active immunization is based on the use of an immunogen to generate a host response aimed at eliminating malignant clones in a controlled way. Several strategies have been developed.

5.3.1. Adoption of Cytokines

A first approach regards the adoption of cytokines (e.g., IFN-γ, IL-10, IL-2) as relevant component of immune response. Indeed, they can directly act on immune cells and modulating their proliferation and signaling against cancer cells. It is well known that cytokines, such as IL-10, are mainly released because of HP-associated chronic inflammation which is implicated in upper GI cancer onset and progression [180]. In this perspective, several ongoing trials are under investigation with both diagnostic and therapeutic purposes. The NCT00197470 study is focused on evaluating the association of the host genetics with the susceptibility to various gastroduodenal disorders, including HP-associated gastric cancer in Japanese population. The study aims at identifying polymorphisms in the IL-1, tumor necrosis factor-alpha (TNF-α) and IL-10 coding genes to clarify the association between those changes and cancer risks to early locate those individuals at higher risks for gastrointestinal malignancies development. Another strategy that is now active in solid cancers among which upper GI tumors regards early detection of cancer recurrence by monitoring changes in a panel of circulating inflammatory cytokines (IL-1, 6, 8, 10, 12 and TNF-α) before and after chemo-radiation (NCT00502502). The phase II randomized clinical trial NCT03554395 compares activated CIK (cytokine induced killer cells) armed with anti-CD3-MUC1 bispecific antibody for advanced GCs to evaluate its safety and clinical efficacy. Another ongoing trial (NCT01783951) has been designed with a similar goal, namely, to evaluate the antitumor effect and safety of activated dendritic cell CIKs (DC-CIK) plus S-1-based chemotherapy for advanced gastric cancer. Interestingly, it has been reported that PD-L1 in human GC inhibits cells to cancer progression and improves cytotoxic sensitivity of cancer cells to CIK therapy [181].

5.3.2. Cancer Vaccines

A second promising strategy is related to cancer vaccination. Cancer is a disease of genes and the occurrence of somatic mutations in oncogenes and tumor suppressor genes drives malignant transformation. However, the accumulation of passenger and driver genetic changes generate cancer-specific neoepitopes that are recognized by autologous T cells as not-self: these molecules on the surface of cancer cells identify ideal targets for vaccines [182]. Great interest in addressed towards clinical development of such therapeutic approach. Well known cancer peptides/proteins recognized by CD8+ and CD4+ lymphocytes are, for instance, melanoma-associated antigen (MAGE-3) [183] and HER-2/neu [184]. Several studies are ongoing. The NCT02276300 study is phase I clinical trial which investigates vaccination against HER2-derived peptide in advanced breast and gastric cancer. BVAC-B is immunotherapeutic vaccine, which uses B cell and monocytes as antigen presenting cell and is under investigation in patients with progressive or recurrent HER2/neu positive GCs (NCT03425773 study). The NCT00023634 trial has been designed to determine toxicity of EGFRvIII peptide vaccine with sargramostim (GM-CSF) or keyhole limpet hemocyanin (KLH) as adjuvant approach in patients carrying EGFRvIII-expressing upper GI cancer. Although not fully documented in upper GI cancers, the variant III of the EGFR receptor seems to behave as oncogene in several solid tumors [185]. Another vaccination strategy aims at using epitope peptide restricted to HLA-A*0201 and a first I trial has confirmed the feasibility and safety of this approach [186]. Subsequent phase II trial is ongoing (NCT00681252). Vaccination using survivin epitope peptide might induce cytotoxic T lymphocytes (CTL) from peripheral blood mononuclear cells of healthy donors. It exhibited specific lysis against HLA-A2 matched tumor cells in vitro and in primary cell cultures derived from GC patients [187]. Vaccination with autologous tumor-derived heat shock proteins (HSPs) is another novel promising approach in GC. The HSP gp96-peptide complexes, as chaperone, can specifically interact with antigen-presenting cells (APCs) and induce their activation. This process allows the secretion of several cytokines and chemokines which, in turn, promote CD4+ and CD8+ T-cell antitumor immune response [188]. This approach resulted safe and advantageous in neoadjuvant settings when combined with conventional chemotherapy in patients affected by les aggressive diseases [189]. Some trials have investigated the use of vaccines against dendritic cells (DCs), which infiltrate tumor stroma. Importantly, the DC density predicts GC prognosis, being higher levels associated to improved OS [190]. An ongoing trial (NCT03185429) aims at learning about the safety and tolerance of autologous TSA-DC cell and evaluates the efficacy and feasibility of the cell therapy compared to standard regimens. Preclinical [191,192] and clinical studies [193,194] have demonstrated that DCs transfected with stabilized mRNA coding for tumor-associated antigen/whole tumor RNA can generate potent anticancer immune responses. In theory, RNA-based vaccines present some potential benefits if compared to classical vaccination approaches: (i) they are pharmaceutically safer, since they cannot integrate with DNA and seem to be active in absence of serious adverse event; (ii) they can target multiple tumor-associated epitopes; (iii) they are not MHC-restricted. However, their clinical application has been limited, until now, by difficulties in obtaining stable and efficient mRNA delivery and a technical improvement is required before fully reaching the clinical scenario [195,196]. More integrated strategies encompass combination of vaccines with standard chemotherapy, which aims at exploiting the above-mentioned potentiality of chemotherapy to upregulate tumor immunogenicity. Notably, a preliminary treatment with conventional chemotherapeutic agents can promote ICI sensitivity, as widely demonstrated in NSCLC [197] and in BRCA1-deficient triple-negative breast cancer models [198]. In adjuvant setting in GC, several combinatorial trials are ongoing. The combination of an adjuvant bacille Calmette-Guérin (BCG) vaccine with chemotherapy can improve OS when compared to chemotherapy alone [199]. Similar results have been obtained with vaccination with gastrin-17 diphtheria toxoid (G17DT)-targeting gastrin peptide combined with chemotherapy [200]. Chemotherapy treatment can sensitize to vaccine against tyrosine kinase receptors, as well. For instance, vaccination using peptides derived from human VEGFR 1 and 2 combined with standard chemotherapy can significantly increase the OS of patients carrying advanced GCs [201]. Preliminary results from vaccination with IMU-13, a structure made of three individual B-cell epitope peptide sequences selected from HER2/neu receptor, plus chemotherapy vs. chemotherapy alone is ongoing on upper GI cancer patients [202]. Finally, attempts of combinations of different novel immunotherapeutic strategies are under investigation. In vitro and in vivo strategies have been adopted to enhance immune response to a low immunogenic tumor cell line obtained from a spontaneous gastric tumor of a CEA424-SV40 large T antigen (CEA424-SV40 TAg) transgenic mouse. In detail, lymphodepletion has been obtained by treating animals with cyclophosphamide and then reconstructed by using syngeneic spleen cells. Subsequently mice underwent effective vaccination with a whole tumor cell vaccine combined with GM-CSF. However, recurrence of Tregs should reduce efficacy of this kind of vaccine in long-term perspective [203].

5.4. Passive Immunization Strategies

Passive immunization is—by definition—induced artificially when antibodies are given as a therapy to a nonimmune individual. Within respect to cancer, this concept refers to the administration of active humoral immunity in the form of pre-formed antibodies or effector lymphocytes against neoplastic clones. Several approaches are under investigation.

Adoptive Cell Therapy

The most promising approach of passive immunization regards adoptive cell therapy. The latter provides T cells isolated from a patient, manipulated and expanded in vitro and then re-infused into the patient itself [204]. Adoptive cell therapy (ACT) using TILs refers to the passive transfer into a patient of antitumor T lymphocytes which can virtually destroy the tumor mass. Similarly, to active immunization contexts, concomitant treatment with chemotherapy can increase ACT efficacy in GCs. To sustain this hypothesis, it has been shown that oxaliplatin, by stimulating high-mobility group box 1 (HMGB1) protein to induce anti-cancerous T lymphocytes, can promote immune-mediated apoptosis of cancer cells [205]. Several in vitro and in vivo studies on drug-resistant GCs, demonstrated that the combination of alkylating-like agents with CIK cells induces the release of a high amount of cytokines. It seemed that the T lymphocyte reduction obtained by chemotherapy, can improve the efficacy of ACT therapy by stimulating the persistence of endogenous T cells in circulation, in parallel with a reduction of immune reactions in non-transformed organs. However, these encouraging results were associated with the occurrence of severe infectious adverse events and this point seriously limited the clinical development of this strategy. A more promising type of adoptive T cell immunotherapy is related the use of chimeric antigen receptor (CAR) T cells. The latter are synthetic receptors that can re-program T cells. Their signaling domain enables the CAR T cells to activate effector functions and expand upon recognition of antigens on cancer cells [206]. Results from preclinical studies of the clinical use of CAR T cells against upper GI cancers are encouraging, although this approach requires complex technologies. Moreover, an important issue is the identification of the surface antigen. Targeting therapeutic tumor markers, such as HER2, CEA and DF2, have been carried out in basic and clinical studies. The recently designed bispecific T-cell engagers (BiTEs) identify a class of artificial bi-specific antibodies that are made of two single-chain variable fragments (scFv): the first specific for a T-cell (typically CD3) molecule and the second specific for a tumor-related antigen. The novel secretable BiTE, αHER2/CD3, consists of HER2-specific scFv 4D5, CD3-specific scFv OKT3 and flexible linkers can specifically target HER2+ tumor cells, such as those found in gastric cancer and CD3+ human T cells [207]. Folate receptor 1 (FOLR1), also known as folate receptor alpha and folate binding protein, is a glycosylphosphatidylinositol-linked protein is frequently overexpressed on the GC cell surface and it cannot be found in health areas [208]. Both FOLR1-CAR KHYG-1, a natural killer cell line and FOLR1-CAR T cells has been demonstrated to recognized FOLR1-expressing GC cells in a MHC-independent manner: this fact promotes the release of several cytokines and induce cancer cell apoptosis [209]. PSCA, formerly named as prostate stem cell antigen, is a glycosylphosphatidylinositol (GPI)-anchored cell surface protein belonging to the Thy-1/Ly-6 family. Notably, anti-PSCA CAR-T cells exert strong anti-tumor cytotoxicity in vitro and can impair tumor dissemination in in vivo animal models [210]. Interestingly, CAR T cell approach has been exploited also against mesothelin, that is expressed in GC tissue, both in vitro and in vivo with favorable results defined by strong cytotoxicity and significant regression of GC subcutaneous masses [211]. Within respect to esophageal cancer, EphA2 (erythropoietin-producing hepatocellular receptor A2), which is one of the Ephrin receptor family, is a frequently overexpressed surface antigen. CAR-T cells designed against EphA2 induce the secretion of many cytokines and display a dose-dependent capacity of cancer cell death in vitro [212].

Moreover, it is well known that PD-1 can trigger or inhibit signals, which play a main role in the tumor environment, through combining with PD-L1. This combination can not only block the activation of T cells by blocking the first and second T cell signal but can also assist regulatory T cells (Tregs) to play an inhibitory function and induce helper T cells (Ths) convert to Tregs. The widespread presence of immune checkpoints in a variety of solid tumors, among which upper GI cancers, may be one of the main reasons for the poor effect of CAR-T technology in solid tumors. Recent indications show that bi-specific Trop2/PD-L1 CAR-T cells have the high therapeutic potential against GC [213]. Several clinical studies are ongoing. Among them, the combined phase I and II NCT03706326 trial in advanced EC, aims at assessing the safety and efficacy exploiting combination of immune checkpoint blockade and CAR T cells. In detail, the study evaluates and compares the effects of anti- MUC1 CAR T cells alone, anti- MUC1 CAR T combining PD-1 knockout engineered T cells and PD-1 knockout engineered T cells. The efficacy of this approach is now under investigation also in several trials in gastric cancer patients (NCT02862028, NCT03615313 and NCT03182803).

6. Conclusions and Remarks

Although a relevant number of genomic alterations are known to be active in upper GI cancers, few actionable targets can be effectively exploited for diagnostic and therapeutic purposes. Growing evidence suggests that immunotherapy could play a relevant therapeutic role alone and in combination with chemo-radiotherapy and other systemic therapies. Viral infection, mutational burden and MSI status are specific players into constant interconnection between tumor and microenvironment, which modulates response to immune checkpoint inhibitors. The therapeutic landscape is rapidly evolving due to constant refinement and validation of molecular biomarkers. The unique context-related malignant behavior that characterizes upper GI cancers drives responses to novel immune and cell therapies. It remains to be clarified if the genetic and immunological heterogeneity may be somehow related to the different anatomic districts that globally defines the upper GI tract. A deep understating of these processes is challenging and requires a multidisciplinary approach. This will lead—in the near future—to more durable clinical responses in a perspective of full treatment personalization.

Supplementary Materials: The following are available online at http://www.mdpi.com/2072-6694/12/8/2105/s1, Table S1: TNM staging for oesophageal cancer, Table S2: TNM stage grouping for oesophageal cancer, Table S3: Post-neoadjuvant pathologic stage grouping, Table S4: Tumor cell grading for oesophageal cancer, Table S5: TNM staging for oesophageal cancer, Table S6: Pathologic TNM staging (A) and grouping (B) for gastric cancer, Table S7: Pathologic staging following neoadjuvant therapy in gastric cancer.

Author Contributions: All the authors contribute to manuscript concept and design; G.A., S.L., C.B. and G.M.S. drafted the manuscript; G.M.S. supervised the work. All authors have read and agreed to the published version of the manuscript.

Funding: Ricerca Corrente-IRCCS Fondazione Policlinico San Matteo to G.M.S.

Acknowledgments: G.M.S. would like to thank the invaluable support received from Benedetta Marchelli and Elena Morganti.

Conflicts of Interest: The authors declare no conflict of interest.

References

1. SEER Cancer Stat Facts. *Esophageal Cancer Bethesda*; National Cancer Institute (NCI): Rockville, MD, USA, 2019. Available online: https://seer.cancer.gov/statfacts/html/esoph.html (accessed on 1 June 2020).
2. Abnet, C.C.; Arnold, M.; Wei, W.Q. Epidemiology of Esophageal Squamous Cell Carcinoma. *Gastroenterology* **2018**, *154*, 360–373. [CrossRef] [PubMed]
3. Siegel, R.L.; Miller, K.D.; Jemal, A. Cancer statistics, 2018. *CA Cancer J. Clin.* **2018**, *68*, 7–30. [CrossRef] [PubMed]
4. Rawla, P.; Barsouk, A. Epidemiology of gastric cancer: Global trends, risk factors and prevention. *Prz. Gastroenterol.* **2019**, *14*, 26–38. [CrossRef] [PubMed]

5. GBD 2017 Stomach Cancer Collaborators. The global, regional and national burden of stomach cancer in 195 countries, 1990–2017: A systematic analysis for the Global Burden of Disease study 2017. *Lancet Gastroenterol. Hepatol.* **2020**, *5*, 42–54. [CrossRef]
6. Bornschein, J.; Selgrad, M.; Warnecke, M.; Kuester, D.; Wex, T.; Malfertheiner, P. H. Pylori infection is a key risk factor for proximal gastric cancer. *Dig. Dis. Sci.* **2010**, *55*, 3124–3131. [CrossRef] [PubMed]
7. Power, D.G.; Kelsen, D.P.; Shah, M.A. Advanced gastric cancer—Slow but steady progress. *Cancer Treat. Rev.* **2010**, *36*, 384–392. [CrossRef] [PubMed]
8. Kanat, O.; O'Neil, B.; Shahda, S. Targeted therapy for advanced gastric cancer: A review of current status and future prospects. *World J. Gastrointest. Oncol.* **2015**, *7*, 401–410. [CrossRef]
9. Bilici, A. Treatment options in patients with metastatic gastric cancer: Current status and future perspectives. *World J. Gastroenterol.* **2014**, *20*, 3905–3915. [CrossRef]
10. Testa, U.; Castelli, G.; Pelosi, E. Esophageal Cancer: Genomic and Molecular Characterization, Stem Cell Compartment and Clonal Evolution. *Medicines* **2017**, *4*, 67. [CrossRef]
11. Kim, J.G. Molecular targeted therapy for advanced gastric cancer. *Korean J. Intern. Med.* **2013**, *28*, 149–155. [CrossRef]
12. Bang, Y.J.; Van Cutsem, E.; Feyereislova, A.; Chung, H.C.; Shen, L.; Sawaki, A.; Lordick, F.; Ohtsu, A.; Omuro, Y.; Satoh, T.; et al. Trastuzumab in combination with chemotherapy versus chemotherapy alone for treatment of HER2-positive advanced gastric or gastro-oesophageal junction cancer (ToGA): A phase 3, open-label, randomised controlled trial. *Lancet* **2010**, *376*, 687–697. [CrossRef]
13. Apicella, M.; Corso, S.; Giordano, S. Targeted therapies for gastric cancer: Failures and hopes from clinical trials. *Oncotarget* **2017**, *8*, 57654–57669. [CrossRef] [PubMed]
14. Hayakawa, Y.; Sethi, N.; Sepulveda, A.R.; Bass, A.J.; Wang, T.C. Oesophageal adenocarcinoma and gastric cancer: Should we mind the gap? *Nat. Rev. Cancer* **2016**, *16*, 305–318. [CrossRef] [PubMed]
15. Stella, G.M.; Senetta, R.; Cassenti, A.; Ronco, M.; Cassoni, P. Cancers of unknown primary origin: Current perspectives and future therapeutic strategies. *J. Transl. Med.* **2012**, *10*, 12. [CrossRef]
16. Zhang, Y.; Li, C.; Chen, M. Prognostic value of immunohistochemical factors in esophageal small cell carcinoma (ESCC): Analysis of clinicopathologic features of 73 patients. *J. Thorac. Dis.* **2018**, *10*, 4023–4031. [CrossRef] [PubMed]
17. Jain, S.; Dhingra, S. Pathology of esophageal cancer and Barrett's esophagus. *Ann. Cardiothorac. Surg.* **2017**, *6*, 99–109. [CrossRef]
18. Lauren, P. The two histological main types of gastric carcinoma: Diffuse and so-called intestinal-type carcinoma. An attempt at a histo-clinical classification. *Acta Pathol. Microbiol. Scand.* **1965**, *64*, 31–49. [CrossRef]
19. Wong, H.H.; Chu, P. Immunohistochemical features of the gastrointestinal tract tumors. *J. Gastrointest. Oncol.* **2012**, *3*, 262–284. [CrossRef]
20. Hirota, S. Differential diagnosis of gastrointestinal stromal tumor by histopathology and immunohistochemistry. *Transl. Gastroenterol. Hepatol.* **2018**, *3*, 27. [CrossRef]
21. Schuchter, L.M.; Green, R.; Fraker, D. Primary and metastatic diseases in malignant melanoma of the gastrointestinal tract. *Curr. Opin. Oncol.* **2000**, *12*, 181–185. [CrossRef]
22. Chen, Y.C.; Fang, W.L.; Wang, R.F.; Liu, C.A.; Yang, M.H.; Lo, S.S.; Wu, C.W.; Li, A.F.; Shyr, Y.M.; Huang, K.H.; et al. Clinicopathological Variation of Lauren Classification in Gastric Cancer. *Pathol. Oncol. Res.* **2016**, *22*, 197–202. [CrossRef] [PubMed]
23. Thorban, S.; Böttcher, K.; Etter, M.; Roder, J.D.; Busch, R.; Siewert, J.R. Prognostic factors in gastric stump carcinoma. *Ann. Surg.* **2000**, *231*, 188–194. [CrossRef]
24. Sons, H.U.; Borchard, F. Gastric carcinoma after surgical treatment for benign ulcer disease: Some pathologic-anatomic aspects. *Int. Surg.* **1987**, *72*, 222–226. [PubMed]
25. Sinning, C.; Schaefer, N.; Standop, J.; Hirner, A.; Wolff, M. Gastric stump carcinoma—Epidemiology and current concepts in pathogenesis and treatment. *Eur. J. Surg. Oncol.* **2007**, *33*, 133–139. [CrossRef] [PubMed]
26. Brusselaers, N.; Vall, A.; Mattsson, F.; Lagergren, J. Tumour staging of oesophageal cancer in the Swedish Cancer Registry: A nationwide validation study. *Acta Oncol.* **2015**, *54*, 903–908. [CrossRef]
27. Birla, R.; Gandea, C.; Hoara, P.; Caragui, A.; Marica, C.; Vasiliu, E.; Constantinoiu, S. Clinical and Therapeutic Implications of the 8th Edition TNM Classification of Adenocarcinomas of the Esophagogastric Junction. *Chirurgia* **2018**, *113*, 747–757. [CrossRef]

28. Wittekind, C. The development of the TNM classification of gastric cancer. *Pathol. Int.* **2015**, *65*, 399–403. [CrossRef]
29. Li, Z.; Xiao, Q.; Wang, Y.; Wang, W.; Li, S.; Shan, F.; Zhou, Z.; Ji, J. A Modified ypTNM Staging System-Development and External Validation of a Nomogram Predicting the Overall Survival of Gastric Cancer Patients Received Neoadjuvant Chemotherapy. *Cancer Manag. Res.* **2020**, *12*, 2047–2055. [CrossRef]
30. Chmelo, J.; Phillips, A.W. ASO Author Reflections: Gastric Cancer Staging: More than Just TNM? *Ann. Surg. Oncol.* **2020**. [CrossRef]
31. Morita, M.; Kumashiro, R.; Kubo, N.; Nakashima, Y.; Yoshida, R.; Yoshinaga, K.; Saeki, H.; Emi, Y.; Kakaji, Y.; Sakaguchi, Y.; et al. Alcohol drinking, cigarette smoking and the development of squamous cell carcinoma of the esophagus: Epidemiology, clinical findings and prevention. *Int. J. Clin. Oncol.* **2010**, *15*, 126–134. [CrossRef]
32. Bucchi, D.; Stracci, F.; Buonora, N.; Masanotti, G. Human papillomavirus and gastrointestinal cancer: A review. *World J. Gastroenterol.* **2016**, *22*, 7415–7430. [CrossRef]
33. Zang, B.; Huang, G.; Wang, X.; Zheng, S. HPV-16 E6 promotes cell growth of esophageal cancer via downregulation of miR-125b and activation of Wnt/β-catenin signaling pathway. *Int. J. Clin. Exp. Pathol.* **2015**, *8*, 13687–13694. [PubMed]
34. Agalliu, I.; Chen, Z.; Wang, T.; Hayes, R.B.; Freedman, N.D.; Gapstur, S.M.; Burk, R.D. Oral Alpha, Beta and Gamma HPV Types and Risk of Incident Esophageal Cancer. *Cancer Epidemiol. Biomark. Prev.* **2018**, *27*, 1168–1175. [CrossRef] [PubMed]
35. Gillies, C.L.; Farrukh, A.; Abrams, K.R.; Mayberry, J.F. Risk of esophageal cancer in achalasia cardia: A meta-analysis. *JGH Open* **2019**, *3*, 196–200. [CrossRef] [PubMed]
36. Coleman, H.G.; Xie, S.H.; Lagergren, J. The Epidemiology of Esophageal Adenocarcinoma. *Gastroenterology* **2018**, *154*, 390–405. [CrossRef] [PubMed]
37. Sawas, T.; Azad, N.; Killcoyne, S.; Iyer, P.G.; Wang, K.K.; Fitzgerald, R.C.; Katzka, D.A. Comparison of Phenotypes and Risk Factors for Esophageal Adenocarcinoma at Present vs Prior Decades. *Clin. Gastroenterol. Hepatol.* **2019**, S1542-3565(19)31269-8. [CrossRef] [PubMed]
38. Wang, R.H. From reflux esophagitis to Barrett's esophagus and esophageal adenocarcinoma. *World J. Gastroenterol.* **2015**, *21*, 5210–5219. [CrossRef] [PubMed]
39. Bleaney, C.W.; Barrow, M.; Hayes, S.; Ang, Y. The relevance and implications of signet-ring cell adenocarcinoma of the oesophagus. *J. Clin. Pathol.* **2018**, *71*, 201–206. [CrossRef] [PubMed]
40. Xie, F.J.; Zhang, Y.P.; Zheng, Q.Q.; Jin, H.C.; Wang, F.L.; Chen, M.; Shao, L.; Zou, D.H.; Yu, X.M.; Mao, W.M. Helicobacter pylori infection and esophageal cancer risk: An updated meta-analysis. *World J. Gastroenterol.* **2013**, *19*, 6098–6107. [CrossRef]
41. Gao, H.; Li, L.; Zhang, C.; Tu, J.; Geng, X.; Wang, J.; Zhou, X.; Jing, J.; Pan, W. Systematic Review with Meta-analysis: Association of Helicobacter pylori Infection with Esophageal Cancer. *Gastroenterol. Res. Pract.* **2019**, 1953497. [CrossRef]
42. ZurHausen, A.; van Rees, B.P.; van Beek, J.; Craanen, M.E.; Bloemena, E.; Offerhaus, G.J.; Meijer, C.J.; van den Brule, A.J. Epstein-Barr virus in gastric carcinomas and gastric stump carcinomas: A late event in gastric carcinogenesis. *J. Clin. Pathol.* **2004**, *57*, 487–491. [CrossRef] [PubMed]
43. Weston, A.P.; Badr, A.S.; Hassanein, R.S. Prospective multivariate analysis of clinical, endoscopic and histological factors predictive of the development of Barrett's multifocal high-grade dysplasia or adenocarcinoma. *Am. J. Gastroenterol.* **1999**, *94*, 3413–3419. [CrossRef] [PubMed]
44. Anaparthy, R.; Sharma, P. Progression of Barrett oesophagus: Role of endoscopic and histological predictors. *Nat. Rev. Gastroenterol. Hepatol.* **2014**, *11*, 525–534. [CrossRef]
45. Urabe, M.; Ushiku, T.; Shinozaki-Ushiku, A.; Iwasaki, A.; Yamazawa, S.; Yamashita, H.; Seto, Y.; Fukayama, M. Adenocarcinoma of the esophagogastric junction and its background mucosal pathology: A comparative analysis according to Siewert classification in a Japanese cohort. *Cancer Med.* **2018**, *7*, 5145–5154. [CrossRef] [PubMed]
46. Sitarz, R.; Skierucha, M.; Mielko, J.; Offerhaus, G.J.A.; Maciejewski, R.; Polkowski, W.P. Gastric cancer: Epidemiology, prevention, classification and treatment. *Cancer Manag. Res.* **2018**, *10*, 239–248. [CrossRef] [PubMed]

47. Cancer Genome Atlas Research Network; Analysis Working Group: Asan University; BC Cancer Agency; Brigham and Women's Hospital; Broad Institute; Brown University; Case Western Reserve University; Dana-Farber Cancer Institute; Duke University; Greater Poland Cancer Centre. Integrated genomic characterization of oesophageal carcinoma. *Nature* **2017**, *541*, 169–175. [CrossRef]
48. Agrawal, N.; Jiao, Y.; Bettegowda, C.; Hutfless, S.M.; Wang, Y.; David, S.; Cheng, Y.; Twaddell, W.S.; Latt, N.L.; Shin, E.J.; et al. Comparative genomic analysis of esophageal adenocarcinoma and squamous cell carcinoma. *Cancer Discov.* **2012**, *2*, 899–905. [CrossRef]
49. Abidali, H.; Muna-Aguon, P.; Vela, S.; Nanda, R. Palmoplantar Hyperkeratosis and Strong Family History of Esophageal Cancer: Tylosis or Not? *Am. J. Gastroenterol.* **2018**, *113*, 1733–1734. [CrossRef]
50. Hosur, V.; Farley, M.L.; Low, B.E.; Burzenski, L.M.; Shultz, L.D.; Wiles, M.V. RHBDF2-Regulated Growth Factor Signaling in a Rare Human Disease, Tylosis With Esophageal Cancer: What Can We Learn From Murine Models? *Front. Genet.* **2018**, *9*, 233. [CrossRef]
51. Donner, I.; Katainen, R.; Tanskanen, T.; Kaasinen, E.; Aavikko, M.; Ovaska, K.; Artama, M.; Pukkala, E.; Aaltonen, L.A. Candidate susceptibility variants for esophageal squamous cell carcinoma. *Genes Chromosomes Cancer* **2017**, *56*, 453–459. [CrossRef]
52. Wild, C.P.; Hardie, L.J. Reflux, Barrett's oesophagus and adenocarcinoma: Burning questions. *Nat. Rev. Cancer* **2003**, *3*, 676–684. [CrossRef] [PubMed]
53. Galipeau, P.C.; Prevo, L.J.; Sanchez, C.A.; Longton, G.M.; Reid, B.J. Clonal expansion and loss of heterozygosity at chromosomes 9p and 17p inpremalignant esophageal (Barrett's) tissue. *J. Natl. Cancer Inst.* **1999**, *91*, 2087–2095. [CrossRef] [PubMed]
54. Gu, J.; Ajani, J.A.; Hawk, E.T.; Ye, Y.; Lee, J.H.; Bhutani, M.S.; Hofstetter, W.L.; Swisher, S.G.; Wang, K.K.; Wu, X. Genome-wide catalogue of chromosomal aberrations in barrett'sesophagus and esophageal adenocarcinoma: A high-density single nucleotide polymorphism array analysis. *Cancer Prev. Res.* **2010**, *3*, 1176–1186. [CrossRef] [PubMed]
55. Ross-Innes, C.S.; Becq, J.; Warren, A.; Cheetham, R.K.; Northen, H.; O'Donovan, M.; Malhotra, S.; di Pietro, M.; Ivakhno, S.; He, M.; et al. Whole-genome sequencing provides new insights into the clonal architecture of Barrett's esophagus and esophageal adenocarcinoma. *Nat. Genet.* **2015**, *47*, 1038–1046. [CrossRef] [PubMed]
56. Dulak, A.M.; Stojanov, P.; Peng, S.; Lawrence, M.S.; Fox, C.; Stewart, C.; Bandla, S.; Imamura, Y.; Schumacher, S.E.; Shefler, E.; et al. Exome and whole-genome sequencing of esophageal adenocarcinoma identifies recurrent driver events and mutational complexity. *Nat. Genet.* **2013**, *45*, 478–486. [CrossRef]
57. Stachler, M.D.; Taylor-Weiner, A.; Peng, S.; McKenna, A.; Agoston, A.T.; Odze, R.D.; Davison, J.M.; Nason, K.S.; Loda, M.; Leshchiner, I.; et al. Paired exome analysis of Barrett's esophagus and adenocarcinoma. *Nat. Genet.* **2015**, *47*, 1047–1055. [CrossRef]
58. Li, D.; Zhang, L.; Liu, Y.; Sun, H.; Onwuka, J.U.; Zhao, Z.; Tian, W.; Xu, J.; Zhao, Y.; Xu, H. Specific DNA methylation markers in the diagnosis and prognosis of esophageal cancer. *Aging* **2019**, *11*, 11640–11658. [CrossRef]
59. Oliveira, C.; Pinheiro, H.; Figueiredo, J.; Seruca, R.; Carneiro, F. Familial gastric cancer: Genetic susceptibility, pathology and implications for management. *Lancet Oncol.* **2015**, *16*, e60–e70. [CrossRef]
60. Van der Post, R.S.; Oliveira, C.; Guilford, P.; Carneiro, F. Hereditary gastric cancer: What's new? Update 2013–2018. *Fam. Cancer* **2019**, *18*, 363–367. [CrossRef]
61. Colvin, H.; Yamamoto, K.; Wada, N.; Mori, M. Hereditary Gastric Cancer Syndromes. *Surg. Oncol. Clin. N. Am.* **2015**, *24*, 765–777. [CrossRef]
62. Ossa, C.A.; Molina, G.; Cock-Rada, A.M. Li-Fraumeni syndrome. *Biomedica* **2016**, *36*, 182–187. [CrossRef] [PubMed]
63. Svec, J.; Schwarzová, L.; Janošíková, B.; Stekrová, J.; Mandys, V.; Kment, M.; Vodička, P. Synchronousgastric and sebaceouscancers, a rare manifestation of MLH1-related Muir-Torre syndrome. *Int. J. Clin. Exp. Pathol.* **2014**, *7*, 5196–5202. [PubMed]
64. Wu, M.; Krishnamurthy, K. Peutz-Jeghers Syndrome. In *StatPearls [Internet]*; StatPearls Publishing: Treasure Island, FL, USA, 2020.
65. Syngal, S.; Brand, R.E.; Church, J.M.; Giardiello, F.M.; Hampel, H.L.; Burt, R.W.; American College of Gastroenterology. ACG clinical guideline: Genetic testing and management of hereditary gastrointestinal cancer syndromes. *Am. J. Gastroenterol.* **2015**, *110*, 223–263. [CrossRef] [PubMed]

66. Polom, K.; Marrelli, D.; D'Ignazio, A.; Roviello, F. Hereditary diffuse gastric cancer: How to look for and how to manage it. *Updates Surg.* **2018**, *70*, 161–166. [CrossRef]
67. Ang, Y.L.; Yong, W.P.; Tan, P. Translating gastric cancer genomics into targeted therapies. *Crit. Rev. Oncol. Hematol.* **2016**, *100*, 141–146. [CrossRef]
68. Jácome, A.A.; Coutinho, A.K.; Lima, E.M.; Andrade, A.C.; Dos Santos, J.S. Personalized medicine in gastric cancer: Where are we and where are we going? *World J. Gastroenterol.* **2016**, *22*, 1160–1171. [CrossRef]
69. Jou, E.; Rajdev, L. Current and emerging therapies in unresectable and recurrent gastric cancer. *World J. Gastroenterol.* **2016**, *22*, 4812–4823. [CrossRef]
70. Farran, B.; Muller, S.; Montenegro, R.C. Gastric cancer management: Kinases as a target therapy. *Clin. Exp. Pharmacol. Physiol.* **2017**, *44*, 613–622. [CrossRef] [PubMed]
71. Cancer Genome Atlas Research Network. Comprehensive molecular characterization of gastric adenocarcinoma. *Nature* **2014**, *513*, 202–209. [CrossRef]
72. Liu, X.; Meltzer, S.J. Gastric Cancer in the Era of Precision Medicine. *Cell Mol. Gastroenterol. Hepatol.* **2017**, *3*, 348–358. [CrossRef] [PubMed]
73. Saisana, M.; Griffin, S.M.; May, F.E. Importance of the type I insulin-like growth factor receptor in HER2, FGFR2 and MET-unamplified gastric cancer with and without Ras pathway activation. *Oncotarget* **2016**, *7*, 54445–54462. [CrossRef] [PubMed]
74. Meric-Bernstam, F.; Johnson, A.M.; Dumbrava, E.E.I.; Raghav, K.; Balaji, K.; Bhatt, M.; Murthy, R.K.; Rodon, J.; Piha-Paul, S.A. Advances in HER2-Targeted Therapy: Novel Agents and Opportunities Beyond Breast and Gastric Cancer. *Clin. Cancer Res.* **2019**, *25*, 2033–2041. [CrossRef] [PubMed]
75. Tomizawa, K.; Suda, K.; Onozato, R.; Kosaka, T.; Endoh, H.; Sekido, Y.; Shigematsu, H.; Kuwano, H.; Yatabe, Y.; Mitsudomi, T. Prognostic and predictive implications of HER2/ERBB2/neu gene mutations in lung cancers. *Lung Cancer* **2011**, *74*, 139–144. [CrossRef]
76. Wang, H.B.; Liao, X.F.; Zhang, J. Clinicopathological factors associated with HER2-positive gastric cancer: A meta-analysis. *Medicine* **2017**, *96*, e8437. [CrossRef]
77. Yoshioka, T.; Shien, K.; Namba, K.; Torigoe, H.; Sato, H.; Tomida, S.; Yamamoto, H.; Asano, H.; Soh, J.; Tsukuda, K.; et al. Antitumor activity of pan-HER inhibitors in HER2-positive gastric cancer. *Cancer Sci.* **2018**, *109*, 1166–1176. [CrossRef]
78. Lordick, F.; Kang, Y.K.; Chung, H.C.; Salman, P.; Oh, S.C.; Bodoky, G.; Kurteva, G.; Volovat, C.; Moiseyenko, V.M.; Gorbunova, V.; et al. Arbeitsgemeinschaft Internistische Onkologie and EXPAND Investigators. Capecitabine and cisplatin with or without cetuximab for patients with previously untreated advanced gastric cancer (EXPAND): A randomised, open-label phase 3 trial. *Lancet Oncol.* **2013**, *14*, 490–499. [CrossRef]
79. Waddell, T.; Chau, I.; Cunningham, D.; Gonzalez, D.; Okines, A.F.; Okines, C.; Wotherspoon, A.; Saffery, C.; Middleton, G.; Wadsley, J.; et al. Epirubicin, oxaliplatin and capecitabine with or without panitumumab for patients with previously untreated advanced oesophagogastric cancer (REAL3): A randomised, open-label phase 3 trial. *Lancet Oncol.* **2013**, *14*, 481–489. [CrossRef]
80. Ohtsu, A.; Shah, M.A.; Van Custem, E.; Rha, S.Y.; Sawaki, A.; Park, S.R.; Lim, H.Y.; Yamada, Y.; Wu, J.; Langer, B.; et al. Bevacizumab in combination with chemotherapy as first-line therapy in advanced gastric cancer: A randomized, double blind, placebo-controlled phase III study. *J. Clin. Oncol.* **2011**, *29*, 3968–3976. [CrossRef] [PubMed]
81. Fuchs, C.S.; Shitara, K.; Di Bartolomeo, M.; Lonardi, S.; Al-Batran, S.E.; Van Cutsem, E.; Ilson, D.H.; Alsina, M.; Chau, I.; Lacy, J.; et al. RAINFALL Study Group. Ramucirumab with cisplatin and fluoropyrimidine as first-line therapy in patients with metastatic gastric or junctional adenocarcinoma (RAINFALL): A double-blind, randomised, placebo-controlled, phase 3 trial. *Lancet Oncol.* **2019**, *20*, 420–435. [CrossRef]
82. Wilke, H.; Muro, K.; Van Cutsem, E.; Oh, S.C.; Bodoky, G.; Shimada, Y.; Hironaka, S.; Sugimoto, N.; Lipatov, O.; Kim, T.Y.; et al. Ramucirumab plus paclitaxel versus placebo plus paclitaxel in patients with previously treated advanced gastric or gastro-oesophageal junction adenocarcinoma (RAINBOW): A double-blind, randomised phase 3 trial. *Lancet Oncol.* **2014**, *15*, 1224–1235. [CrossRef]
83. Fuchs, C.S.; Tomasek, J.; Yong, C.J.; Dumitru, F.; Passalacqua, R.; Goswami, C.; Safran, H.; dos Santos, L.V.; Aprile, G.; Ferry, D.R.; et al. REGARD Trial Investigators. Ramucirumab monotherapy for previously treated advanced gastric or gastro-oesophageal junction adenocarcinoma (REGARD): An international, randomised, multicentre, placebo-controlled, phase 3 trial. *Lancet* **2014**, *383*, 31–39. [CrossRef]

84. Catenacci, D.V.; Ang, A.; Liao, W.L.; Shen, J.; O'Day, E.; Loberg, R.D.; Cecchi, F.; Hembrough, T.; Ruzzo, A.; Graziano, F. MET tyrosine kinase receptor expression and amplification as prognostic biomarkers of survival in gastroesophageal adenocarcinoma. Version 2. *Cancer* **2017**, *123*, 1061–1070. [CrossRef]
85. Kim, H.S.; Chon, H.J.; Kim, H.; Shin, S.J.; Wacheck, V.; Gruver, A.M.; Kim, J.S.; Rha, S.Y.; Chung, H.C. MET in gastric cancer with liver metastasis: The relationship between MET amplification and Met overexpression in primary stomach tumors and liver metastasis. *J. Surg. Oncol.* **2018**, *117*, 1679–1686. [CrossRef] [PubMed]
86. Migliore, C.; Giordano, S. Molecular cancer therapy: Can our expectation be MET? *Eur. J. Cancer* **2008**, *44*, 641–651. [CrossRef] [PubMed]
87. Smolen, G.A.; Sordella, R.; Muir, B.; Mohapatra, G.; Barmettler, A.; Archibald, H.; Kim, W.J.; Okimoto, R.A.; Bell, D.W.; Sgroi, D.C.; et al. Amplification of MET may identify a subset of cancers with extreme sensitivity to the selective tyrosine kinase inhibitor PHA-665752. *Proc. Natl. Acad. Sci. USA* **2006**, *103*, 2316–2321. [CrossRef]
88. Oue, N.; Sentani, K.; Sakamoto, N.; Uraoka, N.; Yasui, W. Molecular carcinogenesis of gastric cancer: Lauren classification, mucin phenotype expression and cancer stem cells. *Int. J. Clin. Oncol.* **2019**, *24*, 771–778. [CrossRef] [PubMed]
89. Keller, S.; Kneissl, J.; Grabher-Meier, V.; Heindl, S.; Hasenauer, J.; Maier, D.; Mattes, J.; Winter, P.; Luber, B. Evaluation of epidermal growth factor receptor signaling effects in gastric cancer cell lines by detailed motility-focused phenotypic characterization linked with molecular analysis. *BMC Cancer* **2017**, *17*, 845. [CrossRef]
90. Apicella, M.; Migliore, C.; Capelôa, T.; Menegon, S.; Cargnelutti, M.; Degiuli, M.; Sapino, A.; Sottile, A.; Sarotto, I.; Casorzo, L.; et al. Dual MET/EGFR therapy leads to complete response and resistance prevention in a MET-amplified gastroesophageal xenopatient cohort. *Oncogene* **2017**, *36*, 1200–1210. [CrossRef]
91. Ha, S.Y.; Lee, J.; Jang, J.; Hong, J.Y.; Do, I.G.; Park, S.H.; Park, J.O.; Choi, M.G.; Sohn, T.S.; Bae, J.M.; et al. HER2-positive gastric cancer with concomitant MET and/or EGFR overexpression: A distinct subset of patients for dual inhibition therapy. *Int. J. Cancer* **2015**, *136*, 1629–1635. [CrossRef]
92. Chen, W.; Wang, J.; Li, X.; Li, J.; Zhou, L.; Qiu, T.; Zhang, M.; Liu, P. Prognostic significance of BRCA1 expression in gastric cancer. *Med. Oncol.* **2013**, *30*, 423. [CrossRef]
93. Lord, C.; Ashworth, A. BRCAness revisited. *Nat. Rev. Cancer* **2016**, *16*, 110–120. [CrossRef]
94. Bang, Y.J.; Xu, R.H.; Chin, K.; Lee, K.W.; Park, S.H.; Rha, S.Y.; Shen, L.; Qin, S.; Xu, N.; Im, S.A.; et al. Olaparib in combination with paclitaxel in patients with advanced gastric cancer who have progressed following first-line therapy (GOLD): A double-blind, randomised, placebo-controlled, phase 3 trial. *Lancet Oncol.* **2017**, *18*, 1637–1651. [CrossRef]
95. Lee, Y.; Ahn, C.; Han, J.; Choi, H.; Kim, J.; Yim, J.; Lee, J.; Provost, P.; Rådmark, O.; Kim, S.; et al. The nuclear RNase III Drosha initiates microRNA processing. *Nature* **2003**, *425*, 415–419. [CrossRef] [PubMed]
96. Van Roosbroeck, K.; Calin, G.A. Cancer Hallmarks and MicroRNAs: The Therapeutic Connection. *Adv. Cancer Res.* **2017**, *135*, 119–149. [CrossRef] [PubMed]
97. Ruan, K.; Fang, X.; Ouyang, G. MicroRNAs: Novel regulators in the hallmarks of human cancer. *Cancer Lett.* **2009**, *285*, 116–126. [CrossRef]
98. Chen, F.; Zhou, H.; Wu, C.; Yan, H. Identification of miRNA profiling in prediction of tumor recurrence and progress and bioinformatics analysis for patients with primary esophageal cancer: Study based on TCGA database. *Pathol. Res. Pract.* **2018**, *214*, 2081–2086. [CrossRef] [PubMed]
99. Luo, H.S.; Wu, D.H. Identification of miR-375 as a potential prognostic biomarker for esophageal squamous cell cancer: A bioinformatics analysis based on TCGA and meta-analysis. *Pathol. Res. Pract.* **2019**, *215*, 512–518. [CrossRef]
100. Zhang, H.C.; Tang, K.F. Clinical value of integrated-signature miRNAs in Esophageal cancer. *Cancer Med.* **2017**, *6*, 1893–1903. [CrossRef]
101. Zhang, Z.; Li, Z.; Gao, C.; Chen, P.; Chen, J.; Liu, W.; Xiao, S.; Lu, H. miR-21 plays a pivotal role in gastric cancer pathogenesis and progression. *Lab. Investig.* **2008**, *88*, 1358–1366. [CrossRef]
102. Löffler, D.; Brocke-Heidrich, K.; Pfeifer, G.; Stocsits, C.; Hackermüller, J.; Kretzschmar, A.K.; Burger, R.; Gramatzki, M.; Blumert, C.; Bauer, K.; et al. Interleukin-6 dependent survival of multiple myeloma cells involves the Stat3-mediated induction of microRNA-21 through a highly conserved enhancer. *Blood* **2007**, *110*, 1330–1333. [CrossRef]

103. Shin, V.Y.; Jin, H.; Ng, E.K.; Cheng, A.S.; Chong, W.W.; Wong, C.Y.; Leung, W.K.; Sung, J.J.; Chu, K.M. NF-κB targets miR-16 and miR-21 in gastric cancer: Involvement of prostaglandin E receptors. *Carcinogenesis* **2011**, *32*, 240–245. [CrossRef]
104. Bloomston, M.; Frankel, W.L.; Petrocca, F.; Volinia, S.; Alder, H.; Hagan, J.P.; Liu, C.G.; Bhatt, D.; Taccioli, C.; Croce, C.M. MicroRNA expression patterns to differentiate pancreatic adenocarcinoma from normal pancreas and chronic pancreatitis. *JAMA* **2007**, *297*, 1901–1908. [CrossRef] [PubMed]
105. Shin, V.Y.; Chu, K.M. MiRNA as potential biomarkers and therapeutic targets for gastric cancer. *World J. Gastroenterol.* **2014**, *20*, 10432–10439. [CrossRef] [PubMed]
106. Li, X.; Luo, F.; Li, Q.; Xu, M.; Feng, D.; Zhang, G. Identification of new aberrantly expressed miRNAs in intestinal-type gastric cancer and its clinical significance. *Oncol. Rep.* **2011**, *26*, 1431–1439. [CrossRef] [PubMed]
107. Michael, M.Z.; O'Connor, S.M.; van Holst Pellekaan, N.G.; Young, G.P.; James, R.J. Reduced accumulation of specific microRNAs in colorectal neoplasia. *Mol. Cancer Res.* **2003**, *1*, 882–889. [PubMed]
108. Takagi, T.; Iio, A.; Nakagawa, Y.; Naoe, T.; Tanigawa, N.; Akao, Y. Decreased expression of microRNA-143 and -145 in human gastric cancers. *Oncology* **2009**, *77*, 12–21. [CrossRef]
109. Luo, H.; Zhang, H.; Zhang, Z.; Zhang, X.; Ning, B.; Guo, J.; Nie, N.; Liu, B.; Wu, X. Down-regulated miR-9 and miR-433 in human gastric carcinoma. *J. Exp. Clin. Cancer Res.* **2009**, *28*, 82. [CrossRef] [PubMed]
110. Smyth, M.J.; Ngiow, S.F.; Ribas, A.; Teng, M.W. Combination cancer immunotherapies tailored to the tumor microenvironment. *Nat. Rev. Clin. Oncol.* **2016**, *13*, 143–158. [CrossRef]
111. Joyce, J.A.; Pollard, J.W. Microenvironmental regulation of metastasis. *Nat. Rev. Cancer* **2009**, *9*, 239–252. [CrossRef]
112. Radojicic, J.; Zaravinos, A.; Spandidos, D.A. HPV, KRAS mutations, alcohol consumption and tobacco smoking effects on esophageal squamous-cell carcinoma carcinogenesis. *Int. J. Biol. Markers* **2012**, *27*, 1–12. [CrossRef]
113. Kubo, N.; Morita, M.; Nakashima, Y.; Kitao, H.; Egashira, A.; Saeki, H.; Oki, E.; Kakeji, Y.; Oda, Y.; Maehara, Y. Oxidative DNA damage in human esophageal cancer: Clinicopathological analysis of 8-hydroxydeoxyguanosine and its repair enzyme. *Dis. Esophagus* **2014**, *27*, 285–293. [CrossRef]
114. Walker, M.M.; Talley, N.J. Review article: Bacteria and pathogenesis of disease in the upper gastrointestinal tract–beyond the era of Helicobacter pylori. *Aliment. Pharmacol. Ther.* **2014**, *39*, 767–779. [CrossRef] [PubMed]
115. Klaunig, J.E.; Kamendulis, L.M.; Hocevar, B.A. Oxidative stress and oxidative damage in carcinogenesis. *Toxicol. Pathol.* **2010**, *38*, 96–109. [CrossRef] [PubMed]
116. Hodge, D.R.; Hurt, E.M.; Farrar, W.L. The role of IL-6 and STAT3 in inflammation and cancer. *Eur. J. Cancer* **2005**, *41*, 2502–2512. [CrossRef] [PubMed]
117. O'Sullivan, K.E.; Michielsen, A.J.; O'Regan, E.; Cathcart, M.C.; Moore, G.; Breen, E.; Segurado, R.; Reynolds, J.V.; Lysaght, J.; O'Sullivan, J. pSTAT3 Levels Have Divergent Expression Patterns and Associations with Survival in Squamous Cell Carcinoma and Adenocarcinoma of the Oesophagus. *Int. J. Mol. Sci.* **2018**, *19*, 1720. [CrossRef] [PubMed]
118. Abdel-Latif, M.M.; Kelleher, D.; Reynolds, J.V. Potential role of NF-kappaB in esophageal adenocarcinoma: As an emerging molecular target. *J. Surg. Res.* **2009**, *153*, 172–180. [CrossRef] [PubMed]
119. Łukaszewicz-Zając, M.; Pączek, S.; Muszyński, P.; Kozłowski, M.; Mroczko, B. Comparison between clinical significance of serum CXCL-8 and classical tumor markers in esophageal cancer (OC) patients. *Clin. Exp. Med.* **2019**, *19*, 191–199. [CrossRef] [PubMed]
120. Chen, M.F.; Lu, M.S.; Chen, P.T.; Chen, W.C.; Lin, P.Y.; Lee, K.D. Role of interleukin 1 beta in esophageal squamous cell carcinoma. *J. Mol. Med.* **2012**, *90*, 89–100. [CrossRef]
121. Piazuelo, E.; Jimenez, P.; Lanas, A. COX-2 inhibition in esophagitis, Barrett's esophagus and esophageal cancer. *Curr. Pharm. Des.* **2003**, *9*, 2267–2280. [CrossRef]
122. Ostrand-Rosenberg, S.; Sinha, P. Myeloid-derived suppressor cells: Linking inflammation and cancer. *J. Immunol.* **2009**, *182*, 4499–4506. [CrossRef]
123. Ha, T.Y. The role of regulatory T cells in cancer. *Immune Netw.* **2009**, *9*, 209–235. [CrossRef]
124. Curiel, T.J.; Coukos, G.; Zou, L.; Alvarez, X.; Cheng, P.; Mottram, P.; Evdemon-Hogan, M.; Conejo-Garcia, J.R.; Zhang, L.; Burow, M.; et al. Specific recruitment of regulatory T cells in ovarian carcinoma fosters immune privilege and predicts reduced survival. *Nat. Med.* **2004**, *10*, 942–949. [CrossRef] [PubMed]

125. Gomez-Rodriguez, J.; Wohlfert, E.A.; Handon, R.; Meylan, F.; Wu, J.Z.; Anderson, S.M.; Kirby, M.R.; Belkaid, Y.; Schwartzberg, P.L. Itk-mediated integration of T cell receptor and cytokine signaling regulates the balance between Th17 and regulatory T cells. *J. Exp. Med.* **2014**, *211*, 529–543. [CrossRef] [PubMed]
126. Ohigashi, Y.; Sho, M.; Yamada, Y.; Tsurui, Y.; Hamada, K.; Ikeda, N.; Mizuno, T.; Yoriki, R.; Kashizuka, H.; Yane, K.; et al. Clinical significance of programmed death-1 ligand-1 and programmed death-1 ligand-2 expression in human esophageal cancer. *Clin. Cancer Res.* **2005**, *11*, 2947–2953. [CrossRef]
127. Huang, T.X.; Fu, L. The immune landscape of esophageal cancer. *Cancer Commun.* **2019**, *39*, 79. [CrossRef] [PubMed]
128. Koide, N.; Nishio, A.; Sato, T.; Sugiyama, A.; Miyagawa, S. Significance of macrophage chemoattractant protein-1 expression and macrophage infiltration in squamous cell carcinoma of the esophagus. *Am. J. Gastroenterol.* **2004**, *99*, 1667–1674. [CrossRef] [PubMed]
129. Noma, K.; Smalley, K.S.; Lioni, M.; Naomoto, Y.; Tanaka, N.; El-Deiry, W.; King, A.J.; Nakagawa, H.; Herlyn, M. The essential role of fibroblasts in esophageal squamous cell carcinoma-induced angiogenesis. *Gastroenterology* **2008**, *134*, 1981–1993. [CrossRef]
130. Wang, J.; Zhang, G.; Wang, J.; Wang, L.; Huang, X.; Cheng, Y. The role of cancer-associated fibroblasts in esophageal cancer. *J. Transl. Med.* **2016**, *14*, 30. [CrossRef]
131. Higashino, N.; Koma, Y.I.; Hosono, M.; Takase, N.; Okamoto, M.; Kodaira, H.; Nishio, M.; Shigeoka, M.; Kakeji, Y.; Yokozaki, H. Fibroblast activation protein-positive fibroblasts promote tumor progression through secretion of CCL2 and interleukin-6 in esophageal squamous cell carcinoma. *Lab. Investig.* **2019**, *99*, 777–792. [CrossRef]
132. Lazăr, D.C.; Avram, M.F.; Romoșan, I.; Cornianu, M.; Tăban, S.; Goldiș, A. Prognostic significance of tumor immune microenvironment and immunotherapy: Novel insights and future perspectives in gastric cancer. *World J. Gastroenterol.* **2018**, *24*, 3583–3616. [CrossRef]
133. Liu, X.; Xu, D.; Huang, C.; Guo, Y.; Wang, S.; Zhu, C.; Xu, J.; Zhang, Z.; Shen, Y.; Zhao, W.; et al. Regulatory T cells and M2 macrophages present diverse prognostic value in gastric cancer patients with different clinicopathologic characteristics and chemotherapy strategies. *J. Transl. Med.* **2019**, *17*, 192. [CrossRef]
134. Fu, M.; Gu, J.; Jiang, P.; Qian, H.; Xu, W.; Zhang, X. Exosomes in gastric cancer: Roles, mechanisms and applications. *Mol. Cancer* **2019**, *18*, 41. [CrossRef] [PubMed]
135. Ohshima, K.; Inoue, K.; Fujiwara, A.; Hatakeyama, K.; Kanto, K.; Watanabe, Y.; Muramatsu, K.; Fukuda, Y.; Ogura, S.; Yamaguchi, K.; et al. Let-7 microRNA family is selectively secreted into the extracellular environment via exosomes in a metastatic gastric cancer cell line. *PLoS ONE* **2010**, *5*, e13247. [CrossRef] [PubMed]
136. Pan, L.; Liang, W.; Fu, M.; Huang, Z.H.; Li, X.; Zhang, W.; Zhang, P.; Qian, H.; Jiang, P.C.; Xu, W.R.; et al. Exosomes-mediated transfer of long noncoding RNA ZFAS1 promotes gastric cancer progression. *J. Cancer Res. Clin. Oncol.* **2017**, *143*, 991–1004. [CrossRef]
137. Zhang, H.; Deng, T.; Liu, R.; Bai, M.; Zhou, L.; Wang, X.; Li, S.; Wang, X.; Yang, H.; Li, J.; et al. Exosome-delivered EGFR regulates liver microenvironment to promote gastric cancer liver metastasis. *Nat. Commun.* **2017**, *8*, 15016. [CrossRef] [PubMed]
138. Comoglio, P.M.; Trusolino, L.; Boccaccio, C. Known and novel roles of the MET oncogene in cancer: A coherent approach to targeted therapy. *Nat. Rev. Cancer* **2018**, *18*, 341–358. [CrossRef]
139. McGee, H.M.; Jiang, D.; Soto-Pantoja, D.R.; Nevler, A.; Giaccia, A.J.; Woodward, W.A. Targeting the Tumor Microenvironment in Radiation Oncology: Proceedings from the 2018 ASTRO-AACR Research Workshop. *Clin. Cancer Res.* **2019**, *25*, 2969–2974. [CrossRef] [PubMed]
140. Leblond, M.M.; Pérès, E.A.; Helaine, C. M2 Macrophages Are More Resistant Than M1 Macrophages Following Radiation Therapy in the Context of Glioblastoma. *Oncotarget* **2017**, *8*, 72597–72612. [CrossRef]
141. Vrána, D.; Matzenauer, M.; Neoral, Č.; Aujeský, R.; Vrba, R.; Melichar, B.; Rušarová, N.; Bartoušková, M.; Jankowski, J. From Tumor Immunology to Immunotherapy in Gastric and Esophageal Cancer. *Int. J. Mol. Sci.* **2018**, *20*, 13. [CrossRef]
142. Dittrich, C.; Kosty, M.; Jezdic, S.; Pyle, D.; Berardi, R.; Bergh, J.; El-Saghir, N.; Lotz, J.P.; Österlund, P.; Pavlidis, N.; et al. ESMO/ASCO Recommendations for a Global Curriculum in Medical Oncology Edition 2016. *ESMO Open* **2016**, *1*, e000097. [CrossRef]

143. Guideline Committee of the Korean Gastric Cancer Association (KGCA), Development Working Group & Review Panel. Korean Practice Guideline for Gastric Cancer 2018, An Evidence-based, Multi-disciplinary Approach. *J. Gastric Cancer* **2019**, *19*, 1–48, Erratum in **2019**, *19*, 372–373. [CrossRef]
144. Wang, F.H.; Shen, L.; Li, J.; Zhou, Z.W.; Liang, H.; Zhang, X.T.; Tang, L.; Xin, Y.; Jin, J.; Zhang, Y.J.; et al. The Chinese Society of Clinical Oncology (CSCO): Clinical guidelines for the diagnosis and treatment of gastric cancer. *Cancer Commun.* **2019**, *39*, 10. [CrossRef] [PubMed]
145. Kitagawa, Y.; Uno, T.; Oyama, T.; Kato, K.; Kato, H.; Kawakubo, H.; Kawamura, O.; Kusano, M.; Kuwano, H.; Takeuchi, H.; et al. Esophageal cancer practice guidelines 2017 edited by the Japan Esophageal Society: Part 1. *Esophagus* **2019**, *16*, 1–24. [CrossRef] [PubMed]
146. Kitagawa, Y.; Uno, T.; Oyama, T.; Kato, K.; Kato, H.; Kawakubo, H.; Kawamura, O.; Kusano, M.; Kuwano, H.; Takeuchi, H.; et al. Esophageal cancer practice guidelines 2017 edited by the Japan esophageal society: Part 2. *Esophagus* **2019**, *16*, 25–43. [CrossRef] [PubMed]
147. Thompson, E.D.; Zahurak, M.; Murphy, A.; Cornish, T.; Cuka, N.; Abdelfatah, E.; Yang, S.; Duncan, M.; Ahuja, N.; Taube, J.M.; et al. Patterns of PD-L1 expression and CD8 T cell infiltration in gastric adenocarcinomas and associated immune stroma. *Gut* **2017**, *66*, 794–801. [CrossRef]
148. Chuang, J.; Chao, J.; Hendifar, A.; Klempner, S.J.; Gong, J. Checkpoint inhibition in advanced gastroesophageal cancer: Clinical trial data, molecular subtyping, predictive biomarkers and the potential of combination therapies. *Transl. Gastroenterol. Hepatol.* **2019**, *4*, 63. [CrossRef]
149. Taieb, J.; Moehler, M.; Boku, N.; Ajani, J.A.; Yañez Ruiz, E.; Ryu, M.H.; Guenther, S.; Chand, V.; Bang, Y.J. Evolution of checkpoint inhibitors for the treatment of metastatic gastric cancers: Current status and future perspectives. *Cancer Treat. Rev.* **2018**, *66*, 104–113. [CrossRef]
150. Ono Pharmaceutical Co Ltd. Opdivo®(Nivolumab) Intravenous Infusion Approved in Taiwan for Supplemental Indication of Advanced or Recurrent Gastric Cancer or Gastro-Esophageal Junction Cancer. Available online: https://www.ono.co.jp/eng/news/pdf/sm_cn180123.pdf (accessed on 17 May 2019).
151. Ono Pharmaceutical Co Ltd. Opdivo®(Nivolumab) Intravenous Infusion Approved for Supplemental Indication of Advanced or Recurrent Gastric or Gastroesophageal Junction Adenocarcinoma and for Expanded use in Recurrent or Advanced Classical Hodgkin Lymphoma in South Korea. Available online: https://www.ono.co.jp/eng/news/pdf/sm_cn180326.pdf (accessed on 17 May 2019).
152. Shitara, K.; Özgüroğlu, M.; Bang, Y.J.; Di Bartolomeo, M.; Mandalà, M.; Ryu, M.H.; Fornaro, L.; Olesiński, T.; Caglevic, C.; Chung, H.C.; et al. KEYNOTE-061 investigators. Pembrolizumab versus paclitaxel for previously treated, advanced gastric or gastro-oesophageal junction cancer (KEYNOTE-061): A randomised, open-label, controlled, phase 3 trial. *Lancet* **2018**, *392*, 123–133. [CrossRef]
153. Wang, F.; Wei, X.L.; Wang, F.H.; Xu, N.; Shen, L.; Dai, G.H.; Yuan, X.L.; Chen, Y.; Yang, S.J.; Shi, J.H.; et al. Safety, efficacy and tumor mutational burden as a biomarker of overall survival benefit in chemo-refractory gastric cancer treated with toripalimab, a PD-1 antibody in phase Ib/II clinical trial NCT02915432. *Ann. Oncol.* **2019**, *30*, 1479–1486. [CrossRef]
154. Bang, Y.J.; Ruiz, E.Y.; Van Cutsem, E.; Lee, K.W.; Wyrwicz, L.; Schenker, M.; Alsina, M.; Ryu, M.H.; Chung, H.C.; Evesque, L.; et al. Phase III, randomised trial of avelumab versus physician's choice of chemotherapy as third-line treatment of patients with advanced gastric or gastro-oesophageal junction cancer: Primary analysis of JAVELIN Gastric 300. *Ann. Oncol.* **2018**, *29*, 2052–2060. [CrossRef]
155. Kelly, R.J.; Lee, J.; Bang, Y.J.; Almhanna, K.; Blum-Murphy, M.; Catenacci, D.V.T.; Chung, H.C.; Wainberg, Z.A.; Gibson, M.K.; Lee, K.W.; et al. Safety and Efficacy of Durvalumab and Tremelimumab Alone or in Combination in Patients with Advanced Gastric and Gastroesophageal Junction Adenocarcinoma. *Clin. Cancer Res.* **2020**, *26*, 846–854. [CrossRef]
156. Janjigian, Y.Y.; Bendell, J.; Calvo, E.; Kim, J.W.; Ascierto, P.A.; Sharma, P.; Ott, P.A.; Peltola, K.; Jaeger, D.; Evans, J.; et al. CheckMate-032 Study: Efficacy and Safety of Nivolumab and Nivolumab Plus Ipilimumab in Patients with Metastatic Esophagogastric Cancer. *J. Clin. Oncol.* **2018**, *36*, 2836–2844. [CrossRef]
157. Wind-Rotolo, M.; Gupta, M.; Comprelli, A.; Reilly, T.P.; Cassidy, J. The Fast Real-time Assessment of Combination Therapies in Immuno-ONcology (FRACTION) program: Innovative, high-throughput clinical screening of immunotherapies. *Eur. J. Cancer* **2018**, *103*, 259–266. [CrossRef]

158. Smyth, E.; Knödler, M.; Giraut, A.; Mauer, M.; Nilsson, M.; Van Grieken, N.; Wagner, A.D.; Moehler, M.; Lordick, F. VESTIGE: Adjuvant Immunotherapy in Patients With Resected Esophageal, Gastroesophageal Junction and Gastric Cancer Following Preoperative Chemotherapy With High Risk for Recurrence (N+ and/or R1): An Open Label Randomized Controlled Phase-2-Study. *Front. Oncol.* **2020**, *9*, 1320. [CrossRef] [PubMed]

159. Bang, Y.J.; Van Cutsem, E.; Fuchs, C.S.; Ohtsu, A.; Tabernero, J.; Ilson, D.H.; Hyung, W.J.; Strong, V.E.; Goetze, T.O.; Yoshikawa, T.; et al. KEYNOTE-585, Phase III study of perioperative chemotherapy with or without pembrolizumab for gastric cancer. *Future Oncol.* **2019**, *15*, 943–952. [CrossRef]

160. Al-Batran, S.; Pauligk, C.; Hofheinz, R.; Lorenzen, S.; Wicki, A.; Rheinhard Siebenhuener, A.; Schenk, M.; Welslau, M.; Heuer, V.; Goekkurt, E.; et al. Perioperative atezolizumab in combination with FLOT versus FLOT alone in patients with resectable esophagogastric adenocarcinoma: DANTE.; a randomized, open-label phase II trial of the German Gastric Group of the AIO and the SAKK. *J. Clin. Oncol.* **2019**, *37* (Suppl. 15), TPS4142. [CrossRef]

161. Arai, H.; Nakajima, T.E. Recent Developments of Systemic Chemotherapy for Gastric Cancer. *Cancers* **2020**, *12*, 1100. [CrossRef]

162. Beeharry, M.K.; Zhang, T.Q.; Liu, W.T.; Gang, Z.Z. Optimization of perioperative approaches for advanced and late stages of gastric cancer: Clinical proposal based on literature evidence, personal experience and ongoing trials and research. *World J. Surg. Oncol.* **2020**, *18*, 51. [CrossRef] [PubMed]

163. Bang, Y.J.; Kaufman, B.; Geva, R.; Stemmer, S.M.; Hong, S.H.; Lee, J.S.; Domchek, S.M.; Lanasa, M.C.; Tang, M.; Gresty, C.; et al. An open-label, phase II basket study of olaparib and durvalumab (MEDIOLA): Results in patients with relapsed gastric cancer. *J. Clin. Oncol.* **2019**, *37* (Suppl. 4), 140. [CrossRef]

164. Bang, Y.J.; Golan, T.; Lin, C.C.; Kang, Y.K.; Wainberg, Z.A.; Wasserstrom, H.; Jin, J.; Mi, G.; McNeely, S.; Laing, N.; et al. Interim safety and clinical activity in patients (pts) with locally advanced and unresectable or metastatic gastric or gastroesophageal junction (G/GEJ) adenocarcinoma from a multicohort phase I study of ramucirumab (R) plus durvalumab (D). *J. Clin. Oncol.* **2018**, *36* (Suppl. 4), 92. [CrossRef]

165. Kudo, T.; Hamamoto, Y.; Kato, K.; Ura, T.; Kojima, T.; Tsushima, T.; Hironaka, S.; Hara, H.; Satoh, T.; Iwasa, S.; et al. Nivolumab treatment for oesophageal squamous-cell carcinoma: An open-label, multicentre, phase 2 trial. *Lancet Oncol.* **2017**, *18*, 631–639. [CrossRef]

166. Kang, Y.K.; Boku, N.; Satoh, T.; Ryu, M.H.; Chao, Y.; Kato, K.; Chung, H.C.; Chen, J.S.; Muro, K.; Kang, W.K.; et al. Nivolumab in patients with advanced gastric or gastro-oesophageal junction cancer refractory to or intolerant of, at least two previous chemotherapy regimens (ONO-4538-12, ATTRACTION-2): A randomised, double-blind, placebo-controlled, phase 3 trial. *Lancet* **2017**, *390*, 2461–2471. [CrossRef]

167. Kato, K.; Cho, B.C.; Takahashi, M.; Okada, M.; Lin, C.Y.; Chin, K.; Kadowaki, S.; Ahn, M.J.; Hamamoto, Y.; Doki, Y.; et al. Nivolumab versus chemotherapy in patients with advanced oesophageal squamous cell carcinoma refractory or intolerant to previous chemotherapy (ATTRACTION-3): A multicentre, randomised, open-label, phase 3 trial. *Lancet Oncol.* **2019**, *20*, 1506–1517. [CrossRef]

168. Boku, N.; Ryu, M.H.; Kato, K.; Chung, H.C.; Minashi, K.; Lee, K.W.; Cho, H.; Kang, W.K.; Komatsu, Y.; Tsuda, M.; et al. Safety and efficacy of nivolumab in combination with S-1/capecitabine plus oxaliplatin in patients with previously untreated, unresectable, advanced or recurrent gastric/gastroesophageal junction cancer: Interim results of a randomized, phase II trial (ATTRACTION-4). *Ann. Oncol.* **2019**, *30*, 250–258. [CrossRef] [PubMed]

169. Muro, K.; Chung, H.C.; Shankaran, V.; Geva, R.; Catenacci, D.; Gupta, S.; Eder, J.P.; Golan, T.; Le, D.T.; Burtness, B.; et al. Pembrolizumab for patients with PD-L1-positive advanced gastric cancer (KEYNOTE-012): A multicentre, open-label, phase 1b trial. *Lancet Oncol.* **2016**, *17*, 717–726. [CrossRef]

170. Fuchs, C.S.; Doi, T.; Jang, R.W.; Muro, K.; Satoh, T.; Machado, M.; Sun, W.; Jalal, S.I.; Shah, M.A.; Metges, J.P.; et al. Safety and Efficacy of Pembrolizumab Monotherapy in Patients with Previously Treated Advanced Gastric and Gastroesophageal Junction Cancer: Phase 2 Clinical KEYNOTE-059 Trial. *JAMA Oncol.* **2018**, *4*, e180013. [CrossRef]

171. Shah, M.A.; Kojima, T.; Hochhauser, D.; Enzinger, P.; Raimbourg, J.; Hollebecque, A.; Lordick, F.; Kim, S.B.; Tajika, M.; Kim, H.T.; et al. Efficacy and Safety of Pembrolizumab for Heavily Pretreated Patients With Advanced, Metastatic Adenocarcinoma or Squamous Cell Carcinoma of the Esophagus: The Phase 2 KEYNOTE-180 Study. *JAMA Oncol.* **2019**, *5*, 546–550. [CrossRef] [PubMed]

172. Tabernero, J.; Van Cutsem, E.; Bang, Y.J.; Fuchs, C.S.; Wyrwicz, L.; Lee, K.W.; Kudaba, I.; Garrido, M.; Chung, H.C.; Salguero, C.H.R.; et al. Pembrolizumab with or without chemotherapy versus chemotherapy for advanced gastric or gastroesophageal junction (G/GEJ) adenocarcinoma: The phase III KEYNOTE-062 study. *J. Clin. Oncol.* **2019**, *37* (Suppl. 18), LBA4007. [CrossRef]

173. Gu, L.; Chen, M.; Guo, D.; Zhu, H.; Zhang, W.; Pan, J.; Zhong, X.; Li, X.; Qian, H.; Wang, X. PD-L1 and gastric cancer prognosis: A systematic review and meta-analysis. *PLoS ONE* **2017**, *12*, e0182692. [CrossRef]

174. Kim, J.; Kim, B.; Kang, S.Y.; Heo, Y.J.; Park, S.H.; Kim, S.T.; Kang, W.K.; Lee, J.; Kim, K.M. Tumor Mutational Burden Determined by Panel Sequencing Predicts Survival After Immunotherapy in Patients with Advanced Gastric Cancer. *Front. Oncol.* **2020**, *10*, 314. [CrossRef]

175. Yang, B.; Bai, J.; Shi, R.; Shao, X.; Yang, Y.; Jin, Y.; Che, X.; Zhang, Y.; Qu, X.; Liu, Y.; et al. TGFB2 serves as a link between epithelial-mesenchymal transition and tumor mutation burden in gastric cancer. *Int. Immunopharmacol.* **2020**, *84*, 106532. [CrossRef]

176. Qu, X.; Zhao, L.; Zhang, R.; Wei, Q.; Wang, M. Differential microRNA expression profiles associated with microsatellite status reveal possible epigenetic regulation of microsatellite instability in gastric adenocarcinoma. *Ann. Transl. Med.* **2020**, *8*, 484. [CrossRef] [PubMed]

177. Giampieri, R.; Maccaroni, E.; Mandolesi, A.; Del Prete, M.; Andrikou, K.; Faloppi, L.; Bittoni, A.; Bianconi, M.; Scarpelli, M.; Bracci, R.; et al. Mismatch repair deficiency may affect clinical outcome through immune response activation in metastatic gastric cancer patients receiving first-line chemotherapy. *Gastric. Cancer* **2017**, *20*, 156–163. [CrossRef] [PubMed]

178. Le, D.T.; Uram, J.N.; Wang, H.; Bartlett, B.R.; Kemberling, H.; Eyring, A.D.; Skora, A.D.; Luber, B.S.; Azad, N.S.; Laheru, D.; et al. PD-1 blockade in tumors with mismatch-repair deficiency. *N. Engl. J. Med.* **2015**, *372*, 2509–2520. [CrossRef] [PubMed]

179. Liu, X.; Choi, M.G.; Kim, K.; Kim, K.M.; Kim, S.T.; Park, S.H.; Cristescu, R.; Peter, S.; Lee, J. High PD-L1 expression in gastric cancer (GC) patients and correlation with molecular features. *Pathol. Res. Pract.* **2020**, *216*, 152881. [CrossRef]

180. Liu, S.; Liu, J.W.; Sun, L.P.; Gong, Y.H.; Xu, Q.; Jing, J.J.; Yuan, Y. Association of IL10 gene promoter polymorphisms with risks of gastric cancer and atrophic gastritis. *J. Int. Med. Res.* **2018**, *46*, 5155–5166. [CrossRef]

181. Li, J.; Chen, L.; Xiong, Y.; Zheng, X.; Xie, Q.; Zhou, Q.; Shi, L.; Wu, C.; Jiang, J.; Wang, H. Knockdown of PD-L1 in Human Gastric Cancer Cells Inhibits Tumor Progression and Improves the Cytotoxic Sensitivity to CIK Therapy. *Cell Physiol. Biochem.* **2017**, *41*, 907–920. [CrossRef]

182. Sahin, U.; Türeci, Ö. Personalized vaccines for cancer immunotherapy. *Science* **2018**, *359*, 1355–1360. [CrossRef]

183. Tanaka, F.; Fujie, T.; Tahara, K.; Mori, M.; Takesako, K.; Sette, A.; Celis, E.; Akiyoshi, T. Induction of antitumor cytotoxic T lymphocytes with a MAGE-3-encoded synthetic peptide presented by human leukocytes antigen-A24. *Cancer Res.* **1997**, *57*, 4465–4468.

184. Kono, K.; Rongcun, Y.; Charo, J.; Ichihara, F.; Celis, E.; Sette, A.; Appella, E.; Sekikawa, T.; Matsumoto, Y.; Kiessling, R. Identification of HER2/neu-derived peptide epitopes recognized by gastric cancer-specific cytotoxic T lymphocytes. *Int. J. Cancer* **1998**, *78*, 202–208. [CrossRef]

185. Rutkowska, A.; Stoczyńska-Fidelus, E.; Janik, K.; Włodarczyk, A.; Rieske, P. EGFRvIII: An Oncogene with Ambiguous Role. *J. Oncol.* **2019**, *2019*, 1092587. [CrossRef]

186. Higashihara, Y.; Kato, J.; Nagahara, A.; Izumi, K.; Konishi, M.; Kodani, T.; Serizawa, N.; Osada, T.; Watanabe, S. Phase I clinical trial of peptide vaccination with URLC10 and VEGFR1 epitope peptides in patients with advanced gastric cancer. *Int. J. Oncol.* **2014**, *44*, 662–668. [CrossRef] [PubMed]

187. Gang, Y.; Zhang, X.; He, Y.; Zheng, J.; Wu, K.; Ding, J.; Fan, D. Efficient induction of specific cytotoxic T lymphocytes against gastric adenocarcinoma by a survivin peptide. *Biochem. Cell Biol.* **2012**, *90*, 701–708. [CrossRef] [PubMed]

188. Lu, W.W.; Zhang, H.; Li, Y.M.; Ji, F. Gastric cancer-derived heat shock protein-gp96 peptide complex enhances dendritic cell activation. *World J. Gastroenterol.* **2017**, *23*, 4390–4398. [CrossRef] [PubMed]

189. Zhang, K.; Peng, Z.; Huang, X.; Qiao, Z.; Wang, X.; Wang, N.; Xi, H.; Cui, J.; Gao, Y.; Huang, X.; et al. Phase II Trial of Adjuvant Immunotherapy with Autologous Tumor-derived Gp96 Vaccination in Patients with Gastric Cancer. *J. Cancer* **2017**, *8*, 1826–1832. [CrossRef]

190. Ishigami, S.; Natsugoe, S.; Tokuda, K.; Nakajo, A.; Xiangming, C.; Iwashige, H.; Aridome, K.; Hokita, S.; Aikou, T. Clinical impact of intratumoral natural killer cell and dendritic cell infiltration in gastric cancer. *Cancer Lett.* **2000**, *159*, 103–108. [CrossRef]
191. Kreiter, S.; Selmi, A.; Diken, M.; Koslowski, M.; Britten, C.M.; Huber, C.; Türeci, O.; Sahin, U. Intranodal vaccination with naked antigen-encoding RNA elicits potent prophylactic and therapeutic antitumoral immunity. *Cancer Res.* **2010**, *70*, 9031–9040. [CrossRef]
192. Fotin-Mleczek, M.; Duchardt, K.M.; Lorenz, C.; Pfeiffer, R.; Ojkić-Zrna, S.; Probst, J.; Kallen, K.J. Messenger RNA-based vaccines with dual activity induce balanced TLR-7 dependent adaptive immune responses and provide antitumor activity. *J. Immunother.* **2011**, *34*, 1–15. [CrossRef]
193. Weide, B.; Carralot, J.P.; Reese, A.; Scheel, B.; Eigentler, T.K.; Hoerr, I.; Rammensee, H.G.; Garbe, C.; Pascolo, S. Results of the first phase I/II clinical vaccination trial with direct injection of mRNA. *J. Immunother.* **2008**, *31*, 180–188. [CrossRef]
194. Weide, B.; Pascolo, S.; Scheel, B.; Derhovanessian, E.; Pflugfelder, A.; Eigentler, T.K.; Pawelec, G.; Hoerr, I.; Rammensee, H.G.; Garbe, C. Direct injection of protamine-protected mRNA: Results of a phase 1/2 vaccination trial in metastatic melanoma patients. *J. Immunother.* **2009**, *32*, 498–507. [CrossRef]
195. Briquez, P.S.; Hauert, S.; de Titta, A.; Gray, L.T.; Alpar, A.T.; Swartz, M.A.; Hubbell, J.A. Engineering Targeting Materials for Therapeutic Cancer Vaccines. *Front. Bioeng. Biotechnol.* **2020**, *8*, 19. [CrossRef]
196. Pardi, N.; Hogan, M.J.; Porter, F.W.; Weissman, D. mRNA vaccines—A new era in vaccinology. *Nat. Rev. Drug Discov.* **2018**, *17*, 261–279. [CrossRef] [PubMed]
197. Pfirschke, C.; Engblom, C.; Rickelt, S.; Cortez-Retamozo, V.; Garris, C.; Pucci, F.; Yamazaki, T.; Poirier-Colame, V.; Newton, A.; Redouane, Y.; et al. Immunogenic Chemotherapy Sensitizes Tumors to Checkpoint Blockade Therapy. *Immunity* **2016**, *44*, 343–354. [CrossRef]
198. Nolan, E.; Savas, P.; Policheni, A.N.; Darcy, P.K.; Vaillant, F.; Mintoff, C.P.; Dushyanthen, S.; Mansour, M.; Pang, J.B.; Fox, S.B.; et al. Combined immune checkpoint blockade as a therapeutic strategy for BRCA1-mutated breast cancer. *Sci. Transl. Med.* **2017**, *9*, eaal4922. [CrossRef] [PubMed]
199. Ochiai, T.; Sato, H.; Hayashi, R.; Asano, T.; Sato, H.; Yamamura, Y. Postoperative adjuvant immunotherapy of gastric cancer with BCG-cell wall skeleton. 3- to 6-year follow up of a randomized clinical trial. *Cancer Immunol. Immunother.* **1983**, *14*, 167–171. [CrossRef] [PubMed]
200. Ajani, J.A.; Hecht, J.R.; Ho, L.; Baker, J.; Oortgiesen, M.; Eduljee, A.; Michaeli, D. An open-label, multinational, multicenter study of G17DT vaccination combined with cisplatin and 5-fluorouracil in patients with untreated, advanced gastric or gastroesophageal cancer: The GC4 study. *Cancer* **2006**, *106*, 1908–1916. [CrossRef] [PubMed]
201. Masuzawa, T.; Fujiwara, Y.; Okada, K.; Nakamura, A.; Takiguchi, S.; Nakajima, K.; Miyata, H.; Yamasaki, M.; Kurokawa, Y.; Osawa, R.; et al. Phase I/II study of S-1 plus cisplatin combined with peptide vaccines for human vascular endothelial growth factor receptor 1 and 2 in patients with advanced gastric cancer. *Int. J. Oncol.* **2012**, *41*, 1297–1304. [CrossRef]
202. Chao, Y.; Yau, T.; Maglakelidze, M.; Bulat, I.; Tanasanvimon, S.; Charoentum, C.; Arpornwirat, W.; Maneechavakajorn, J.; Dechaphunkul, A.; Ungtrakul, T.; et al. A phase Ib study of IMU-131 HER2/neu peptide vaccine plus chemotherapy in patients with HER2/neu overexpressing metastatic or advanced adenocarcinoma of the stomach or gastroesophageal junction. *J. Clin. Oncol.* **2019**, *37* (Suppl. 15), 4030. [CrossRef]
203. Van den Engel, N.K.; Rüttinger, D.; Rusan, M.; Kammerer, R.; Zimmermann, W.; Hatz, R.A.; Winter, H. Combination immunotherapy and active-specific tumor cell vaccination augments anti-cancer immunity in a mouse model of gastric cancer. *J. Transl. Med.* **2011**, *9*, 140. [CrossRef]
204. Maus, M.V.; Fraietta, J.A.; Levine, B.L.; Kalos, M.; Zhao, Y.; June, C.H. Adoptive immunotherapy for cancer or viruses. *Annu. Rev. Immunol.* **2014**, *32*, 189–225. [CrossRef]
205. Kono, K.; Mimura, K.; Kiessling, R. Immunogenic tumor cell death induced by chemoradiotherapy: Molecular mechanisms and a clinical translation. *Cell Death Dis.* **2013**, *4*, e688. [CrossRef]
206. Martinez, M.; Moon, E.K. CAR T Cells for Solid Tumors: New Strategies for Finding, Infiltrating and Surviving in the Tumor Microenvironment. *Front. Immunol.* **2019**, *10*, 128. [CrossRef] [PubMed]
207. Luo, F.; Qian, J.; Yang, J.; Deng, Y.; Zheng, X.; Liu, J.; Chu, Y. Bifunctional αHER2/CD3 RNA-engineered CART-like human T cells specifically eliminate HER2(+) gastric cancer. *Cell Res.* **2016**, *26*, 850–853. [CrossRef] [PubMed]

208. Low, P.S.; Kularatne, S.A. Folate-targeted therapeutic and imaging agents for cancer. *Curr. Opin. Chem. Biol.* **2009**, *13*, 256–262. [CrossRef] [PubMed]
209. Kim, M.; Pyo, S.; Kang, C.H.; Lee, C.O.; Lee, H.K.; Choi, S.U.; Park, C.H. Folate receptor 1 (FOLR1) targeted chimeric antigen receptor (CAR) T cells for the treatment of gastric cancer. *PLoS ONE* **2018**, *13*, e0198347. [CrossRef] [PubMed]
210. Wu, D.; Lv, J.; Zhao, R.; Wu, Z.; Zheng, D.; Shi, J.; Lin, S.; Wang, S.; Wu, Q.; Long, Y.; et al. PSCA is a target of chimeric antigen receptor T cells in gastric cancer. *Biomark. Res.* **2020**, *8*, 3. [CrossRef]
211. Lv, J.; Zhao, R.; Wu, D.; Zheng, D.; Wu, Z.; Shi, J.; Wei, X.; Wu, Q.; Long, Y.; Lin, S.; et al. Mesothelin is a target of chimeric antigen receptor T cells for treating gastric cancer. *J. Hematol. Oncol.* **2019**, *12*, 18. [CrossRef]
212. Shi, H.; Yu, F.; Mao, Y.; Ju, Q.; Wu, Y.; Bai, W.; Wang, P.; Xu, R.; Jiang, M.; Shi, J. EphA2 chimeric antigen receptor-modified T cells for the immunotherapy of esophageal squamous cell carcinoma. *J. Thorac. Dis.* **2018**, *10*, 2779–2788. [CrossRef]
213. Zhao, W.; Jia, L.; Zhang, M.; Huang, X.; Qian, P.; Tang, Q.; Zhu, J.; Feng, Z. The killing effect of novel bi-specific Trop2/PD-L1 CAR-T cell targeted gastric cancer. *Am. J. Cancer Res.* **2019**, *9*, 1846–1856.

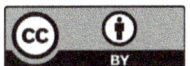

© 2020 by the authors. Licensee MDPI, Basel, Switzerland. This article is an open access article distributed under the terms and conditions of the Creative Commons Attribution (CC BY) license (http://creativecommons.org/licenses/by/4.0/).

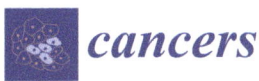

Article

Preservation of Organ Function in Locally Advanced Non-Metastatic Gastrointestinal Stromal Tumors (GIST) of the Stomach by Neoadjuvant Imatinib Therapy

Nikolaos Vassos [1,2], Jens Jakob [3], Georg Kähler [2], Peter Reichardt [4], Alexander Marx [5], Antonia Dimitrakopoulou-Strauss [6], Nils Rathmann [7], Eva Wardelmann [8] and Peter Hohenberger [1,*]

1. Mannheim University Medical Center, Division of Surgical Oncology and Thoracic Surgery, University of Heidelberg, 68167 Mannheim, Germany; nikolaos.vassos@umm.de
2. Mannheim University Medical Center, Department of Surgery, University of Heidelberg, 68167 Mannheim, Germany; georg.kaehler@umm.de
3. Department of General, Visceral and Pediatric Surgery, University Medical Center Göttingen, 37073 Göttingen, Germany; jens.jakob@med.uni-goettingen.de
4. Department of Oncology and Palliative Care, Helios Klinikum Berlin-Buch, 13125 Berlin, Germany; peter.reichardt@helios-gesundheit.de
5. Mannheim University Medical Center, Institute of Pathology, University of Heidelberg, 68167 Mannheim, Germany; alexander.marx@umm.de
6. German Cancer Research Center (DKFZ), Clinical Cooperation Unit Nuclear Medicine, 69210 Heidelberg, Germany; a.dimitrakopoulou-strauss@dkfz.de
7. Institute of Clinical Radiology and Nuclear Medicine, Mannheim University Medical Center Mannheim, University of Heidelberg, 68167 Mannheim, Germany; nils.rathmann@umm.de
8. Gerhard-Domagk-Institute of Pathology, University Hospital Münster, 48149 Münster, Germany; eva.wardelmann@ukmuenster.de
* Correspondence: peter.hohenberger@umm.de; Tel.: +49-621-383-2609 or +49-621-383-2447; Fax: +49-621-383-1479

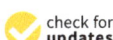

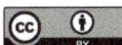

Simple Summary: This study reports a single-center analysis of 55 patients with primary, locally advanced gastric GIST treated with imatinib mesylate (IM) preoperatively for a median of 10 months. The therapy yielded shrinkage of median tumor size from 113 mm to 62 mm. This facilitated 50 patients to undergo significantly less-extensive surgical procedures and resulted in a stomach preservation rate of 96%. The rate of R0 resections was 94% and was followed by a mean recurrence-free-survival time of 132 months with the median not reached. The approach was successful even for patients starting IM during an episode of upper gastrointestinal bleeding. Neoadjuvant IM therapy for locally advanced, non-metastatic gastrointestinal stromal tumors (GIST) of the stomach may play an important role in preserving organ function which might be important for IM plasma levels in an adjuvant or metastatic setting.

Abstract: Background: Neoadjuvant imatinib mesylate (IM) for advanced, non-metastatic gastrointestinal stromal tumors (GIST) of stomach is recommended to downsize the tumor prompting less-extensive operations and preservation of organ function. Methods: We analyzed the clinical-histopathological profile and oncological outcome of 55 patients (median age 58.2 years; range, 30–86 years) with biopsy-proven, cM0, gastric GIST who underwent IM therapy followed by surgery with a median follow-up of 82 months. Results: Initial median tumor size was 113 mm (range, 65–330 mm) and 10 patients started with acute upper GI bleeding. After a median 10 months (range, 2–21 months) of treatment, tumor size had shrunk to 62 mm (range, 22–200 mm). According to Response Evaluation Criteria In Solid Tumors version 1.0 and version 1.1 (RECIST 1.1), 39 (75%) patients had partial response and 14 patients had stable disease, with no progressive disease. At plateau response, 50 patients underwent surgery with an R0 resection rate of 94% and pathological complete response in 24%. In 12 cases (24%), downstaging allowed laparoscopic resection. The mean recurrence-free survival (RFS) was 123 months (95%CI; 99–147) and the estimated 5-year RFS was 84%. Conclusions: Neoadjuvant IM allowed stomach preservation in 96% of our patients with excellent long-term RFS, even when starting treatment during an episode of upper GI bleeding.

Preservation of the stomach provides the physiological basis for the use of oral IM in the adjuvant or metastatic setting.

Keywords: gastrointestinal stromal tumor; GIST; stomach; neoadjuvant therapy; imatinib; organ preservation

1. Introduction

Gastrointestinal stromal tumors (GISTs) are the most common mesenchymal tumors of the gastrointestinal tract, arising mostly in the stomach [1,2]. GISTs exhibit a broad spectrum of clinical behavior [2–4] and are characteristically driven by activating mutations of KIT- or platelet-derived growth factor receptor-a (PDGFR-a) gene in approximately 85–90% of cases [5,6]. Surgery was the mainstay of curative treatment of GIST [7,8]. Since 2001, the natural history of GISTs has been dramatically altered through the use of imatinib mesylate (IM), a receptor tyrosine kinase inhibitor of KIT [9–11]. Imatinib is approved for treatment of metastatic or unresectable GISTs and for adjuvant therapy after R0 resection of GIST with significant risk of metastatic spread [11,12].

Although the majority of GISTs are resectable at presentation, a significant number of GISTs are either locally advanced, requiring challenging and complex operations which can lead to postoperative morbidity [3], or the tumors also might present as primarily not resectable with clear margins; however, debulking procedures are difficult to perform due to the high vascularity of growing GIST lesions [13]. In GIST of the stomach, adopting the standard therapy of epithelial gastric cancer, i.e., total gastrectomy may produce a conflict with adjuvant therapy as imatinib plasma levels are significantly below the therapeutic threshold [14].

The use of IM in the neoadjuvant setting can play an important role by downsizing the tumor, in this way decreasing the extent of resection (i.e., organ-preserving operation) [15–25]. Particularly in cases of gastric GISTs, neoadjuvant IM therapy may also convert surgical procedures from an open to a laparoscopic approach.

The purpose of this study was to evaluate the clinic-pathological profile and the surgical and oncological outcomes of patients with gastric GIST who underwent a neoadjuvant IM therapy followed by surgery from a prospectively kept database. We particularly were interested in analyzing a subgroup of patients who had started neoadjuvant therapy in the clinical setting of acute upper GI bleeding from imatinib-sensitive gastric GIST.

2. Material and Methods

2.1. Patient Selection

From November 2002 to December 2019, 989 patients with histologically proven GIST were treated by one therapeutic surgical team (PH). Of these, 476 patients had the primary GIST originating from the stomach(Figure 1). In addition to a prospective phase II neoadjuvant study (NCT00112632) [23], we subjected patients who had locally advanced, histopathologically proven gastric GISTs to the similar protocol. The indication was given when patients would have required extensive surgeries (total gastrectomy or multivisceral resection) for curative treatment or when the tumors were ill-located (e.g., GIST at the esophagogastric junction) requiring an abdomino-thoracic approach [26]. Patients with metastatic disease at time of diagnosis or patients treated because of local recurrence of gastric GIST were not included in this analysis.

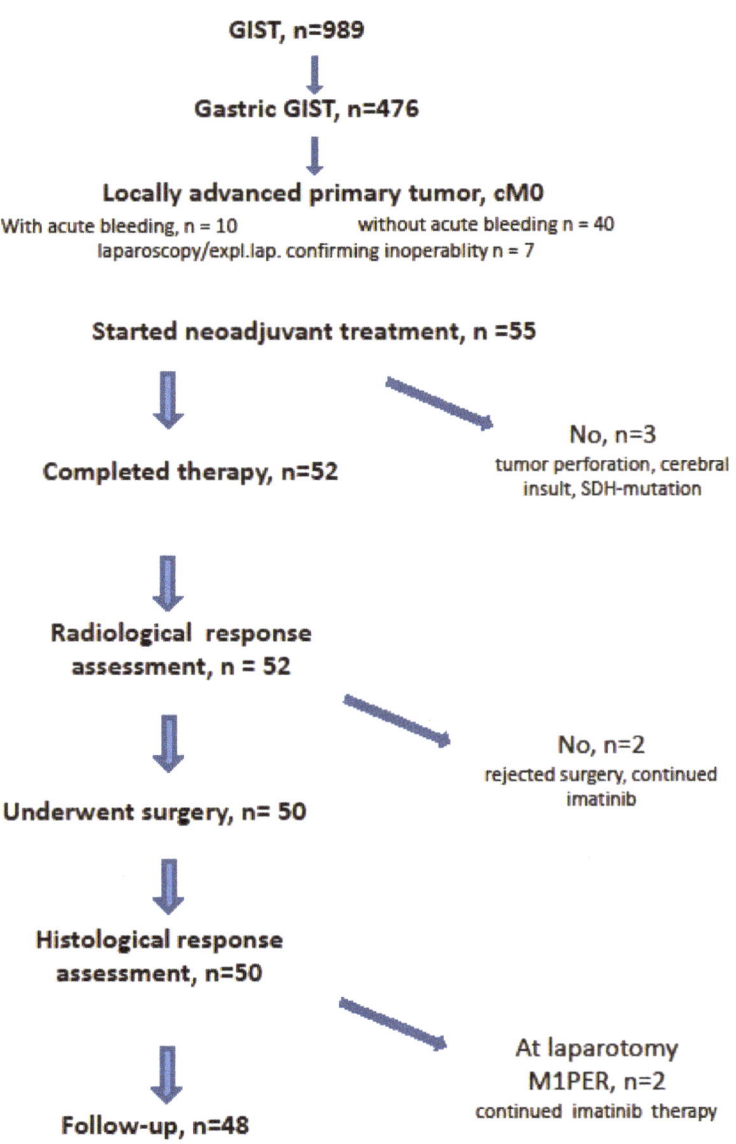

Figure 1. CONSORT statement.

2.2. Clinical Condition

Only seven patients (12.7%) were asymptomatic and the tumor was detected incidentally (Figure 2). Seven patients had already undergone an exploration (exploratory laparotomy ($n = 3$) or diagnostic laparoscopy ($n = 4$)) at another hospital declaring inoperability or tumor resection with only multivisceral procedure and therefore had been referred to our institution.

It is of note that in 10 patients (18.2%), the GIST was diagnosed due to an acute upper GI bleeding. When there was suspicion on endoscopy and abdominal CT scan, we immediately started with imatinib after endoscopical control of the bleeding and tumor biopsy. Patients who suffered from subacute melena or occult fecal bleeding prompting the diagnosis of GIST were subsumed in the subgroup of tumor-specific symptoms.

Gender and Age

Males   n=33, median 56.3 yrs (range, 33-78 yrs.)

Females   n=22, median 61.5 yrs (range, 30-86 yrs.)

Symptoms at diagnosis

Asymptomatic (incidental finding)   n= 7 (12.7%)

Unspecific symptoms   n=23 (41.8%)

Tumor-specific symptoms   n=15 (27.3%)

Urging (acute upper GI bleeding)   n=10 (18.2%)

Operability

Prior laparotomy/laparoscopy rendering the patient inoperable   n=7

Mutational status   exon 11 deletion involving codon 557/558   n=16

exon 11 point mutation   n=13

exon 11 duplications, insertions and combinations n=16

exon 13 K642E   n= 1

exon 9 mutation   n= 1

no mutation detectable on biopsy/resection specimen   n= 8

Response monitoring by 18F-FDG-PET

yes   n=17

no   n=38

Figure 2. Demographic, clinical and histopathological data.

2.3. Imatinib Mesylate Therapy and Response Assessment

The treatment plan of each patient was managed by a multidisciplinary GIST team consisting of surgical oncologists, medical oncologists, pathologists and radiologists. Before treatment started, tumor biopsy was obtained and all patients had confirmed diagnosis of GIST. Mutation analysis was always carried-out when enough tissue material was available. Risk stratification into very low, low, intermediate and high risk followed the NIH-Fletcher criteria for GIST risk assessment [1].

Imatinib was given orally at 400 mg per day, as a single daily dosing; one patient with KIT exon 9 mutation received 800 mg of imatinib. The duration of IM therapy was intended to last 6 months or as long as the tumor was still shrinking in size.

Response to neoadjuvant IM therapy was evaluated 1 month after the treatment start and then every 3 months either with positron emission computed tomography (PET-CT), dual-energy computed tomography (DE-CT) or contrast-enhanced magnetic resonance imaging (CE-MRI). PET imaging was only used to make sure that the tumor would respond to imatinib. Thus, it was of importance in the earlier patients when the results of mutational analysis took longer than it does today. Response was determined according to the Response Evaluation Criteria In Solid Tumors version 1.0 and version 1.1 (RECIST 1.1) as a complete response (CR), partial response (PR), stable disease (SD) or progressive disease (PD) [27].

2.4. Conduct of Surgery

Based on the imaging data, removal of the residual tumor was indicated when the maximum therapeutic response was reached (no further reduction in tumor diameters in consecutive imagings of 3 months) or when no further influence on the resectional strategy was expected. A margin of safety of 1 cm was considered enough to spare organ function [28]. The type of surgery was classified according to EORTC STBSG classification: local excision (wedge resection), limited resection (partial resection of the stomach), typical organ resection (total gastrectomy) and multivisceral resection (including adjacent organs) or other (with verbal specification) [29]. Postoperative complications were classified using the Clavien–Dindo classification [30].

The extent of tumor regression was measured at the resection specimen. Complete remission was defined as 100% necrosis (complete absence of viable tumor cells), a near total remission was defined as 95–99% necrosis, subtotal 90–95%, partial remission with 50–90% necrosis and stable disease with <50% necrosis. Resection margin status was defined as R0, R1 and R2 [31].

2.5. Postoperative Drug Therapy

There was no stringent policy regarding drug treatment after residual tumor resection. We did not continue imatinib in patients with >95% regression of the tumor and discussed further drug therapy on an individual basis.

2.6. Follow-Up

Postoperative follow-up consisted of a physical examination and acquisition of DE-CT at 3-month intervals for the first 2 years, every 6 months for the next 3 years and yearly thereafter for the next 5 years. Recurrence was defined as recurrent disease in the region of the previously located tumor. Metastasis was defined as disease in distant sites, predominantly liver and peritoneum. All patients were followed-up for a median of 82 months (range, 3–182 months) and were last updated in June 2020.

2.7. Statistical Analysis

The statistical analysis of the prospectively maintained database was performed with SPSS (version 21). Survival outcomes in terms of RFS was analyzed. RFS was calculated from the date of surgical resection to the date of clinical or radiological evidence of disease relapse, last follow-up or death, whichever occurred first. RFS percentages and treatment effect comparisons were obtained from the Kaplan–Meier method [32] and log-rank test [33]. Date is given as median with range or mean +/− standard deviation. Correlative analytics were obtained by Pearson and Spearman rank-coefficient tests. Differences were considered statistically significant when $p \leq 0.05$.

3. Results
3.1. Demographic and Clinicopathological Data

Fifty-five patients (22f, 33m) with a median age of 58.2 years, (range, 30–86 years) were included in this study (Table 1). Detailed demographic, clinical and histopathological data are listed in Table 1. The median tumor size before start of imatinib was 113 mm (range, 65–330 mm). Mitotic index could be determined in 41 patients (75%); in the remaining patients the size of the biopsy did not allow us to count enough high-power fields (HPFs). According to National Institutes of Health (NIH) consensus [1], the risk classification was "high risk" in 26 patients (48%), "intermediate risk" in 15 patients (28%) and "low risk" in 13 patients (24%).

Table 1. Analysis of Response Data.

Tumor Size			
Tumor size at start of treatment:	113 mm (range, 65–330 mm) (measured by CT/MRI)		
Tumor size prior to surgery:	69 mm (range, 25–228 mm) (measured by CT/MRI)		
Tumor size at resection specimen:	62 mm (range, 22–200 mm) (measured by pathology)		
Pathology Review of the Resection Specimen			
Complete necrosis (no viable tumor cells)	n = 12 (24%)		
Near total (>95% necrosis)	n = 10 (20%)		
Subtotal (>90% necrosis)	n = 7 (14%)		
Partial remission (>50% necrosis)	n = 14 (28%)		
Stable disease (<50% necrosis)	n = 7 (14%)		
Correlation of Response to Therapy (Pearson, Two-Sided; Spearman)			
Δtumor diameter pre vs. post		$p = 0.078$	$p = 0.089$
RECIST 1.1		$p = 0.2$	$p = 0.21$
Mutational type exon 11		$p = 0.04$	$p = 0.037$
	point mutation del involving codons 557_558 others		

3.2. Mutational Data

Mutation analysis was performed in 49 patients and showed exon 11 mutation in 47 patients with the majority of the mutations consisting of deletions involving codons 557 and 558 (n = 15) or point mutation (n = 12) (Table 1). In one patient, a SDHB mutation was determined after 2 months of imatinib and the patient was operated on immediately. In six patients mutation analysis could not be carried out from the biopsy and even at the resection specimen it was not feasible due to complete tumor necrosis and significant tumor shrinkage. In another patient who had significant tumor shrinkage, a K642E mutation at KIT exon 13 was found with NGS-sequencing from the residual tumor mass.

3.3. Imatinib Therapy and Clinical Response

The median time of preoperative imatinib therapy was 10 months (range, 2–21 months) and 52 patients (94.5%) completed the expected treatment duration. Among the patients who did not complete therapy there was the patient with the SDHB mutation whose treatment had to be stopped and a male patient of 69 years (with a history of vascular occlusive disease) who died from a cerebral insult 3 weeks after start of imatinib. Another patient developed perforation of the tumor, located at the posterior part of the stomach, 8 weeks after start of treatment due to extensive tumor regression. He underwent emergency subtotal gastrectomy, partial resection of the diaphragm and splenectomy. Another patient experienced grade 3 skin toxicity which could be resolved by switching therapy to nilotinib. Grade 2 side effects included skin toxicity (n = 1) and depression (n = 2).

The median tumor size prior to surgery shrank to 62 mm (range, 22–200 mm). According to RECIST 1.1, 39 patients had a PR (75%) while 14 patients had SD (25%) and no patient had progressive disease, see Table 1.

All 10 patients who started neoadjuvant therapy with acute upper GI bleeding experienced no further episode of bleeding and completed their drug schedule until surgery.

3.4. Surgical Data

Fifty patients underwent surgery after achieving the plateau response. Except for the patient who experienced tumor perforation, all others were operated on at the intended date. Two patients refused surgery. Of these two, one patient preferred to continue with imatinib while another one committed suicide.

At laparotomy, in two patients previously undetected peritoneal metastases were found at the bursa omentalis and the omentum. In 48 patients, total gastrectomy or abdomino-thoracic resection could be avoided, resulting in a stomach preservation rate of 96% (see Figures 3 and 4). The details of the surgical procedures are illustrated in Figure 4 (e.g., treatment option before IM vs. surgical procedure after IM). In 12 cases (24%), the downstaging of the tumor allowed a laparoscopic procedure instead of open laparotomy.

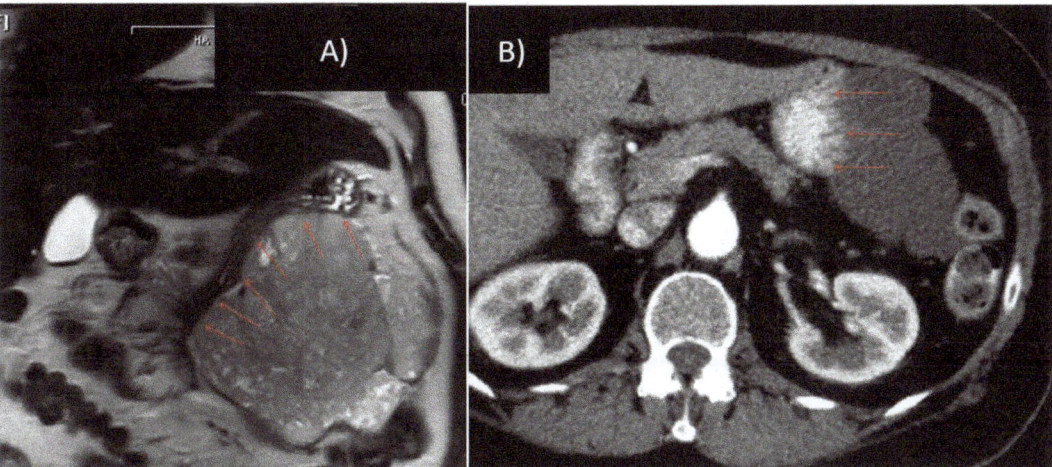

Figure 3. 76 year old female, gastrointestinal stromal tumors (GIST) with broad contact to the greater curvature, scheduled for total gastrectomy, left hemicolectomy and left-sided pancreatico-/splenectomy (**A**) prior to and (**B**) after 10 months of imatinib therapy.

All patients having undergone prior exploratory laparotomy and declared inoperable ($n = 3$) could be resected with clear margins by multivisceral (MVR) total gastrectomy, total gastrectomy alone and subtotal gastrectomy in one patient each. In the four patients who had prior diagnostic laparoscopy (MVR only), segmental resection with Merendino reconstruction ($n = 1$), subtotal ($n = 1$) or segmental ($n = 1$) gastric resection, and MVR ($n = 1$) had to carried out for R0 tumor removal.

Surgical complications were observed in seven patients (14%) and included postoperative pancreatic fistula ($n = 2$), surgical site hemorrhage ($n = 2$), prolonged pleural effusion ($n = 2$) and wound infection ($n = 1$). Of them, three patients required intervention (grade 3 Clavien–Dindo). None of these patients required reoperation and there was no postoperative mortality.

3.5. Histopathological Data

Except for the two patients with peritoneal metastases (R2 resection), only in one patient was an R1 resection stated by the pathologist, resulting in an R0 resection rate of 47/50 patients (94%).

The final histopathological report showed no residual viable tumor (pCR) in 12 cases (24%); for details see Table 1. Interestingly, in seven cases there was a less than 50% necrosis observed, despite the fact that even in this subgroup the median tumor size shrank from 84 mm (range, 65–122 mm) to 60 mm (range, 22–115 mm).

Only the mutational type correlates significantly ($p = 0.037$) with the extent of tumor regression. There was no significant relationship of RECIST classification to the difference in tumor size from prior to imatinib vs. post-imatinib (Table 1). The difference between tumor size prior to imatinib vs. at the resection specimen exceeded $p = 0.05$.

Patients scheduled for total gastrectomy/multivisceral resection (n=24)
- multivisceral TG   n= 2
- multivisceral PG   n= 6
- segmental resection of the stomach   n= 10
- laparoscopic partial gastric resection   n= 6

Patients scheduled for abdomino-thoracic gastric-esophageal resection (n=13)
- abd.-thoracic proximal gastric/esophageal resection   n= 1
- segmental resection + Merendino reconstruction   n= 4
- resection of the gastric fundus   n= 6
- laparoscopic wedge gastric resection   n= 2

Patients scheduled for subtotal/near-total gastrectomy (n=13)
- segmental gastric resection + transverse mesocolon   n= 2
- segmental gastric resection + liver segment 2   n= 1
- open segmental or transgastric resection   n= 4
- laparoscopic wedge gastric resection   n= 6

*TG=total gastrectomy, sTG = subtotal gastrectomy, PG=partial/segmental gastrectomy, multivisceral means left-sided resection of the pancreas +/- splenectomy +/- colonic segment +/- partial resection of the diaphragm (without allograft replacement)

Figure 4. Comparison of scheduled surgery prior to imatinib vs. surgical procedure performed after neoadjuvant therapy.

3.6. Recurrence-Free Survival

Of the 50 patients operated, 34 (68%) are alive with no evidence of disease. The most common sites at detection of distant metastases were peritoneum ($n = 7$) and liver ($n = 6$), both combined ($n = 2$), while one patient developed a locoregional recurrence at the surgical site. Three patients have died from their disease, and another four patients from other causes.

Kaplan–Meier curve (Figure 5) demonstrates a mean recurrence-free survival of 123 months (95%CI 99–147 months) with the median not yet reached.

We evaluated prognostic factors with respect to the influence on RFS. However, no statistically significant result could be obtained from initial tumor size ($p = 0.34$), mutational type ($p = 0.86$) and mitotic count ($p = 0.12$). Furthermore, the most logical factor (extent of tumor necrosis) was not proven to be of significant influence ($p = 0.33$, all log-rank).

With respect to adjuvant imatinib therapy after residual tumor removal, the single patient who experienced tumor perforation continued with imatinib and is free from recurrence after 12 years. Another seven patients were recommended to continue with imatinib therapy in order to complete a 36 months total duration of neoadjuvant plus adjuvant drug therapy. Of these, three patients developed hepatic and/or peritoneal metastases and died from their disease after multiple lines of therapy. Another two patients completed 3 years with no evidence of recurrence, one patient chose to stick with the drug until now and one patient is still in the completion phase.

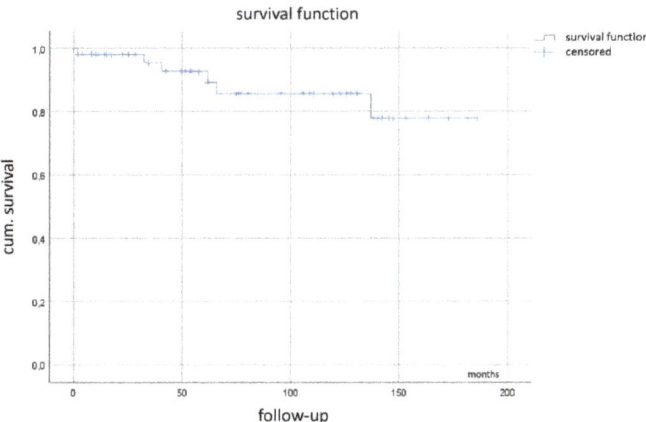

Figure 5. Recurrence-free survival.

4. Discussion

Surgery for primary GIST of the stomach is different from surgery for epithelial gastric cancer. Detailed lymphadenectomy, the mainstay to treat gastric carcinoma, is not required except in a subgroup of patients with Carney–Stratakis syndrome or SDH-deficient tumors presenting typically in young females [34]. On the other hand, GISTs originating from the muscularis layer of the intestine tend to grow luminally with potential acute bleeding or exophytically towards the surrounding organs. As GIST may be a fragile mass and often represents a highly vascularized lesion, larger gastric GIST may require more extended surgery with major morbidity and functional deficits due to the proximity to vital structures or the location in difficult sites (e.g., gastroesophageal junction). This may be the indication for imatinib therapy prior to surgery as recommended by several guidelines [35]. The neoadjuvant administration of IM turns out to be beneficial for patients with locally advanced or marginally resectable, non-metastatic GIST. Proper selection of candidates for neoadjuvant therapy is the prerequisite for successful therapy and requires tumor genotyping based on preoperative biopsy with the mutational spectrum not different from the metastatic situation [36]. In our study, all patients were either diagnosed with imatinib-sensitive mutations of *KIT* or we used ^{18}F-FDG-PET to make sure the expected efficacy would really take place. This was particularly the case in the earlier patients when mutational analysis took more time than today [37,38].

The few formal trials on preoperative imatinib therapy often include both locally advanced and metastatic patients with GIST arising from the whole GI tract [15,21,24,36,39–42]. In the RTOG study [24] only 15 patients were truly treated under neoadjuvant conditions across all locations. Thus, our series comprises the largest patient cohort of locally advanced, non-metastatic gastric GIST patients treated with neoadjuvant IM therapy followed by surgery. Large GISTs carry an increased risk of intraoperative tumor rupture and dissemination because of their fragility and hypervascularity which has a detrimental effect on disease-free status and overall survival [43–46]. Beyond the organ-saving approach through objective tumor downsizing, preoperative imatinib also improves the integrity of tumor capsule and decreases the risk of intraperitoneal bleeding/tumor perforation, leading to a very high rate of R0 resections [21,46]. We demonstrate a significant regression of median tumor size from 11.3 cm to 6.2 cm, which reflects the main advantage of imatinib as induction therapy in patients with locally advanced GIST. Particularly the subgroup of 10 patients (18.2%) with upper GI bleeding from the tumor profited from this approach. None of them had to be operated on prematurely due to a recurrent bleeding episode and the surgical tumor resection could be moved from an emergency procedure to an elective operation. No postoperative imatinib-related complications were observed.

The approach provided an excellent oncological long-term result. Based on the NIH consensus criteria [1], 48% of the patients could be classified as high risk for tumor recurrence. Even if one uses the contour maps by Joensuu et al. [47], providing a better assessment tool and eliminating the dichotomous threshold of 5 cm and 5 mitoses pro 50 HPF, the mean recurrence-free survival of more than 10 years looks very promising. The basis probably is laid by the fact that 44% of the resection specimen showed >95% necrosis and 94% of the patients have undergone R0 resection. This is due to patient selection with *KIT* exon 11 mutations almost exclusively. It is also known from treating metastatic patients that KIT deletions involving codons 557 and 558 respond very well to imatinib [48] (Figure 2). Our data are in line with a multicenter study including 161 patients with locally advanced non-metastatic GISTs pooled from 10 EORTC-STBSG sarcoma centers showing that >80% of the tumors responded to imatinib, facilitating R0 resection in >80% of the cases [24]. After a median 40 weeks of imatinib, the R0 resection rate was 83% and the 5-year DFS was 65% with median OS of 104 months [24].

Another recently published series on 150 patients with GIST treated on a neoadjuvant basis across all tumor sites reports an overall survival rate of 81% at 5 years [49]. The difference might be due to shorter treatment duration (median 7.1 months with a range starting at 0.2 months) and a clearly lower rate of partial tumor remissions of 40% which was 75% in our series. Furthermore, the resection margins with 63.3% R0 resections and 18% each of R1 and R2 resection are inferior to our study [49]. It has been noted from further studies that patients after R0 resection have a significantly lower risk of developing tumor progression compared to patients with R1/R2 resection (60% vs. 23.8%, $p = 0.11$, [22,40]).

The duration of neoadjuvant imatinib administration may be important to obtain adequate tumor response. An early compilation of case reports by Haller et al. [50] suggested that the longer the treatment the better the remission. We indicated surgery after having reached a plateau with no further tumor shrinkage and the risk of developing secondary resistance to therapy still remaing low [39]. At this time point, all our patients showed either PR or SD and no patient showed any progression during imatinib therapy. The rate of partial responses in our patients is higher compared with the phase II RTOG 0132 trial, in which 83% of patients had stable disease after 12 months of imatinib [15].

A strength of this study is that it demonstrates that laparoscopic procedures more and more can be successfully used in this setting of locally advanced GIST with median tumor size of more than 10 cm after downstaging with tyrosine kinase inhibitors. The study, however, also has limitations referring mainly to patient selection which is hardly avoidable. Patients can easily be convinced to swallow a pill per day and avoid total gastrectomy or multivisceral resection. A randomized trial does not look feasible at all under these circumstances and therefore the formal evidence of using neoadjuvant imatinib is not better than grade 2+ according to SIGN^{+1} [51].

Given the fact that in small tumor biopsies the number of mitoses could not be counted per 5 mm^2 or 50 HPF, the risk classification of patients according to NIH or Miettinen/Lasota is doubtful in some cases. This also influences the decision of whether or not to subject patients to postoperative adjuvant imatinib therapy. Using the extent of regression from the resection specimen in the seven mentioned patients does not allow us to draw conclusions. The willingness of the patients to continue with the drug also influenced the administration of adjuvant imatinib therapy. Several patients felt relief from the drug and the tumor after surgery and were not willing to continue. Our individualized approach does not allow us to draw further conclusions.

In gastric GIST a problem is the rather high rate of tumors without mutations in KIT or with mutations in PDGFRA. We tried to overcome this with ^{18}F-FDG-PET scanning to eliminate patients who would not respond adequately. We also postponed patients with epitheloid GIST until mutation analysis had been performed, as this feature is often associated with PDGFRA mutations not being sensitive to imatinib.

5. Conclusions

In conclusion, neoadjuvant imatinib in our series of locally advanced gastric GIST proved to allow organ-sparing surgical procedures with a very high rate of R0 resections and excellent long-term recurrence-free survival. This holds true also for patients starting their treatment during an episode of upper gastrointestinal bleeding. Toxicity was mild and tolerable and in 96% of the patients major parts of the stomach could be preserved, maintaining the physiological basis for the use of oral tyrosine kinase inhibitors in the adjuvant or metastatic setting.

Author Contributions: Conceptualization, N.V., J.J., G.K. and P.H.; methodology, N.V. and P.H.; software, N.V. and P.H.; validation, P.H.; formal analysis, N.V. and P.H.; investigation, N.V., P.H. and G.K.; resources, G.K., A.M., N.R., E.W. and P.H.; data curation, N.V., A.M., A.D.-S., N.R., E.W. and P.H.; writing—original draft preparation, N.V. and P.H.; writing—review and editing, N.V., J.J., G.K., P.R., A.M., A.D.-S., N.R., E.W. and P.H.; supervision, P.H. All authors have read and agreed to the published version of the manuscript.

Funding: This research received no external funding.

Institutional Review Board Statement: The Medical Ethics Commission II, Medical Faculty Mannheim of the University of Heidelberg, Maybachstr. 14, 68169 Mannheim, Reference 2020-827R.

Informed Consent Statement: All patients consented to the use of their tissues and data for research purposes.

Data Availability Statement: The data that support the findings of this study are available from the corresponding author upon reasonable request.

Conflicts of Interest: The authors declare no conflict of interest.

References

1. Fletcher, C.D.; Berman, J.J.; Corless, C.; Gorstein, F.; Lasota, J.; Longley, B.J.; Miettinen, M.; O'Leary, T.J.; Remotti, H.; Rubin, B.P.; et al. Diagnosis of gastrointestinal stromal tumors: A consensus approach. *Hum. Pathol.* **2002**, *33*, 459–465. [CrossRef] [PubMed]
2. Nilsson, B.; Bümming, P.; Meis-Kindblom, J.M.; Oden, A.; Dortok, A.; Gustavsson, B.; Sablinska, K.; Kindblom, L.G. Gastrointestinal stromal tumors: The incidence, prevalence, clinical course, and prognostication in the preimatinib mesylate era—A population-based study in western Sweden. *Cancer* **2005**, *103*, 821–829. [CrossRef] [PubMed]
3. DeMatteo, R.P.; Lewis, J.J.; Leung, D.; Mudan, S.S.; Woodruff, J.M.; Brennan, M.F. Two hundred gastrointestinal stromal tumors: Recurrence patterns and prognostic factors for survival. *Ann. Surg.* **2000**, *231*, 51–58. [CrossRef]
4. Miettinen, M.; Lasota, J. Gastrointestinal stromal tumors: Review on morphology, molecular pathology, prognosis, and differential diagnosis. *Arch. Pathol. Lab. Med.* **2006**, *130*, 1466–1478.
5. Hirota, S. Gain-of-function Mutations of c-kit in human gastrointestinal stromal tumors. *Science* **1998**, *279*, 577–580. [CrossRef]
6. Heinrich, M.C.; Corless, C.L.; Duensing, A.; McGreevey, L.; Chen, C.J.; Joseph, N.; Singer, S.; Griffith, D.J.; Haley, A.; Town, A.; et al. PDGFRA activating mutations in gastrointestinal stromal tumors. *Science* **2003**, *299*, 708–710. [CrossRef]
7. Roberts, P.J.; Eisenberg, B. Clinical presentation of gastrointestinal stromal tumors and treatment of operable disease. *Eur. J. Cancer* **2002**, *38*, 37–38. [CrossRef]
8. Dematteo, R.P.; Heinrich, M.C.; El-Rifai, W.M.; Demetri, G. Clinical management of gastrointestinal stromal tumors: Before and after STI-571. *Hum. Pathol.* **2002**, *33*, 466–477. [CrossRef]
9. Joensuu, H.; Roberts, P.J.; Sarlomo-Rikala, M.; Andersson, L.C.; Tervahartiala, P.; Tuveson, D.; Silberman, S.; Capdeville, R.; Dimitrijevic, S.; Druker, B.; et al. Effect of the tyrosine kinase inhibitor STI571 in a patient with a metastatic gastrointestinal stromal tumor. *N. Engl. J. Med.* **2001**, *344*, 1052–1056. [CrossRef]
10. Heinrich, M.C.; Blanke, C.D.; Druker, B.J.; Corless, C.L. Inhibition of KIT Tyrosine Kinase Activity: A Novel Molecular Approach to the Treatment of KIT-Positive Malignancies. *J. Clin. Oncol.* **2002**, *20*, 1692–1703. [CrossRef]
11. Demetri, G.D.; Demetri, G.D.; von Mehren, M.; Blanke, C.D.; Van den Abbeele, A.D.; Eisenberg, B.; Roberts, P.J.; Heinrich, M.C.; Tuveson, D.A.; Singer, S.; et al. Efficacy and safety of imatinib mesylate in advanced gastrointestinal stromal tumors. *N. Engl. J. Med.* **2002**, *347*, 472–480. [CrossRef] [PubMed]
12. van Oosterom, A.T.; Judson, I.; Verweij, J.; Stroobants, S.; Donato di Paola, E.; Dimitrijevic, S.; Martens, M.; Webb, A.; Sciot, R.; van Glabbeke, M.; et al. Safety and efficacy of imatinib (STI571) in metastatic gastrointestinal stromal tumours: A phase I study. *Lancet* **2001**, *358*, 1421–1423. [CrossRef]

13. Demetri, G.D.; von Mehren, M.; Antonescu, C.R.; DeMatteo, R.P.; Ganjoo, K.N.; Maki, R.G.; Pisters, P.W.T.; Raut, C.P.; Riedel, R.F.; Schuetze, S.; et al. NCCN Task Force report: Update on the management of patients with gastrointestinal stromal tumors. *J. Natl. Compr. Cancer Netw.* **2010**, *8* (Suppl. 2), 1–41. [CrossRef]
14. Demetri, G.D.; Wang, Y.; Wehrle, E.; Racine, A.; Nikolova, Z.; Blanke, C.D.; Joensuu, H.; von Mehren, M. Imatinib plasma levels are correlated with clinical benefit in patients with unresectable/metastatic gastrointestinal stromal tumors. *J. Clin. Oncol.* **2009**, *27*, 3141–3147. [CrossRef]
15. Eisenberg, B.L.; Harris, J.; Blanke, C.D.; Demetri, G.D.; Heinrich, M.C.; Watson, J.C.; Hoffman, J.P.; Okuno, S.; Kane, J.M.; von Mehren, M. Phase II trial of neoadjuvant/adjuvant imatinib mesylate (IM) for advanced primary and metastatic/recurrent operable gastrointestinal stromal tumor (GIST): Early results of RTOG 0132/ACRIN 6665. *J. Surg. Oncol.* **2009**, *99*, 42–47. [CrossRef]
16. Shrikhande, S.V.; Marda, S.S.; Suradkar, K.; Arya, S.; Shetty, G.S.; Bal, M.; Shukla, P.J.; Goel, M.; Mohandas, K.M. Gastrointestinal stromal tumors: Case series of 29 patients defining the role of imatinib prior to surgery. *World J. Surg.* **2012**, *36*, 864–871. [CrossRef]
17. Koontz, M.Z.; Visser, B.M.; Kunz, P.L. Neoadjuvant imatinib for borderline resectable GIST. *J. Natl. Compr. Cancer Netw.* **2012**, *10*, 1477–1482. [CrossRef]
18. Tielen, R.; Verhoef, C.; van Coevorden, F.; Gelderblom, H.; Sleijfer, S.; Hartgrink, H.H.; Bonenkamp, J.J.; van der Graaf, W.T.; de Wilt, J.H. Surgical treatment of locally advanced, non-metastatic, gastrointestinal stromal tumours after treatment with imatinib. *Eur. J. Surg. Oncol.* **2013**, *39*, 150–155. [CrossRef]
19. Fiore, M.; Palassini, E.; Fumagalli, E.; Pilotti, S.; Tamborini, E.; Stacchiotti, S.; Pennacchioli, E.; Casali, P.G.; Gronchi, A. Preoperative imatinib mesylate for unresectable or locally advanced primary gastrointestinal stromal tumors (GIST). *Eur. J. Surg. Oncol.* **2009**, *35*, 739–745. [CrossRef]
20. Andtbacka, R.H.; Ng, C.S.; Scaife, C.L.; Cormier, J.N.; Hunt, K.K.; Pisters, P.W.T.; Pollock, R.E.; Benjamin, R.S.; Burgess, M.A.; Chen, L.L.; et al. Surgical resection of gastrointestinal stromal tumors after treatment with imatinib. *Ann. Surg. Oncol.* **2007**, *14*, 14–24. [CrossRef] [PubMed]
21. Raut, C.P.; Posner, M.; Desai, J.; Morgan, J.A.; George, S.; Zahrieh, D.; Fletcher, C.D.M.; Demetri, G.D.; Bertagnolli, M.M. Surgical management of advanced gastrointestinal stromal tumors after treatment with targeted systemic therapy using kinase inhibitors. *J. Clin. Oncol.* **2006**, *24*, 2325–2331. [CrossRef] [PubMed]
22. Blesius, A.; Cassier, P.A.; Bertucci, F.; Fayette, J.; Ray-Coquard, I.; Bui, B.; Adenis, A.; Rios, M.; Didier, C.; Perol, D.; et al. Neoadjuvant imatinib in patients with locally advanced non metastatic GIST in the prospective BFR14 trial. *BMC Cancer* **2011**, *11*, 72. [CrossRef] [PubMed]
23. Hohenberger, P.; Langer, C.; Wendtner, C.M.; Hohenberger, W.; Pustowka, A.; Wardelmann, E.; Andre, E.; Licht, T. Neoadjuvant treatment of locally advanced GIST: Results of APOLLON, a prospective, open label phase II study in KIT- or PDGFRA-positive tumors. *J. Clin. Oncol.* **2012**, *30*, abstr 10031. [CrossRef]
24. Rutkowski, P.; Gronchi, A.; Hohenberger, P.; Bonvalot, S.; Schoffski, P.; Bauer, S.; Fumagalli, E.; Nyckowski, P.; Nguyen, B.P.; Kerst, J.M.; et al. Neoadjuvant Imatinib in Locally Advanced Gastrointestinal Stromal Tumors (GIST): The EORTC STBSG Experience. *Ann. Surg. Oncol.* **2013**, *20*, 2937–2943. [CrossRef]
25. Wang, S.Y.; Wu, C.E.; Lai, C.C.; Chen, J.S.; Tsai, C.Y.; Cheng, C.T.; Yeh, T.S.; Yeh, C.N. Prospective evaluation of preoperative IM use in locally advanced gastrointestinal stromal tumors: Emphasis on the optimal duration of preoperative IM use, safety, and oncological outcome. *Cancers* **2019**, *11*, 424. [CrossRef]
26. Staiger, W.I.; Ronellenfitsch, U.; Kaehler, G.; Schildhaus, H.U.; Dimitrakopoulou-Strauss, A.; Schwarzbach, M.H.; Hohenberger, P. The Merendino procedure following preoperative imatinib mesylate for locally advanced gastrointestinal stromal tumor of the esophagogastric junction. *World J. Surg. Oncol.* **2008**, *6*, 37. [CrossRef]
27. Eisenhauer, E.A.; Therasse, P.; Bogaerts, J.; Schwartz, L.H.; Sargent, D.; Ford, R.; Dancey, J.; Arbuck, S.; Gwyther, S.; Mooney, M.; et al. New response evaluation criteria in solid tumours: Revised RECIST guideline (version 1.1). *Eur. J. Cancer* **2009**, *45*, 228–247. [CrossRef]
28. Rutkowski, P.; Skoczylas, J.; Wisniewski, P. Is the surgical margin in gastrointestinal stromal tumors different? *Visc. Med.* **2018**, *34*, 347–352. [CrossRef]
29. Hohenberger, P.; Bonvalot, S.; van Coevorden, F.; Rutkowski, P.; Stoeckle, E.; Olungu, C.; Litiere, S.; Wardelmann, E.; Gronchi, A.; Casali, P. Quality of surgery and surgical reporting for patients with primary gastrointestinal stromal tumors participating in the EORTC STBSG 62024 adjuvant imatinib study. *Eur. J. Cancer* **2019**, *120*, 47–53. [CrossRef]
30. Dindo, D.; Demartines, N.; Clavien, P.A. Classification of Surgical Complications: A New Proposal With Evaluation in a Cohort of 6336 Patients and Results of a Survey. *Ann. Surg.* **2004**, *240*, 205–213. [CrossRef]
31. Hermanek, P.; Wittekind, C. The pathologist and the residual tumor (R) classification. *Pathol. Res. Pract.* **1994**, *190*, 115–123. [CrossRef]
32. Kaplan, E.L.; Meier, P. Nonparametric estimation from incomplete observations. *J. Am. Stat. Assoc.* **1958**, *53*, 457–481. [CrossRef]
33. Mantel, N. Evaluation of survival data and two new rank order statistics arising in its consideration. *Cancer Chemother. Rep.* **1966**, *50*, 163–170. [PubMed]
34. Bachet, J.B.; Landi, B.; Laurent-Puig, P.; Italiano, A.; Le Cesne, A.; Levy, P.; Safar, V.; Duffaud, F.; Blay, J.Y.; Emile, J.F. Diagnosis, prognosis and treatment of patients with gastrointestinal stromal tumour (GIST) and germline mutation of KIT exon 13. *Eur. J. Cancer* **2013**, *49*, 2531–2541. [CrossRef] [PubMed]

35. Casali, P.G.; Abecassis, N.; Aro, H.T.; Bauer, S.; Biagini, R.; Bielack, S.; Boukovinas, I.; Bovee, J.V.M.G.; Brodowicz, T.; Brotto, J.M.; et al. Gastrointetinal stromal tumors: ESMO-EURACAN clinical practice guidelines for diagnosis, treatment and follow-up. *Ann. Oncol.* **2018**, *29*, 267. [CrossRef]
36. Jakob, J.; Hohenberger, P. Neoadjuvant therapy to downstage the extent of resection of gastrointestinal stromal tumors. *Visc. Med.* **2018**, *34*, 359–365. [CrossRef]
37. Choi, H. Response evaluation of gastrointestinal stromal tumors. *Oncologist* **2008**, *13* (Suppl. 2), 4–7. [CrossRef]
38. Van den Abbeele, A.D. The lessons of GIST–PET and PET/CT: A new paradigm for imaging. *Oncologist* **2008**, *13* (Suppl. 2), 8–13. [CrossRef]
39. Bonvalot, S.; Eldweny, H.; Pechoux, C.L.; Vanel, D.; Terrier, P.; Cavalcanti, A.; Robert, C.; Lassau, N.; Cesne, A.L. Impact of Surgery on Advanced Gastrointestinal Stromal Tumors (GIST) in the Imatinib Era. *Ann. Surg. Oncol.* **2006**, *13*, 1596–1603. [CrossRef]
40. Wang, D.; Zhang, Q.; Blanke, C.D.; Demetri, G.D.; Heinrich, M.C.; Watson, J.C.; Hoffman, J.P.; Okuno, S.; Kane, J.M.; von Mehren, M.; et al. Phase II Trial of Neoadjuvant/adjuvant Imatinib Mesylate for Advanced Primary and Metastatic/recurrent Operable Gastrointestinal Stromal Tumors: Long-term Follow-up Results of Radiation Therapy Oncology Group 0132. *Ann. Surg. Oncol.* **2011**, *19*, 1074–1080. [CrossRef]
41. Gronchi, A.; Fiore, M.; Miselli, F.; Lagonigro, M.S.; Coco, P.; Messina, A.; Pilotti, S.; Casali, P.G. Surgery of residual disease following molecular-targeted therapy with imatinib mesylate in advanced/metastatic GIST. *Ann. Surg.* **2007**, *245*, 341–346. [CrossRef] [PubMed]
42. Rutkowski, P.; Nowecki, Z.; Nyckowski, P.; Dziewirski, W.; Grzesiakowska, U.; Nasierowska-Guttmejer, A.; Krawczyk, M.; Ruka, W. Surgical treatment of patients with initially inoperable and/or metastatic gastrointestinal stromal tumors (GIST) during therapy with imatinib mesylate. *J. Surg. Oncol.* **2006**, *93*, 304–311. [CrossRef] [PubMed]
43. Hohenberger, P.; Ronellenfitsch, U.; Oladeji, O.; Pink, D.; Ströbel, P.; Wardelmann, E.; Reichardt, P. Pattern of recurrence in patients with ruptured primary gastrointestinal stromal tumour. *Br. J. Surg.* **2010**, *97*, 1854–1859. [CrossRef] [PubMed]
44. Gronchi, A.; Raut, C.P. The combination of surgery and imatinib in GIST: A reality for localized tumors at high risk, an open issue for metastatic ones. *Ann. Surg. Oncol.* **2012**, *19*, 1051–1055. [CrossRef] [PubMed]
45. Hohenberger, P.; Eisenberg, B. Role of surgery combined with kinase inhibition in the management of gastrointestinal stromal tumor (GIST). *Ann. Surg. Oncol.* **2010**, *17*, 2585–2600. [CrossRef] [PubMed]
46. Tang, S.; Yin, Y.; Shen, C.; Chen, J.; Yin, X.; Zhang, B.; Yao, Y.; Yang, J.; Chen, Z. Preoperative imatinib mesylate (IM) for huge gastrointestinal stromal tumors (GIST). *World J. Surg. Oncol.* **2017**, *15*, 79. [CrossRef] [PubMed]
47. Joensuu, H.; Vehtari, A.; Riihimäki, J.; Nishida, T.; Steigen, S.E.; Brabec, P.; Plank, L.; Nilsson, B.; Cirilli, C.; Braconi, C.; et al. Risk of recurrence of gastrointestinal stromal tumour after surgery: An analysis of pooled population-based cohorts. *Lancet Oncol.* **2012**, *13*, 265–274. [CrossRef]
48. McAuliffe, J.C.; Hunt, K.K.; Lazar, A.J.; Choi, H.; Qiao, W.; Thall, P.; Pollock, R.E.; Benjamin, R.S.; Trent, J.C. A randomized, phase II study of preoperative plus postoperative imatinib in GIST: Evidence of rapid radiographic response and temporal induction of tumor cell apoptosis. *Ann. Surg. Oncol.* **2009**, *16*, 910–919. [CrossRef]
49. Cavnar, M.J.; Seier, K.; Gönen, M.; Curtini, C.; Balachandran, V.P.; Tap, W.D.; Antonescu, C.R.; Singer, S.; DeMatteo, R.P. Prognostic factors after neoadjuvant imatinib for newly diagnosed primary gastrointestinal stromal tumor. *J. Gastrointest. Surg.* **2020**. [CrossRef]
50. Haller, F.; Detken, S.; Schulten, H.J.; Happel, N.; Gunawan, B.; Kuhlgatz, J.; Füzesi, L. Surgical management after neoadjuvant imatinib therapy in gastrointestinal stromal tumours (GISTs) with respect to imatinib resistance caused by secondary KIT mutations. *Ann. Surg. Oncol.* **2007**, *14*, 526–532. [CrossRef]
51. Edinburgh: Scottis Intercollegiate Guidelines Network. Available online: http://www.sign.ac.uk/ (accessed on 10 April 2008).

MDPI
St. Alban-Anlage 66
4052 Basel
Switzerland
Tel. +41 61 683 77 34
Fax +41 61 302 89 18
www.mdpi.com

Cancers Editorial Office
E-mail: cancers@mdpi.com
www.mdpi.com/journal/cancers

www.ingramcontent.com/pod-product-compliance
Lightning Source LLC
LaVergne TN
LVHW070505100526
838202LV00014B/1789